Our Adventures During the War of 1870

Our Adventures During the War of 1870
The Experiences of Two British Nurses During the Franco-Prussian War

Emma Maria Pearson

and

Louisa Elisabeth McLaughlin

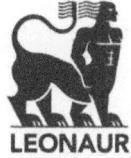

Our Adventures During the War of 1870
The Experiences of Two British Nurses During the Franco-Prussian War
By Emma Maria Pearson and Louisa Elisabeth McLaughlin

First published under the title
Our Adventures During the War of 1870 in two volumes

Leonaur is an imprint of Oakpast Ltd

Copyright in this form © 2021 Oakpast Ltd

ISBN: 978-1-78282-982-9 (hardcover)
ISBN: 978-1-78282-983-6 (softcover)

http://www.leonaur.com

Publisher's Notes

The views expressed in this book are not necessarily those of the publisher.

Contents

Preface	9
The Start for the War	11
An Express Train	17
The Two "Châteaux"	23
The Midnight Drive	31
The Knights of St. John	38
The Rescue	46
The Burning of the Red-Cross Banner	54
The Chase After the King	61
England to the Rescue	70
Alone on the Hills	82
The Last Hours of the Empire	90
The Saddest Scene of All	97
A Miserable Village	108
To England and Back	117
Louise's Letter	124
Caserne Asfelde	132
Under Whose Orders?	139
'La Belle Normandie'	146

The King's Headquarters	154
The Battlefield at Home	162
The Army of the Loire	172
The Only Victory	179
The Week of Battle	187
Le Dimanche Noir	197
Under the Shadow of the Union Jack	205
A Lost Battlefield	216
The Army of the Vosges	226
Convent Life at Orleans	238
A Sad New Year	249
Peace	258
A German Funeral Pyre	270
A Gallant Little Town	277
The Loiret	290

To The
Honourable Georgiana Rushout;
For Whose Generous Aid and Sympathy
In Our Efforts
To Relieve the Sick and Wounded in the Late War,
We Owe a Debt of Gratitude,
This Book is Dedicated
By Her Sincere and Affectionate
Emma Maria Pearson
And
Louisa Elisabeth MacLaughlin.
June 1871

Preface

Our aim in the volume we present to the kindly consideration of our English friends, has been not only to give a simple and truthful sketch of personal experiences, during the campaigns of 1870-71, but to show the evils war inflicts on those who take no active part in it, its degrading influence on national character, and the cruel sufferings of an invaded country.

In speaking of our great National Society for the Relief of the Sick and Wounded in War, we have given a straightforward statement of our transactions with them. No attempt has been made to enter into any discussion as to the causes of what we consider to have been much of failure in carrying out the great work before them.

Their intentions were, undoubtedly, the noblest and best; and if, unfortunately, their services should again be required, they will have learnt wisdom and economy by the past.

That our sympathies were and are French we do not deny. We lived amongst them, and were daily witnesses of their miseries. But we have tried to do justice to all, and to record our gratitude to the officers of the German Army, whose kindness, with a few exceptions, was unvarying.

Emma Maria Pearson,
Louisa Elisabeth McLaughlin.

Boraston Rectory, Tenbury: June 1871.

CHAPTER 1

The Start for the War

Life in an invaded country, overrun by the troops of a foreign power, is in every respect so different from life in our peaceful English land, that the simple record of personal adventures and impressions during a residence in various parts of France in the autumn of 1870, and the winter and early spring of 1871, may help to realise the horrors and the demoralisation of war to the minds of those who happily never knew by occupation of an enemy, the domestic state of their towns and villages, and the sufferings of all classes from details of misery which naturally are overlooked by the military and special war correspondents of the English journals. They record faithfully what they see, but much escapes their notice as they follow the advance or retreat of the contending armies.

Many of these miseries are the necessary consequences of war, but are often aggravated by the violence of the victorious soldiery, and the utter want of comprehension which must exist when an excited trooper endeavours to explain in an unknown tongue to a frightened peasant what is required of him. Whilst wishing to do every justice to both belligerent powers, it must be admitted that the impatience of a German soldier, when his harsh gutturals fail to produce any effect on the understanding of those around him, is something perfectly horrible, and his howls and yells enough to drive an unoffending citizen into a state of distraction. During our sojourn in this unhappy land of France we met with many instances of this, and many lives were lost simply from this unfortunate want of knowledge of a few words of each other's language.

I must premise before fairly starting the story of our lives during this great war, that from the first Louise and myself formed a deep attachment to each other, our sympathies on almost every point were the same, and we became inseparable companions. If in writing this sketch of our adventures I am obliged to use the singular and egotistical pronoun 'I' in many places, it is only to avoid the difficulty of describing scenes in which each took a separate part. There was no danger, no hardship, no adventure, she did not equally share; and as we sit side by side, recalling the events we witnessed, and looking over the diary she kept, whilst we feel it is far better one should act as scribe, we beg it distinctly to be understood our little work is a joint composition.

No idle curiosity brought us to the seat of war: we formed part of what was called, in France, 'the English Column,' sent from 'the British National Society for the Relief of the Sick and Wounded in War,' and consisting, when it started, of four ladies, a paid nurse, a surgeon, and a secretary, and with orders to repair directly to the king's headquarters for service with the Prussian Army.

We left London for Dover on the night of August 16, with all the fresh enthusiasm of untried soldiers, determined not to spend on ourselves a shilling more than we could help of the Society's money; and so sternly resolved to go through any amount of hardship, that we should have been actually annoyed if any amount of decent comfort had been predicted as our lot. On our arrival we went on board the Ostend boat, beginning our course of self-denial by taking second-class tickets; however, the second-class cabin was an utter impossibility: we got ready to bivouac on deck, and commence campaigning experiences by passing a night in the open air.

We did not, I am afraid, reflect sufficiently, as I was afterwards told, on the dignity of the great Society whose pioneers in active personal work we were, or how incumbent it was upon us to keep it up under all circumstances. In harbour the sea was calm, and the night seemed fine. We were undeceived. I believe it rained, I know it blew; but except a consciousness of suffering, we were beyond all speculations on any subject. We had wrapped ourselves up in our railway rugs, and spread our water-proof sheets over us; but it was all in vain: the spray dashed over us, the cold wind chilled us; and the only consolation we had was, that happen what might, we never could be more wretched—we had reached the Ultima Thule of misery.

But morning and Ostend came at last, and we crawled to the custom-house, where our baggage was to be examined. The Red Cross marked upon it saved us all trouble on that score, but the boxes sent out with us by the committee were a great trial. They showed a wonderful facility for coming to pieces on the slightest provocation, and depositing their contents by the way; and we were very glad to register them through to Aix-la-Chapelle, which was our first destination. But from that day to this we never saw them again. They did arrive at last at Aix, but the expense of forwarding them was more than the worth of them, and they were probably opened, and their contents used for the Hospitals there. They contained bandages, linen rags, and some second-hand shirts and socks; also, two pairs of white kid gloves—for what purpose sent is a mystery.

All through the war, much was sent out that was utterly useless, much that was not worth carriage. I mention this to show how much money and labour was wasted in this gigantic effort to alleviate measureless human suffering, from want of practical experience, and a due consideration of the fitness of things. Second-hand under clothing, unless almost new, will not bear one washing. Bandages especially do not answer the expense of sending out; they weigh very heavily; calico can be always purchased near the scene of action, and they cost far less made on the spot.

We lost no time in proceeding to Brussels, where we arrived at noon; and having a letter to deliver to the President of the International Society there, I went at once, accompanied by one of the ladies, to the committee rooms. It was a singular proceeding. A number of letters were read which had no particular bearing on any subject, and the affair was getting dull, when a lady begged permission to address the meeting. The gravity with which the chairman and committee listened to the tale of her grievances was really ludicrous. It seemed some other zealous lady had refused to allow her collection of linen and *charpie* to be added to the general collection, though a special portion of space had been allotted to the contributions of the faubourgs and villages around.

This ambitious village declined to disappear in the general mass of villages, had taken back its bales, had set up for itself under the presidentship of the ambitious lady, and had even presumed to seek for aid in the city. Such insubordination and poaching upon other people's manors could not be allowed: the lady of the village was to be duly admonished that the lady of the city would not stand it, and the village was temporarily excommunicated. How the affair ended, of course I have no means of knowing, but I hope by a reconciliation between city and suburb.

Next morning we duly repaired to the station, where we met the secretary, who had been detained by the charge of bringing out five hundred pounds' worth of very valuable stores for our use: instead of having to wait for his arrival at Aix-la-Chapelle, we were enabled thus to proceed direct to Luxembourg *en route* for Saarbruck and the front.

We arrived early in the evening. It was a sunny August day, and the little town of Luxembourg looked actually sleepy in the light of the setting sun. War might have been a thousand miles away for any signs we could see of it there, but there were rumours that sounds of heavy firing had come on the still summer air to the quiet neutral town, and it was true: only thirty miles away, across the frontier, was Metz, and that day was one of the terrible three days' struggle called by the Germans the Battle of Gravelotte, by the French the Battle of St. Privat. It was the great struggle after which Bazaine retreated within his lines, and the ring of the besiegers closed round him and his army, and left famine to do its work in the doomed city. The battle covered a great space of ground, on which stood many small villages, and it is called by the various names of these by the soldiers of different corps.

Next day we left for Saarbruck, and at the station met a gentlemanly Englishman, evidently a soldier, who entered into conversation with some of our party, and whom we afterwards called 'the General' when he took command of us a few days later. All went well till we reached a way-side station, called Wasserbillig: here the line was cut, and we were transferred to an omnibus, and our baggage to country waggons. As we drove slowly along, we saw on our left an ancient Roman tomb in three storeys. There was sculpture in *bas-relief* still left upon it that showed its occupant had been some great warrior, but its situation was its chief beauty in our eyes.

Its history was then and is still unknown to us—what celebrated chieftain slept there, or what event it was built to record; but there it stood, at the head of a gorge that, opening between, deep-wooded banks, gave a view of the fertile plain below, with the blue Moselle winding through it. Those old Romans knew how to build, and where to place their buildings. They were at once artists and architects.

At last we reached Treves. The station was crowded with soldiers; and, as we lingered on the broad steps leading up to it, and whilst the secretary was enquiring for the waggons, which had not yet come up with us, the General in opening his valise to take out something, showed his papers and his passport, which proved he was the real Simon Pure. Now when he had given his name at Luxembourg, the secretary had chosen to doubt the fact: we had believed in it, and we enjoyed a little triumph in informing him that we were right, and he was wrong. The proof was too clear, and the secretary admitted his error, and permitted us to present the General with a little white shield, on which was a red velvet cross, to place in his hat, like those we had made for the secretary and our surgeon, Mr. Parker, and which the General had admired and wished for.

We had to wait at Treves for the baggage, and we went into the station to try and find a refreshment room; but in war time, as we found, refreshment rooms and waiting rooms are all invaded and taken possession of by the soldiery, and we were obliged to content ourselves with some bread and beer in a large hall, round the centre table of which sat a number of recruits for the Prussian Army, drinking, smoking, and singing. Our entrance was the signal for a burst of delight. 'The English! the English! come to nurse our wounded!' was the cry from all; and directly after, one man gravely advanced from the rest, and begged us to drink their health, which of course we did, and they then sang for us the chorus our entrance had interrupted, and we heard for the first time '*Die Wacht am Rhein.*'

It seems they were all bakers, part of the reserve called out for service, and their uniforms were rough and ill-fitting, very unlike the smart, well-drilled Prussian soldiers we afterwards encountered. They were stupid, heavy looking fellows, and, in spite of all their singing, certainly much depressed. No wonder. Would our gallant volunteers feel more cheerful if ordered from the office, the workshop, and the farm, to hard and dangerous service? From first to last the greater part of the German soldiery we encountered detested the war, and only longed for peace and home. Bavarians, Hessians, and Prussians proper were divided amongst themselves, yet they fought well.

The German Army is a splendid machine, but no English soldier would submit to the treatment the German soldiers endure from the sergeants and corporals of their regiments. They are governed by simple brute force, and that, combined with Schnapps and a good dinner, will always manage the worst of them. Yet it must be confessed that drunkenness is the exception, not the rule. They have enormous appetites, and a great capacity for strong liquors, but they seemed to take both meat and drink in huge quantities with impunity.

At the appointed hour we found ourselves at the train, and were implored to get in, as it was then starting. We remonstrated that the gentlemen had not arrived, and the guard remarked that the train would wait half an hour or so. In time of war it was of no consequence. Having made this comfortable arrangement, we inspected the preparations for receiving the wounded. A staff of Red Cross stretcher bearers was in attendance to carry them from the train to the carriages, waiting to take them to hospital. After experience convinced us it would be far better to carry the seriously wounded on the stretchers to the hospital, instead of transferring them to a carriage, but it is only experience that teaches these details. Trays with glasses of raspberry vinegar and water, bread, biscuits, and fruit, were there ready for the refreshment of the sufferers, and kind and active helpers waiting to distribute it all.

The train which brought them came in at last: there were very few, and they were not badly wounded. There had not been time to bring the mass of wounded from the scene of action. We watched the emptying of the carriages. Our gentlemen had arrived, still our train did not move on, and, at last we discovered we were waiting for some high official who was to act as convoy of a large sum of money for the army. Apparently, it was difficult to get, for two hours elapsed before three or four country carts arrived, and were brought up close to the platform. They were loaded with canvas bags, containing silver coin, which were passed or rather thrown from hand to hand by a line of soldiers to the waggon reserved for them.

It seemed a cumbrous way of sending money, but was probably the easiest distribution in small sums. During this time '*Die Wacht am Rhein*' had been again chanted by the warlike bakers, the chorus being led by our German secretary, who had bought 'a book of the words' in town. Doubts as to the neutrality of this proceeding might be suggested, but as he never professed anything but the most intense Germanism, it was not surprising. At last the train moved on. Treves vanished in the distance. We were fairly started for the Seat of War.

Chapter 2

An Express Train

It was 8 o'clock before we reached Saarlouis, a station on the Saarbruck line. The railroad runs through the lovely valley of the Saar, and in the light of an August evening all looked so still and quiet, that war might have been a thousand miles away. The train had come thus far in a jerky and deliberate manner, apparently for no particular reason except the amusement of the guards and stokers. In time of war, a general disorganisation of the details of every-day life takes place, which induces irregularity even where there is no occasion for it; and though it is most earnestly to be hoped that England will never experience this scourge on her own shores, yet it is a matter of speculation if solid, steady-going English men and women would ever become as 'slipshod' as the French under the same circumstances.

The horrors of war are great: it is one long nightmare of suffering and terror to the miserable inhabitants of the invaded country—one long holiday of recklessness to the conquerors; but its worst feature is, after all, the universal demoralisation to all concerned in it. Peace may be re-established, the invaders may return home in triumph, the suffering people may shake off their sullen despair and set themselves to recover their fallen fortunes; but through long years the evil effects of that demoralisation will be felt on the character of both nations.

We found we should remain some little time at Saarlouis, and whilst walking on the platform several women came up and asked if we were English, and if we had come to nurse the wounded. They seemed surprised to find us on Prussian ground, as they thought all the English were for the French. So delighted were they with our assurances that we were strictly neutral, that they presented us with bunches of delicate pink oleanders, which we placed in our hats to please them.

It was very late before the train arrived at the long suburb of Saarbruck, St. Johann. We had stopped five or six times for an hour, and were fairly worn out. As it was quite dark, we could see nothing but the lights in the various houses: there was a feverish look about the place, from the fact that every house was lighted at midnight. At last Saarbruck station was reached; but what a scene met us there! The broad platform, which extended to a line on the other side of it, was covered with stalls of provisions lighted by pine torches: the keepers of them, wearied with a long day's work, were sleeping here and there by the side; the waiting room was turned into a rough kitchen, and the buildings were much damaged by shells, fired on the celebrated day when the boy, then heir to the Empire of France, received his 'baptism of fire.' No one at that time foresaw by what a baptism of tears it would be followed.

Trains of wounded had been passing all day, another was momentarily expected, and we heard that our convoy would go no farther that night, but might start at any hour in the morning. The best arrangement seemed to be that we should sleep in the carriages, and this was made for us. We then tried to find some supper: here a Mr. Herbert, of the Cologne Ambulance, (field hospitals were called ambulances at that time), was of great use to us; he found a stall where we could get some coffee, bread, and oranges, and this was not the last occasion on which his kindness was of essential service. He showed us where a shell had struck the rooms, but the ruin was nothing compared to the accounts we had read in the newspapers in England, and often since we have read of scenes in which we ourselves took a part, with a sort of puzzled wonder where we could have been not to have seen all this, till we finally decided either that we had no eyes and ears, or newspaper correspondents had sometimes more than the proper allowance, to say nothing of official telegrams and reports, even those of 'the pious King William to his dear Augusta.'

Having finished our exploration, we started for our 'Hôtel du Chemin de Fer,': which we had seen comfortably shunted on to a siding a little way ahead of the station. We blundered over the rails and tried to find a place easy to walk on; and whilst, tired and out of breath with our exertions, we plunged resolutely on, keeping our eyes fixed on the train we had left, we suddenly saw it, to our great dismay, going off at what appeared to be full speed down the line. Now all our 'little baggages' were there, and we commenced the pursuit of our flying hotel in good earnest.

Hunting a moveable lodging over the uneven ground of a junction station at one in the morning, with no other prospect of a bed but overtaking it, is not an exhilarating proceeding, and we were very glad to see the hotel stop, and to climb into it, and compose ourselves for the night, having performed our *toilette* by putting on our wrappers and putting off our boots. Sleeping in a railway carriage as it flies along, with a short halt here and there, and the conviction that one is approaching the desired destination, is even then not a comfortable way of passing the night; but deliberately doing it with the carriage standing still, is more uncomfortable, and none of us felt much refreshed in the morning.

We were fresh from England, and all its profusion of soap and water, and had not got accustomed to sometimes a pint of water amongst us, and sometimes none at all. Dirt had not become our normal condition, and before we looked out for breakfast, we tried to find some dressing room, however rude. Whilst wandering hopelessly about the junction station with its network of lines, we looked up, and on the top of a high green bank, which bounded it, we espied our gentlemen, evidently with water and a towel. We instantly climbed up, cleared the paling, and demanded a share in their luxuries, which included a pump, with a wooden trough; and after this, feeling greatly the better, we descended again and got some coffee and oranges, after which Louise and myself strolled into the town. We amused ourselves by going shopping, woman's sure comfort, and heard amusing tales of the bombardment from the people.

Nothing very terrible had happened: the station being on the heights opposite the French batteries had suffered most. The young Frenchwoman who told us this had passed three days in the cellar, for fear of the bomb-shells. She was one of those who had volunteered, with the rest of her townswomen, to nurse the wounded. They were divided into bands, and each took ten days' duty in turns. She had just returned to her shop, but they had not had many gravely wounded in the town. At that time, it was too near the frontier, and the men were sent farther into Germany. When we returned to the station, we found what may be vaguely called 'a great many trains' going to start.

We knew ours by its having a truck attached to it, on which was the omnibus of the Cologne Ambulance—a light waggonette for two horses, which would hold six inside, with a cover of tarpaulin. It was an admirable vehicle for the purpose, for at night it was a comfortable bedroom for two or three. We discovered it at last, but quite in a different direction; and after reaching it with much difficulty, and establishing ourselves for the journey, we were told we must go in another train which had not yet been formed.

We waited about, were sent from one train to another, and at last, utterly worn out, found the one which was finally decided upon by the authorities, and then to our sorrow heard that our kind friends of the Cologne Ambulance had had their truck and baggage wagon taken off the train to make way for a carriage of soldiers, and must wait, how long no one knew—not very long after all, as it turned out, for they came on an hour or two later, and we all met at St. Avoid, a lonely wayside station, fairly in France. Close by was the battlefield of Forbach, which extended thus far, and traces of the combat were visible as we came along, also of the march of an army, which we learned to track by an unfailing sign—the number of empty bottles.

We passed the station without stopping, and about a quarter of a mile beyond came to a stand-still, and there we remained till eight in the evening, after nine hours' delay. It must not be imagined this was a passenger train—it was entirely for military purposes, and we travelled in it as part of an ambulance, and therefore we were independent of time-tables; but even had it not been so, the line was so blocked that it was impossible to stir. Eight trains were on the road before us, in a space of sixteen miles, between St. Avold and Remilly, where the line ended at a distance of only sixteen miles from Metz itself. Remilly was the station to which all the wounded of the three days' Battle of Vionville and Gravelotte were brought, and during that day and the next, both of which we spent in our carriage on the line, two thousand waggons of wounded passed us, each containing from six to ten men. This may give a truer idea of the German losses on those days, than the official telegrams. There were very few French amongst them.

This 19th of August was a very long day. The train might have started at any moment, and we were afraid to go far. We saw on a high road, which traversed the plain at the distance of a mile, a column of troops; but we could not see the gleam of bayonet or sword, only a bright line of colour above and below, and a few dark spots on either side the column. At last we recognised them—French prisoners—in their red *kepis* and trousers; the first but not the last time we saw so sad a sight. It was too far for us to venture, and we contented ourselves with strolling in the fields, and picking up such relics as we could find, principally torn papers.

In the midst of this occupation we heard a shrill whistle, and off went our train. We immediately began to run over the heavy grass land, as if there was a possibility of catching it, and the proceeding afforded much amusement to the soldiers in the carriages.

Just as we were breathless and despairing, we saw a picturesque dragoon officer, in a silver helmet and long white cloak, who was standing on the line, wave his hand to us to stop, and we slackened our pace. When we came up to him, he told us the train was only going on a few hundred yards, and we had no chance of reaching Remilly that night. He was one of the finest and handsomest Germans I ever saw, with an Italian complexion and jet black hair, a bright smile and a kindly manner. We were told he was a Stolberg, one of the noble family of that name. When the White Cuirassierst fell so thick and fast at Floing, near Sedan, we may hope he escaped from the massacre; for if he was as good as he was handsome, as the old proverb insinuates, he must have been the *enfant gâté*, of his home.

Another and another long hour passed, and finding there was no possibility of getting on, we went back to the little station. It was ruined and roofless: shot and shell had fallen round it all the day of the battle; but in one small engine-house a few French prisoners were lying on the ground, too tired and dispirited even to rise from their straw beds. One was from Clermont Ferrand, and spoke sadly of his native village, and the long imprisonment he feared lay before him. Now we wished we had bread, wine, or tobacco to give them; but such things are not included in 'little baggages,' or were not then. We learned wisdom afterwards, and carried about cigars; and no greater comfort could be given to a sick or captive soldier of either nation than those of tobacco.

It was getting late; coffee and oranges had not been a substantial breakfast, and we had not even a morsel of bread—no water, only a little brandy in our flasks. We began to be very hungry, and at last the General produced a pot of Liebig: a fire was lighted with sticks and dry grass, some ditch water was procured, and we had a little soup. The soldiery began to light fires by pulling up the stakes and paling which bounded the low wood on our left, and some adventurous spirits started off for a potato field in the distance, and came back with a goodly quantity. We were just watching the boiling of the potatoes, and meditating a friendly exchange of brandy for a few of them, when the whistle sounded again, and the poor fellows had to jump in, leaving their fires, and burning their hands in trying to save their half-boiled potatoes, and we had to go without our dinner.

At Faulquemont we stopped again, and this time for the night. It was too early to sleep, and, indeed, something in the shape of supper was most desirable; but as it was pitch dark, and we could see nothing except some bivouac fires, which were being lighted, it seemed hopeless. At last a young German, who had travelled in our carriage from Saarbruck, came up to the window, and informed us that he had found a rough *auberge* in the village, and there was actually '*bifteck*'. It was too tempting a prospect; and as he kindly offered to escort us, two of us started off. It was just midnight when we returned to the train, and the scene was most picturesque.

Under a group of trees, in a green meadow by the side of the line, bivouac fires had been lighted, and crowds of soldiers were assembled round them, singing in chorus the national airs of Germany; and never again shall we hear '*Vaterland*' and '*Die Wacht am Rhein*' sung under such effective circumstances, when all around seemed to add reality to the words of the songs; the watch-fires throwing a lurid light on the groups of soldiers—their deep rich voices rising in chorus on the still air of an August night—and the consciousness that we were, in truth, on the battlefields of this great war. It was early morning before the singing ceased, and we were left to find what rest we could.

But still there were no signs of going on, and the delay was most trying, knowing how much our stores and help were needed at the front. We could get no conveyance of any kind to take us across country, so there was nothing for it but to wait patiently. The General, however, being offered a seat in a private carriage, left his baggage in our charge, and went off straight to headquarters.

If the detail of our journey to reach the scene of action seem somewhat prolonged. let it be remembered that it is in such simple details that the difference is seen between peace and war; the interruption of all ordinary routine, and the little minor miseries which, in the aggregate, amount to so much; and that this sketch is not only of battlefields and scenes of trial and excitement, but would aim to show what daily life is in an invaded country-

CHAPTER 3

The Two "Châteaux"

At the station we heard the sad-reason of our delay, which promised to be so long that the General took a light country cart and pushed on to headquarters at Pont-à-Mousson. As each train ran into the station at Remilly, it was emptied of its load of soldiers and re-filled with the wounded. This necessarily occupied a very long time, and kept the entrance to Remilly blocked with trains. One going back to Saarbruck soon ran into the station of Faulquemont, and the porters divided our train, which was standing there, in two, so that we could cross to the down line and give the poor fellows some bread and water.

There was a little at the station, not much; we gave to all we could, and the carriages, with their burden of suffering, soon went on. We consulted what was best to be done, and an expedition into the village was decided upon, to find provisions. The secretary went off into a violent state of excitement, declaring that it was the duty of the mayor of the place to provide refreshments for the wounded, and if he did not do his duty, he should be made to do it; and taking the law into his own hands, presented himself (at least so ran his tale) to the astounded official, and ordered him to send bread and brandy to the station.

The effect was certainly the arrival of several women with this assistance. We cut up the bread, and the secretary procured some buckets of water, into which he poured brandy. It was not a wise thing to do, as it was probable the wounded would prefer pure water, and so it turned out. Another train came in, and we commenced giving the provisions as fast as we could. The poor fellows were lying on straw, in luggage vans, and one side being left open for air, it was very easy to reach them; but one and all, after a sip of brandy and water, asked for pure water, and we were obliged to empty the buckets and re-fill them from a pump close by. It was hard work carrying the bread and water, and perpetually re-filling the cups of our flasks. The halt was but a short one, and we had to make all the haste we could, while hands were thrust out, and pathetic appeals made to us to be quick and give them some before they were off.

All day long this went on at intervals, and what between running with basket and buckets, and pumping at an impracticable pump, we were fairly worn out, when at five o'clock we started on our way to Remilly. On that day 2,000 waggons passed, averaging 15 wounded in each. It was a very pretty country we ran through, green and pastoral, and showing no signs of war till we reached Herny, a village six miles further on; and there, in the meadows, on either side the way, was an enormous camp of provisions, guarded by comparatively few soldiers. The king's headquarters had been there two days before, and we heard their camp was always that space of time in rear of them.

At last, at eight p.m., we reached Remilly, having been just thirty-four hours coming thirty-nine English miles! The platform was crowded with ambulance-bearers, waiting for the next convoy of country carts bringing wounded, and they were now coming in; but amidst all the confusion a Prussian *aide-de-camp* made way up to our secretary, who presented him as Baron L—, sent from Pont-à-Mousson to meet us. The baron took the reins into his own hands, informed the secretary that from that moment we were under his charge; he had his orders to take us straight to the king, and at ten next morning should be ready to escort us, assuring us at the same time of a warm welcome at headquarters. All seemed now satisfactorily arranged, and finding the carts had arrived, and the miserable sufferers were being laid on heaps of straw on the platform, we piled up our little baggages in a corner, gave them into charge, and went to give what aid we could.

For the first time we were in actual contact with the fearful details of the war. Many of the wounds had been but roughly bandaged needing fresh dressings, from the effect of the jolting over rough roads for eight or ten hours in a burning sun. They were all Germans, and several so fearfully hurt, it seemed impossible to carry them on; yet they were gradually got into the trains, the most seriously wounded into first-class carriages, the rest into the baggage-waggons. Darkness came on, and flaming pitch torches were lighted, and threw a red glare on the scene. Moans of pain, and sudden and sharp cries of agony, added to its fearful effect. Crimson-stained rags and bits of torn clothing, dirty straw, blankets, caps, and guns, were strewed about, and the heat was stifling, whilst the smoke of the torches choked wounded and assistants alike. It was a relief when the train was off, and whilst waiting for more carts, to go out into the village and try to find a shelter; for our 'Hôtel du Chemin de Per' had gone back to Saarbruck, and we were literally 'houseless by night.'

But the little town itself presented a sad sight. Close to the station was an open place with trees, and here were many wounded lying on straw, so that we had difficulty in making our way across it. Piteous appeals were made for water and help, and it seemed bad management not to have taken them on to the platform, now nearly cleared of wounded, to wait for the next train. We wandered up a street with a high wall on one side, and seeing an hotel, or rather *auberge*, I turned into the entrance and civilly asked if rooms were to be had there. A Prussian soldier instantly seized me by the shoulder and commenced pushing me into the street with considerable violence. A *sous-officier*, who was passing, asked what he was doing, and reprimanded him severely, explaining to him that it was impossible for strangers to know that the house was taken up for soldiers' quarters; and he also told us so was every inn in the town, and that it hopeless to search further. We had had nothing since our rough breakfast but a dry crust of rye bread. We had been too busy at Faulquemont to think of our own wants, and the prospect of no bed and no supper was not cheering.

We made our way back to the station amidst groups of noisy soldiers, and found our party assembling and preparing for a similar exploring expedition. It was now pitch dark, and our report was far from encouraging; but someone suggested that the Knights of St. John had always the best house in town, and probably would give us shelter, and we started for the large *château* of which they had taken possession. We looked at the long range of windows, and thought that surely some one small room could be spared us, and full of hope, heard the bell ring, saw the door opened, showing a lighted hall, and were informed that we could not lodge there! We might go over the way, where the Protestant Sisters, working with their Order, had a *château*, and see what they would do for us.

We humbly withdrew, and I suggested a bivouac under the rose-bushes in the garden of the inhospitable Hospitallers; at all, events it was cool and calm and quiet, away from the glare of the station and the noise in the crowded streets; but as a last resource we did go over the way and found an equally large *château*, and here were more fortunate. The kindly Sisters had pity upon us and took us all in, gentlemen and all, only regretting they had nothing but mattresses to offer us, and actually gave us tea, bread and butter, and eggs; and taking us through a room where several severely wounded men were lying, one in the agonies of death, showed us into what in we should call the back drawing-room. As we could be of no use to the poor fellows next door, we at once took possession of our mattresses, which we thoroughly enjoyed, and slept profoundly.

Now as we ran into the Remilly station that evening, not knowing the horrors we should encounter there, we had seen on a high wooded bank on our left a charming white stone *château*, with gardens and shrubberies coming down to the line, and a summer-house overlooking the country, with Indian chairs and matting, and we had drawn fancy pictures of the family sitting round the table in the long dining-room whose windows we could see, and who, hearing of the arrival of houseless and dinnerless strangers in the town, bound on an errand of mercy, would send a polite domestic in gorgeous livery to seek for us, with a courteous invitation to become the honoured guests of that White Château; and great was our surprise and amusement the next morning, when, on descending from our room, we wandered into the garden before breakfast, to find ourselves standing close by the Indian summer-house. We were actually the guests of the White Château, though the happy family and the gorgeous footman had faded with the dreams of the night before into empty air.

The *château*, like so many others we afterwards saw, had been deserted by the happy family of our fancy sketch, and was now occupied as an ambulance by the deaconesses. Far better it should be so than be used as soldiers' quarters. It was the great object then and afterwards to turn every good house into an ambulance where it was possible to do so, and much abuse arose from an unlimited use of the article of the Geneva Convention, which stipulates for the safety of every house in which wounded are nursed.

Persons who had neither the means nor the instruction sufficient to support and nurse the wounded, would beg for a wounded man or two as a security, and the result was much neglect from ignorance, and much suffering from want not only of the luxuries, but the necessaries for a sick or wounded man; and it was a wise rule which was afterwards made that no house should be considered an ambulance unless it could accommodate six wounded.

I myself spoke with an old woman who went to the Prussian *commandant du place* (town mayor) at Orléans to get a brassard stamped and a safe-conduct for her house as an ambulance for one man. I asked her what she could give him to eat and drink, to begin with; she said milk, and a little bread. She had nothing but that for herself, but she could not support the hardship of having four German soldiers in her little cottage. I had much trouble to persuade her it was no use applying for a licence, and I believe I utterly failed in the attempt.

After breakfast we packed up all our little baggage, and waited for our secretary and the *aide-de-camp*. He presently arrived, and told us he thought we should do much better to remain there in the *château*, and establish an ambulance, than go to headquarters; and he had told the *aide-de-camp* so, who had gone off to report it to Prince Pless at Pont-à-Mousson, and that he would make all arrangements with the deaconesses. Now there were twelve deaconesses to thirty wounded, and no prospect of more arriving, as all, however badly hurt, were at this time sent on by train. It was a transgression of our positive orders, which left no discretion to us as to our destination; and besides, the deaconesses did not want us, and plainly said so. Nothing could be kinder or more courteous than they were.

If we were resolved to stay, they would do their best to make us comfortable: give us a wing of the house, the use of all their cooking utensils, anything in their power; but they did not really want or wish for us; and it was an anomalous position for English ladies to be placed in, to force themselves into a house, unasked, and establish themselves there, where they could be of no service, and where even their stores were not required, as the deaconesses were amply supplied by the Order of St. John. We plainly expressed our opinion, and urged compliance with our written orders. The secretary, excited himself; but firmness won the day, and the arrival of Mr. Herberte, who had reached Remilly with his stores three hours after us, settled the question. He offered to take the ladies on to Pont-à-Mousson in his waggonette, if the gentlemen would follow with the baggage; and it was so arranged, and that we were to start at three o'clock.

This being happily settled, we began to enjoy the beauties of the garden, when a great noise and bustle suddenly commenced in the street, below the wall which divided the garden from the town. We went directly on to the raised terrace just inside the wall, and saw four soldiers running from all quarters with their arms, and taking up a position opposite the gate. A long road, leading in a straight line to Metz, was visible, and evidently something was expected down this road. On enquiry, we heard there was a sortie from Metz, that the French were coming straight to the village, and the Prussian outposts were already driven in. The deaconesses were very anxious that a conspicuous Red-Cross flag should be exhibited from the topmost turret, as if the French had artillery, we were in the direct line of fire; though, if the Prussians defended the road, it was difficult to see how, in a military point of view, they could be dislodged by artillery, without the necessity of including the *château* in the fire of their guns.

We were exactly in the position of a bull's eye in a target, and the Red-Cross flag would have been of very little use. However, the Deaconesses and several of our ladies set to work to make one, which, being extended on the floor of the vestibule, the party at work round it in various gave the exact effect of a game of 'Hunt the slipper.' All the Grand Préparations, however, were useless; the report was a false one, and the town settled down into such quietude as a town only sixteen miles from a besieged city, and much closer still to the besieging lines, may be supposed to enjoy.

About three o'clock we were summoned by Mr. Herberte to embark on board his waggonette. The secretary and surgeon had procured waggons for the baggage, and professed their intention of walking, though why they could not have got a little *charrette* or country cart, I do not know. The stores of the Cologne Ambulance and ours were all placed in charge of a troop of cavalry, together with the military stores. Major Siersdorff, the commander, ordered us all to keep together till we reached Cormy, where we were to rest for the night; but it was already late before, to use a naval phrase, the convoy got under weigh. Our waggonette and the light carriage, with the major and three other officers, soon outstripped the heavy waggons, and we had perpetually to stop till they came up.

About this period it appears our gentlemen were seized with the brilliant idea of taking a short cut through the woods; and, disregarding the advice of some gentlemen attached to an Italian Ambulance from Turin, which they were on the way to join near Metz, the rash individuals cut themselves sticks, and set out on a walking tour. The result may be easily guessed: we missed each other. Darkness came on, and we were still far from Cormy, but the lights of a large cavalry camp were glimmering in the distance. The major and Mr. Herberte having consulted together, and finding the baggage waggons still far in the rear, it was resolved that we should push on as fast as possible to the village close by the camp, where was the *château* of Coin-sur-Seille, now occupied by his Excellency General Von der Groeben, as headquarters of the division he commanded. We passed the little huts of the camp, roughly made branches stuck into the ground and interwoven together, for the Germans have no tents; and, turning down a wooded lane, drove into a crowded courtyard, where we halted whilst our kind escort went to ask hospitality for us from the general.

He soon returned with an *aide-de-camp*, who spoke English perfectly, and told us he had an English wife. He was most courteous; said the general only regretted he had not known of our coming sooner, to prepare some rooms for us; but at this time of night we must content ourselves with such rough accommodation as he could offer us. Thankful even for this, we got out of the carriage, and were met on the steps of the *château* by a very gentlemanly officer, who was no less a person than the general himself. He welcomed us with the utmost kindness, and taking a light from the hand of one of the servants, himself preceded us upstairs, showed us into a couple of rooms where we could rest for the night, and withdrew, wishing us good repose.

Two elderly females made their appearance; they were old servants of the family who had left the *château*. They had nothing to offer us, poor things; they had a hard struggle to live themselves; but they got us some hot water, and we made a little soup with Warren's meat biscuits, which refreshed us very much. Louise said she saw at the Remilly station barrels of the same biscuit, for the use of the Prussian Army; and though this little book is not like the Christmas pantomimes now-a-days, a vehicle for advertisements, it is but just to say how very good the soup was which they made, and it was fortunate for the Prussians to have a supply of them.

We were up very early the next morning; and, descending into the large old-fashioned kitchen of the *château*, bribed the servants to give us a little coffee and bread and butter; whilst thus breakfasting, we heard the history of the *château*. It belonged to a 'Madame Windle,' an Englishwoman probably, as she had gone to England. The *château* had been taken possession of and turned into a barrack by the Prussians; but the old ladies spoke in the highest terms of General Von der Groeben and his considerate kindness. There was no wanton mischief or destruction, only several acts of dishonesty on the part of individual soldiers, such as pocketing rich china cups and small articles for use or ornament, and carrying off saucepans and other cooking utensils; but compared with what we saw and heard afterwards, in other places, the *château* had a fortunate escape in being occupied by so true a gentleman as His Excellency.

We wandered about the lovely terraced gardens, and gathered

handfuls of autumn roses! The pears and grapes were not ripe, nor the peaches and apricots, and if they had been, there would have been none left for us. There were too many troopers lounging about not to have spied out the first ripe fruit and appropriate it, if there had been any. But at the best it is a sad sight to see a splendid home so pulled to pieces; drawing-rooms turned into bedrooms; the gilded furniture all displaced and strewn about here and there. Too often far worse scenes occur; and it is sadder still to see a cottage home so desecrated, and the savings of a life-time destroyed in an hour.

We left the *château* about eight o'clock, having thanked the General for his kindness, and Mr. Herberte having told us that his cousin in the *cuirassiers* was most anxious to show us their camp, we drove back a few yards, and then walked through the long line of huts. All looked bright and cheerful in the morning sunlight. Accoutrements were being cleaned; horses were saddling, and the troopers were preparing to mount when the breakfast in the officers' hut was over. There was no difference in this hut, except that it was larger, and a few mats and rugs were on the straw which formed at once bed and carpet. The huts were arranged in streets as in all camps, and the pathways were kept very clean. The regiment was one of the White Cuirassiers. The uniform is the same in all these regiments, a steel breast-plate, a helmet—whose shape is that of the only perfectly graceful helmet I ever saw—white coats and jack-boots. The difference is in the facings: some having blue, some black, brown, yellow, or green.

After this we crossed the road to the Lancers' camp, the other side, and watched the exercises of the cavalry, both light and heavy, for some time, expecting every instant the arrival of the convoy and the missing gentlemen. Intelligence came at last that they had stopped short of Coin-sur-Seille for the night, and gone on to Cormy by another road, and we started off for the same town, where a road branched off to Pont-à-Mousson. There had been a universal agreement amongst us that stragglers were to rendezvous at Cormy, and we felt assured of meeting our friends and baggage there, and being safely taken on to the headquarters before night. We should then receive our orders from Prince Pless, the head of the German Ambulance department, and know our destination; but our wanderings were not fated to terminate so easily, and Cormy was to be the beginning instead of the end of our troubles. But no omen of evil disturbed us as we drove along the high road from Coin-sur-Seille to Cormy, in the sunshine of that lovely August morning.

Chapter 4

The Midnight Drive

The road from Coin-sur-Seille to Cormy was an exceedingly pretty one: trees on each side of it, and a charming view over green fields and patches of wood to a blue distance; and as we drove along, and came suddenly round a corner, a fresh view was disclosed—the houses of a large town and the spire of a splendid cathedral. It looked so cheerful and beautiful, with the quiet fertile country all around; and yet that city was Metz, and the low dull sound we heard now and then the booming of the cannon. We were nearer to the town than the Prussian lines, but the works of defence were hidden by the intervening country. We looked at it with a strange interest. The siege had at that time hardly begun, and its future fate was all uncertain. M'Mahon and the relieving forces were probably on the march, and no one could foretell the dark tale of treason and shame that will go down with the name of Metz to the latest posterity.

It was noon when we reached Cormy, a town of one long street and one cross street, crowded with men attached to various ambulances. We halted just through the town, and looked about for our friends and baggage. Nowhere could we see them. Major Siersdorff told us that he had enquired at the quarters of the Knights of St. John, and had orders for us to go on directly to Ste. Marie-aux-Chênes, near Metz, which was full of wounded. This message had been left by the secretary; but where he was was a mystery; a greater mystery still why he did not wait at Cormy according to agreement, and why he did not make the slightest effort to find us; for at that very time he was in Cormy, as Louise saw the surgeon (Mr. Parker) at a distance, and wanted to speak to him, but was over-persuaded by the lady who was with her to go on to the house where they had been informed another lady and myself had taken refuge from the confusion in the streets.

I had gone to search for our convoy, and meeting a very civil young German gentleman, with the Red-Cross badge on his arm, who directed my companion and myself to the quarters of the Knights of St. John, we had accepted his kind offer to take us to the garden of an hospital, where soup was being boiled, and to give us a basin whilst he sent in search of our companions, who were just at the end of the street.

Louise persisted that she had seen the doctor, and I went back with her to the spot. We found a camp fire, and the gentlemen of the Swiss Ambulance taking a rough dinner by it. They said our friend had been there, and one of them had met the secretary only ten minutes before. They were sure he was still in town. Now it was an important point to find him. There were we, with no roof to shelter us, sitting by a road-side, uncertain what to do and where to go; and to add to our troubles, Mr. Herberte got his orders to go to some other villages, and could not take us to Ste. Marie. We had no vehicle, and were certainly in as awkward a predicament as ever English ladies were placed in. A suspicion of unfair play crossed the minds of Louise and myself at that time, and has never since been dissipated. Why was no note left for us? We had only a vague message; and the secretary, the surgeon, and the valuable stores, had all vanished together.

Now the sympathies of Louise and myself were strongly French; I do not deny it; but that never interfered with our doing all in our power for the German wounded. In that, at least, we were strictly neutral; and so neutral that the secretary might have a guess we should object to the entire appropriation of the society's stores for the benefit of the Knights of St. John or the German use alone. Was this at the bottom of a wish to part the ladies and the stores—in short, to get rid of the female incumbrances, while he clung to the baggage? We shall never know; but there we were; and in a hopeless state I invaded the *sanctum* of the Knights, and requested we might be sent on. We waited awhile, all in vain, still expecting some news. How our heavy waggons got out of town I do not know, unless they went by a cross road, so as to avoid the main street; otherwise we must have seen them.

But at last it was time to depart. Our kind friends of the Cologne Ambulance were off, and we felt very desolate and helpless as we sat on a bench by the road-side to wait for the two rough waggons which were to convey us. They came at last, and with them a most gentlemanly Knight of St. John to act as our escort, and we started. Perhaps very few English have travelled in those bullock-waggons, with their very long poles and sleepy drivers, who, regardless of anything except their nap and pipe, and evidently unaccustomed to travel in long strings of vehicles such as crowded all the roads now-a-days, never thought of pulling up when a stop occurred, so that our pole ran with a sudden jerk into the waggon in front, and the waggon behind ran theirs into us, and a sort of electric shock ran all up and down the line; and as this happened on an average every ten minutes, the progress if slow is exciting; but, except for this, the mode of travelling is delightful. Extended on a heap of sweet-smelling hay, wandering slowly through a lovely country, buried in a soft bed, and sheltered from rain by pulling a water-proof sheet over all, and going to sleep under it, it is a dreamy, idle way of going from place to place, which, if you are not in a hurry, is the perfection of the '*Dolce far niente.*'

The waggons were ready; the Knight of St. John mounted in front had confided to our care his elegant court sword, having evidently more confidence in his revolver; we had arranged ourselves comfortably, and were about to start, when an excited individual, also a Knight of St. John, dashed up and ordered us to stop. We humbly asked why, and who he was; and he replied. Major Baron von Zedlitz. Now I had been warned before I left London, if I did encounter such an individual, to keep clear of him. He had nothing to do with us. We were to obey Prince Pless, and no one else; and I remarked that we were going to Ste. Marie-aux-Chênes, and that, as we were late, I should be obliged by his not detaining us.

On this he grew furious, and declared we were to stay in Cormy. There were so many wounded there, we must remain to nurse them; and he would give us a house and send for our baggage; but stay we should. I declined positively to do so, and he used what I believe might be very bad language, veiled in guttural German; at least it sounded like it, and we thought so, because he added directly afterwards, 'If you were in a drawing-room I should not speak so to you.'

To this I answered, 'A lady is a lady in a hay-waggon as well as a drawing-room; you ought to remember that.' He then said the English Society had sent us. I said 'Yes,' and their orders we were bound to obey. His reply was not very *apropos*: 'That he cared nothing for the Prince of Wales.' This must have been such a dreadful loss to his royal highness that we laughed outright, and our *chevalier* requested the baron to 'go away'—a mild translation, but expressing the sense of what he said; and as the bullocks took it into their heads to go on, we did go on, and left our friend gesticulating in the street.

It was two o'clock when we left Cormy, and a seven hours' journey before us; and just as we got out of the town, and down a steep bank, which would have been the ruin of a respectable carriage, we met a troop of dragoons. The officer stopped us, asked if we were the English ladies, and said an express had been sent to Remilly to bring us to headquarters. Prince Pless was very angry that we had not come on with the *aide-de-camp*, as arranged on our first arrival. We said we must go on to Ste. Marie now as our stores and baggage were there, but we would tell the secretary. I must here remark that our surgeon, Mr. Parker, had gone on with him, on the faith that a gentleman to whom the secretary spoke was Prince Pless.

The description did not accord with the personal appearance of the prince, as we saw him afterwards at Versailles; nor is it clear why the prince should send a messenger from Pont-à-Mousson to bring us on there, and then give orders in Cormy that we should go to Ste. Marie; and why he did not give them some written order? We were thoroughly puzzled; and as Louise and I sat nestling in the hay, discussing the matter with profound gravity, we must have reminded any looker-on of the original owls in an ivy bush. Our sagacious discourse was cut short by a worse jerk than usual, and we saw we were by the bank of a river, across which was thrown a temporary bridge for exit from the town, while the real bridge was reserved for the passage of the carts of wounded which still came on in endless stream from the neighbourhood of the battlefields.

Had we been five minutes sooner we could have crossed, but a German regiment was just ahead of us; after them came all their provision waggons, and they were followed by a pontoon train, the massive iron boats placed on very heavy broad-wheeled trucks, which tried the strength of the bridge. It bore very well, except that every now and then some plank had to be replaced. But it was just at the other end, where the bank of soft sand rose steeply, that all the troubles occurred. The only chance of getting up it was lashing the horses into a gallop, and this only succeeded half way, for the wheels of the heavy trucks invariably sank so deep into the sand that other horses had to be attached in front, and the wheels dug out; and when this was done, and the waggon safely landed on the road the bank had to be re-made, and so on for about twenty waggons.

Two whole hours we waited in despair, watching the proceeding, and thinking how much more simple it would have been to have sent the pontoon trains by the old bridge, and the lighter carts by the new; but the order had been given, and it would have required an application to at least three departments, and three dozen officers, a quire of paper, and a couple of secretaries, to have diverted the course of one waggon. There never were such a people for pens and ink and forms to fill in as the Prussians. Our Circumlocution Office is nothing to it.

But at last we started, and got fairly over the bridge and into the long line of waggons going up one way and coming down the other. It seemed as hopeless as ever; but our gallant Knight aroused himself, called to a dragoon, and we were allowed to break the line and go on. We saw a refractory waggon and driver fairly hunted off the road, down the bank, and into the meadow below. It seemed impossible for it not to go over, but it escaped. At last we came where the waggons were three abreast, and a carriage containing a wounded officer of rank was trying to pass down the road. One resource remained for us, if we would not pass hours in the block, and it was had recourse to. The dragoon, brandishing his drawn sword and shouting fearfully, dashed down the bank and into the field; our driver stood up and urged on his quiet beasts, and to my horror I found we were going after the dragoon. What a jolting and bumping it was!

But the waggon was evidently built on the principle of never losing its equilibrium, and as for the harness breaking, it could not well do that, for the ropes of which it was composed were so loose that the wonder was how the bullocks kept in them, and why they did not catch their feet in the traces which dangled about. Over the meadow we went, till we had headed the line and regained the road. The Knight wrapped himself up in his cloak, and lighted his cigar.

We dug a hole in the hay, in which we could keep ourselves warm (for the sun was setting and the evening was damp and chill), and composed ourselves to sleep. Weary hours passed away, and still the bullocks jogged on. Three times we went the wrong road, and had to retrace our steps. We passed through the town of Ars-sur-Moselle, with its Roman ruin. Night set in, and there we were, between Metz and the Prussian lines, and our destination apparently as far off as ever. We slept and woke, and slept again; we got cold and cramped; and where we were no one knew, not the Knight or the drivers.

Except our two waggons, not a vehicle was to be seen, and the villages were deserted. At last we emerged on a level space of country. It lay white and bare in the darkness, and a fearful smell compelled us to keep our handkerchiefs close to our faces, and even then, it produced a feeling of sickness. The Knight flung away the red end of his last cigar, and turning round, told us this was the battlefield. We could see nothing but the outline of a vast space, over, which we had to pass. The sad details were hidden in the darkness, and we went slowly on till we entered a ruined village, and halted before an almost roofless house, where lights were still gleaming, though a hot steam on the windows hid the occupants. The door opened, and a gentleman came out, his stained apron showing too plainly what had been his occupation. He told us the village was Gravelotte, Ste. Marie was a mile further on, and prayed for bread and wine for his wounded.

We had none to give. The Knight promised to send some back from their stores at Ste. Marie, and we started again. Just beyond and behind the village the hottest fight had been, and the dead had been hastily buried by a hillock between Gravelotte and Ste. Marie, but indeed for miles the whole battlefield was scarred with a thousand graves; not single tombs, but trenches, in which the dead were piled, with a rough wooden cross above them, to point out the place. Catholic and Protestant alike seem to have accepted that holy sign as the most fitting to mark where the soldiers of both nations and all faiths were buried side by side on the field where they fell. Just afterwards we passed a number of blazing watchfires. They were the outposts of the army of Prince Frederick Charles.

In half an hour more we halted again at the entrance of a village. A German sentinel told us it was Ste. Marie, and now where our secretary and the baggage were was the question. We wandered slowly on through the long street, not meeting a living soul, till we found ourselves at the other extreme end of the village. Here a countryman appeared, who suggested that probably the strangers were at a '*château*' which he pointed out, down a very muddy lane. The Knight proposed that before we ventured down it on what might be a useless search he should go and enquire, unless we were afraid to be left; but really we saw no cause for fear in the street of a village, however deserted; and he was about to start when we heard a call, and saw our absconded friends running up the street, professing their great astonishment at seeing us, their wonder at how they could have missed us, and the agonies of mind they had gone through on our account.

Where we were to sleep was the question, and the night being far advanced, it was indeed a serious question. The Knight most courteously suggested that at all events the quarters of the Knights of St. John would doubtless afford us shelter; and there we repaired, and were received by what we might irreverently describe as an elderly party, the very type of a lodging-house keeper; but who, we were informed, was a Mrs. Seeman, who had come from Dresden, with some Alexandrine Sisters, to assist the Knights in their care of the wounded.

We were shown into a most comfortable room, with handsome mahogany bedsteads, feather beds, pillows, and clean sheets. We had not undressed since we left England, nine days before, and the prospect was most inviting. There were two or three Knights there, distinguished by the white enamel cross suspended round the neck, and a young esquire. They regretted that they had but little to offer us, but to that we were welcome; and we gratefully accepted some very weak tea and some slices of rye bread. We wondered what was to become of us. Would the Knights vacate their comfortable beds, and sleep in their cloaks in some other apartment, or were there other apartments as luxuriously furnished; for, in spite of the stores piled about the room, it was comparative luxury. At last Madame S— rose, and said two of the ladies must sleep in the house where the Knights dined, and the others in this house.

We waited till she returned from disposing of them for the night, and she then showed us into a sort of closet, in which was a bed; and how thankful we were to creep into it, even hungry as we were, and to enjoy our first good night's rest! I do not think we should have gone off to sleep so contentedly had we known, as we did afterwards, that the Knights of St. John sat down to a good hot supper, with pale ale and wine. But how they do their work will be seen as we go on. It was enough for us to have tea and bread and a bed; and had our privations been unavoidable, we should have been rather glad of them than otherwise; but it was not so, and Mr. Parker often said afterwards he felt ashamed to sit down and sup with them, knowing how little we had had.

It was well he did. It was his last chance for some days, and hard and trying work lay before him; and often we stinted ourselves to leave a larger portion for one, who, we knew, must require it more than we did; so it was well that he enjoyed a good supper. The name of our kind and courteous escort we never knew; but if ever this book should meet his eye, we beg here to thank him for the trouble he took, and the long journey he underwent, in fulfilment of his Knightly duty of guarding unprotected females over a lonely country, and past the outposts of the besieging and defending forces, where, certainly, it was wholly unfitting for them to venture alone. But our venturous journey was safely ended under his care, and we were ready to commence our duties with the coming day.

CHAPTER 5

The Knights of St. John

The morning of the 23rd of August opened with a downpour of rain, which continued all day. Under such circumstances no lonely village like Ste. Marie could have looked gay; but the brightest sunshine would have failed to give an air of cheerfulness to a place so ruined, so desolate, so full of pain and sorrow. It might have been truly said of it that day 'There was not a house where there was not one dead.' The battles of the 16th, 17th, and 18th. had extended over many miles of country, on which stood several villages, amongst them St. Privat, Vionville, Gravelotte, Briey, and Ste. Marie; and the wounded, who could not be carried to the rear, were dispersed amongst these villages. The inhabitants had mostly fled from them.

Shot and shell had done their work of destruction. All the habitable houses were occupied as ambulances, whilst the churches were also crowded. The miseries endured by the poor fellows, laid down to suffer and die in the first shelter that could be found—their greatest luxury a heap of straw—must be seen to be understood. Too often overlooked in out-of-the-way barns and stables, they long in vain for even bread or water; and death on the battlefield is a happy alternative from such prolonged agony.

It was now our duty to go amidst these scenes of horror, and we prepared ourselves, ready for the arrival of the surgeon-in-chief, who was to allot to us our share in the work. But first some sort of breakfast was desirable, and Mrs. Seeman informed us we should have some bread and coffee when the Knights had finished their repast, and we had ground a certain quantity of coffee-beans. The oldest and crankiest of coffee-mills was produced. We set to work—one of the ladies really was most indefatigable—but imagine our disgust when we found we were grinding for the Knights! We abandoned the coffee-mill, and adjourned to the other house, to wait for what might come.

Coffee and rye bread came at last. I suppose the Knights had eaten all the butter and eggs, for we only saw the shells; and when we returned to the quarters we were shown into an airy loft, without a single article of furniture in it, and informed this was our bedroom, and the gentlemen and the stores were to be stowed in the entrance, which was part of the loft, divided from it by a partition of planks. The windows were all broken, and the shutters hung loose on their hinges. It was lucky it was August. We thought that probably they would find us two or three mattresses, and a table, and a couple of chairs, so that we should be pretty comfortable. As for a *toilette* apparatus, we had been told that morning that there was no water, except for the wounded and for cooking, so that was evidently a superfluity.

Water was doubtless very scarce. The streams and wells were tainted with blood. It was only what was in the cisterns that was available. We had grown very immoral by this time, and regarded the theft of a couple of pints of water as a venial sin, and with this we all made our toilette. It was the greatest hardship of all, and we resolved that, come what might, water we would find, even if the Knights had to grow their beards, and do without the cans of shaving-water we saw carried into their room.

This, however, is a digression. To return to the later events of the day. The surgeon-in-chief came at last, paid us a great many pretty compliments, sent one surgeon to the church with one of the ladies, allotted to another a house in which were all the worst cases of gangrene, to Louise several stables full of wounded, to myself a house with about fifty. Surgeons and orderlies were very scarce. There was not a Sister of Mercy there, and the Alexandrine Sisters remained in the quarters to see to the cookery, and assist Mrs. Seeman. The dinners were to be given out at noon. Our first task was to wash the men as much as possible—a great difficulty with little water, no soap, and no sponges. *Charpie*, however, answered as well; and when their dirty stocks were taken off, and as much of their bloodstained clothes as possible, we commenced to dress the wounds of all, except those whom the surgeons themselves attended to.

In Louise's case she could not undress her poor men. They had only straw, and were obliged to keep on their coats. Nothing is so bad for them as this. The dust and blood, the sensation of dirt, is quite enough to make them feverish. The lady who had the church worked very hard; she put it into splendid order in twenty-four hours; but though the storehouse of the Knights was full of goods, there was immense difficulty in getting anything.

Many of the men were so desperately wounded it was useless to do anything but give them a little water. One man in my house laid grovelling on the floor; he would not keep on his mattress, and tore off even the blanket, his sole covering; he had been shot in the head, and how he had survived was a marvel. His awful appearance, as he rose and staggered about the room, with the blood streaming down, was too much for the nerves of the wounded soldiers. The German orderlies tried to keep him quiet; all in vain; and to finish his sad story, I applied to the surgeon to have him placed somewhere alone. It was twenty-four hours before it was done; and during the night he rose, and trying to get out nearly fell upon a poor Frenchman, the back part of whose right shoulder had been entirely carried away by a piece of shell. He shrieked with terror, and the orderlies declared that, order or no order, the miserable man must be changed, and he was finally taken down into the loose box of a stable below, where next day he died.

The hay-loft over this stable was the operation room, to which patients were brought from the smaller houses, and here the surgeons worked for hours at their sad task. About noon the soup came, no meat, only a morsel of bread, and having seen the dinner finished, I was going up the street to get mine, when I met Louise coming out of her stables. She asked me what time the patients were to have their soup. I said dinner was over, and on going to the quarters she discovered that her men had been quite forgotten. This rectified, we went into the other house, and found some soup, a very small piece of boiled bacon, and no vegetables. On this we dined, and went back to our work, which was more to watch the men, give them water, and change such dressings as required replacing, than the active work of the morning.

No wine was allowed to the French, and no cigars. The Germans had both, and the stores were full of wine and tobacco, so the want of them could not be the excuse. I applied to Mrs. Seeman for a bottle, and with some grumbling she gave me one. Louise also got some, and we gave it equally to both. Nothing can be kinder or more good-natured than German *infirmiers* to friend and foe alike, and when I left the bottle at night I found in the morning they had given it, as I had done, to both. It was but a little each man required, just to flavour and colour the water.

The rain continued as hard as ever, and as I went home to see how our bedroom was furnished, I found exactly what I had left—nothing. I sent for some straw. The German orderly who acted as servant instantly sent half-a-dozen soldiers with a shock a-piece, and half-a-dozen more after them. Louise and I then divided the straw, and laid our waterproof sheet over our heap, and seeing a large chest of '*spongio piline*,' one of those useless things sent out by the committee, we covered the sheet with the squares of *spongio*, and finding some sheets in a box, which said sheets were utterly useless at present in the stables, we laid them over it, and so constructed a bed that was at least clean, if not very soft. We then turned another chest of *spongio* on end, hung a railroad rug gracefully over it, and adorned it with our dressing things and several small books.

We also got a cardboard box of quinine powders, covered that with a small white cloth, stood up a round hand-glass upon it against the wall, and flattered ourselves that we had a *toilette* table of decided elegant appearance. Another box served as a table, chairs we had none, and the loft might have been called chilly on this rainy evening, even though it was August; but our work kept us warm. We then adjourned to the entrance, and in a fit of excessive charity set to work at the surgeon's bed, which was piled up in a recess, and so scientifically did we arrange it, that the unfortunate young man slept, or rather did not sleep, at an angle of forty-five, and passed the night slipping out at what might be called the foot of the bed, only stopped in his career into the centre of the room by the heavy boxes of waterproof sheeting which we had placed at the end of the straw heap to keep him warm and comfortable. His good temper and gaiety were proof even against this trial, and next morning he thanked us for our efforts, but said, if it made no difference to us, he preferred to lie with his head a little lower.

Supper at seven concluded the day, soup and very little *bouillon*, and one bottle of very sour wine. We were not epicures, yet we should have enjoyed a small piece of the chickens in white sauce, and the roast potatoes, and a glass of the port wine or pale ale that we saw go in to the Knights, who dined before us. Alas! bones, and empty bottles were our share of the gorgeous banquet! If we had only been allowed to dine before them, it would have been better; but as it was, we always saw the 'leavings' and never had any! They went to Frau Seeman. We were very hungry, and that is the honest truth. We had no store of food or wine, and we could not make an indigestible meal of *gutta percha* tissue, lint, and bandages. Quinine powders were the only things that we could have had; and under the circumstances, and considering the appetite they stimulate, it was not advisable to dose ourselves with them. If really there had been nothing to eat, we should have been quite contented. In our first enthusiasm, as I have said, luxuries and comforts were distasteful to us; but we were hungry and there were eatables, but none for us, and we went hungry to bed and were famished in the morning.

Breakfast was as scanty as ever, and just as it was over we heard the secretary say something which betrayed his intention of leaving Ste. Marie that day. We instantly asked him where he was going, and he said to England; his task of bringing us out was accomplished, and he should start in an hour. We requested him to take some letters for us, and he got very excited, and declared we ought to have no time to write, even to our relations, if we did our work properly. We could just send a Feld-Post card, but write we could not and should not. Louise most wisely assented to every word he said, fully intending to write a budget all the time by the first opportunity, and not having any intention of confiding her letters to his care; but I incautiously said, 'I have promised Captain Burgess, the Secretary of the Committee, to write to him as soon as we arrived at headquarters, and though we were not there, I should write and say where we were.'

He got more excited than ever; perhaps he was afraid we should write letters for the papers. Now this I had, at the request of the committee, promised not to do myself, and to express this their urgent desire and positive order to the other ladies. I can safely say I never transgressed it, though I was offered a handsome remuneration, neither did Louise. I have reason to believe it was disobeyed by one of the party, but it was unknown and unsanctioned by me. However, this might be, to our writing the secretary decidedly objected, and went off suddenly without any letters from anyone in his charge.

As for the Feld-Post cards, they, at that time, only passed in the German lines, and our English friends would not have been the wiser for any information sent upon them. I think later in the war they did go to England, but of this I am not sure; and before leaving the subject of posts I may remark that the uncertainty of the Feld-Post made it a sort of lottery as to whether any letters would ever reach. Sometimes they did, sometimes not; but we never got a newspaper by it, though German papers came safely to their destination. Had we got one now and then, we should have thought that they were stopped on account of their contents; but as it was, I fancy the weight of newspapers caused a general order to bring no foreign ones, the letter carts for cross country work being light and small.

After breakfast we went to our duty. In the light of a sunny morning, Ste. Marie looked sadder than ever, with its roofless houses, and the dirt and disorder of its only street. There were heaps of shakos, shoes, belts, tins, pots, cartouche boxes, pieces of bombshell, and, worst of all, rags, bandages, and *charpie* thrown out of the windows, and bearing evidence of their having been but lately used.

Not a woman or child was to be seen; a few were crouching in their ruined houses, but not daring to venture out, and every sign of trade or business had vanished. Even the conquering army had passed on, and only a small guard of soldiers was quartered there.

I found one of my wounded soldiers dying, a young Bavarian, and all he longed for was a little beer. How I had seen dozens of pale ale, unpacked, in the Knights' quarters. I saw hampers of 'Bass' in the storehouses, addressed for the use of the sick and wounded, and I went back directly to Mrs. Seeman, who officiated as store-keeper, and asked for a bottle. I was told there was none. I said there was; I had seen it; but the answer was it was for the use of the Knights. I begged in vain, and resolved to wait the return of some one of them to ask for a little.

I went upstairs, and whilst there two entered the house, accompanied by several German Army surgeons, and, coming into the outer room of the loft, requested me to open the stores, that they might select what they wanted, as they were going back to the camp. I told them the stores were in charge of the surgeon. He was at his duties; they must return later. They declined to go without the stores, and I sent for Mr. Parker, remaining myself on the watch. When he came, they wanted almost everything; but, with great tact, he contrived to get off by giving a quarter of what they wanted, and some of the very instruments they took we saw, five months afterwards, unused, to be taken home to Berlin, for service in their private practice there. Surely army surgeons (I call all army surgeons who were serving with the troops) should be supplied with instruments at the expense of their own government, not at the cost of private subscribers to a charitable fund.

After they were courteously bowed off, the surgeon and myself agreed we would hide all the small and valuable things under the straw of our bed in the inner room; we dragged in cases of valuable waterproof sheetings and *gutta-percha* tissue, and buried quinine powders, boxes of oiled silk, and various other articles in the straw. I forgot to mention this to Louise, who passed an uncomfortable night, and the next morning complained how very "knobby" the straw was; she was prepared to find it prickly, but not angular.

When we had finished hiding the valuable stores, I went down and again begged for some beer. Frau Seeman refused to give me anything, except a bottle of syrup to make some lemonade. With this I returned to my hospital, but the poor fellow was disappointed at not obtaining what he longed for, and in half an hour afterwards died. The morning duty being over, I returned back to quarters, and watched the Knights of St. John packing up four or five waggons of stores, to be sent back to Pont-a-Mousson, then the central depot, and resolved that, if they had such a superabundance, they should have none of ours.

After our early dinner Louise and I went our rounds to see that our patients had their dinners, and then resolved to walk just down the street and out of the village, where we could see over a great part of the battlefield. We went through the garden at the back of the house and found ourselves at once upon it, for Ste. Marie had been in the centre of the fight. For several miles the country all around was a barren level plain, on which there grew no single blade of grass. It had been corn and potato fields, divided by low hedges, but now the ground was as hard and bare as the Mall in Saint James's Park; but, unlike that, not a tree, not a shrub. Scattered over it were torn bits of clothing, helmets, swords, guns, tin pots, knives, knapsacks, combs, brushes, bottles, and odds and ends of all sorts here and there. Dark stains showed where some dead or wounded man had fallen; in one place was a huge heap of shakos and belts, guarded by a sentinel, and at intervals mounds of fresh earth showed where the dead were buried.

Nothing could be more depressing than the view over this dry, dusty plain, with a leaden sky lowering above and a chill wind whistling by. A great number of letters, papers, leaves of books, and cards were strewed about. I picked up some, and it was very sad to read the loving words from home, and to think of the hopes all mouldering under those mounds of earth. I will give an extract from one which contained no address, and was simply signed 'Nathalie.'

> *Chaire peti ami.* . . . I thank thee that thou hast sent me thy portrait; when I look at it, it seems as if I saw thee thyself. Alas, how happy I should be, if it would speak to me! Dear friend, I know it is impossible; but after all I wager there will come a happy day when I shall see thee thyself, and thou will never know how happy thy portrait made me. Dear friend, thou askest was I grieved to see thee depart? I was, indeed, though I did not say

so, that I might not vex thy mother, who weeps for thee every day. Charles has left. I gave him thy address; he will tell thee all the news. Eugenie comes not to see me as often as she did. Thou askest me why Stephen, who loves Honorine, does not marry her. I know nothing; they do not tell me. She told him he did not go to see her often enough; only upon a Sunday. Alas, dear friend, she is more greedy than I, who should be happy if I saw thee every Sunday, or even once a month.

Thou askest me did I dance on the feast day of St. Eustache; no, I did not dance. Thou must have been there; I had not spirit to dance and thou not there with me. If I went there at all, it was because I thought I ought not to do wrong, and vex my father and mother. Nevertheless, I did not know, dear friend, it would have displeased thee; but without that, thou seest, it gave me no pleasure. Emile has the umbrella thou didst leave in the little cottage... Paul sends his compliments, and embraces thee with all his heart, so do my father and mother. As for thy little friend, she too embraces thee with all her heart, praying thee not to forget her who loves thee, and will love thee for ever.

Nathalie.

P.S.—Today is the first of the season for the chase. Thy brother has killed one hare, and Louis Michelli two.
August 29, 1869.

There were other letters written by the same loving hand, all dated the same year, and now stained with blood, and trampled underfoot in the mud, lying close by a square of newly-turned earth, the grave of some twenty French soldiers. Poor Nathalie; her letters were carried to the last battlefield of her '*cher petit ami,*' and the happy day never came when he went back to dance with his true-hearted love at the feast of St. Eustache. Louise and I wandered for a short time over this melancholy plain, and then returned by the road, with the stumps of what had once been the poplar trees, which border all those long, straight roads of France, on each side of us, and went to our various duties, till it began to grow dusk, the wounded were dozing away the weary hours, and we went back to our quarters.

CHAPTER 6

The Rescue

After our return, and whilst standing over the kitchen fire, in hopes of being requested to take a cup of the coffee which was boiling, we heard a voice asking, in German, if the good people would boil some eggs for him. The accent was most welcome to our ears—it was English—and turning round I saw a gentleman in a white cap and an English grey tweed coat. I instantly said, 'Are you not from England?' and the answer was, 'Good gracious, are you the English column?'

'Yes,' I said; and before I had time to explain he rushed into the street, shouting 'Here they are!' Louise and I naturally rushed after him, and there, in the middle of the dirty street, stood 'the General,' who commenced a series of the profoundest bows, whilst our friend in the white cap, name then unknown, expressed his delight at having found us. They had been sent from Pont-à-Mousson to look for us, after the return of the messenger who had gone to Remilly with the news that we had left, and no one knew where we were. The said messenger, an English naval officer, had accompanied the other two on the chase, and they had caught an aged Knight of St. John to act as their escort, whose cross was a safe conduct everywhere, and who wanted to get to Bar-le-Duc, and, being utterly ignorant of geography, was being dragged about the country in the most opposite directions.

This elderly individual had retired to rest somewhere, his usual employment, and our three friends were looking out for dinner and shelter. We offered them such hospitality as we could. Mr. Parker begged a loaf of bread; Louise and I procured some hot water. We produced the cups of our flasks and our clasp knives, turned a box of stores on end, put a candle into an empty wine bottle, and prepared for the gorgeous banquet. Whilst I mixed Liebig with the water, Louise stormed the kitchen fire, stole some coffee, and boiled the eggs they had brought, and the gallant General, the naval officer, and the kind-hearted M.P. in the white cap assembled round the festive board, when the M.P. suddenly remembered himself of two Swiss surgeons they had picked up on the way, who had only been offered by the housekeeper, Mrs. Seeman, some soup, as they said, made of dirty water, and nothing else.

A shout into the street brought them up to join the party, and we passed round the cups and one glass; they eat Liebig, and eggs, and bread, and enjoyed themselves. Now both Louise and myself persisted in calling the General 'Mr. Henry,' having been informed by the secretary that it was necessary to do so, as he was strictly *incognito*, he having property in France, which would be forfeit were it known that he was with the German Armies; but hearing Mr. W— (the M.P.) and Mr. A— (the lieutenant) address him by his name, we asked if it was really necessary to alter his army rank. He laughed heartily and said, 'Yes,' and he was much obliged to us for promoting him. The General told us that at the headquarters they had been uncomfortable about us, and Mr. A— had been despatched in search of us; that on his return they were requested to hunt us up, which they had been doing in every village between Pont-à-Mousson and Ste. Marie, and on every part of the battlefields.

There was some political reason, it was believed, why the secretary carefully avoided headquarters, and the General had been placed in charge of us and the stores, and was to take us straight to the king. The army was moving on to Châlons, and we must follow it directly. As for property in France, he had not an acre. We were honestly delighted; not that we wished to leave our work at Ste. Marie, but we had lost all confidence in our leader, and Louise and myself much preferred being under the command of an English officer with a name known and honoured.

No Belgravian saloon was more cheerful than the attic of the Knights' house that afternoon. What did broken windows and medicine chests for chairs matter? Turtle soup and salmon have been served up to *blasé* Londoners, and been less enjoyed than Liebig's soup in cups or flasks and slices of dry bread. Cigars were lighted, affairs medical and military discussed, till darkness closed in, and we actually lighted a second candle, and chatted on till suppertime. We then all adjourned together to the other house

A judicious enumeration of the titles and orders of the General and a description of the wonderful influence exercised over the British government by the illustrious senator induced Frau Seeman to increase the quantity of *bouillon,* and even to add some cold bacon.

The Admiral (we promoted him too for the benefit of Frau Seeman) brought out two bottles of wine, and we supped and sat over it so long that we were fairly turned out by Frau Seeman, whose very comfortable bedroom we were occupying; and as their ideas of bedrooms and sitting-rooms seemed somewhat confused, and the lady showed evident symptoms of taking off her cap, we thought it better to adjourn at once, especially as only the evening before, whilst sitting in the Knights' room, having been invited to take a cup of tea with the *frau*, we had been astounded by the apparition of a Knight in a blanket, reminding me exactly of an illustration in an edition of *Don Quixote*, whose pictures were the delight of my childhood, and who coolly proceeded to get into bed, and request that a cup, *a large one*, of the hottest tea might be immediately administered to him, as he had been taking a bath, and feared to catch cold. Of course, it rained very heavily as we went back. Not a light was to be seen, and we slipped about in the mud in a very uncomfortable way.

The Admiral and Mr. W— had found a room and a mattress. The General shared Mr. Parker's heap of straw, and in spite of the assurance of Frau Seeman that at half-past twelve precisely the French would make a great sortie from Metz, taking Ste. Marie-aux-Chênes on their way to somewhere, we retired to our own straw and a dreamless sleep. Not a gun boomed from the lines of either army, there was neither dog nor cat in the village to disturb us with their howls, the very mice were starved out and had forsaken the garret, there was no excuse for lying awake, and the sun shone in through the holes in the roof before we were roused from our rest.

After coffee the General walked with me to the hospital, and said that he had decided on our leaving for Pont-à-Mousson that day, so as to arrive in time for dinner; that he would require waggons to convey us and the stores, under escort of the surgeon, whilst he and his friends went on to procure quarters for us. Dinner would be at seven o'clock, they would meet us in the Grande Place, and show us our lodgings. The king would be gone on, and we should have to follow him till we overtook him; and he begged me to inform the other ladies that all were to be ready at noon.

He went into the house with me, and took the kindest interest in the poor fellows, especially the few French who were there. 'Wounded' is a claim on the sympathy of everyone; but wounded and a prisoner is a stronger one still; and so, he felt it, as we did afterwards through many a long, sad day. And what a contrast was his tall, upright figure, his clear eye and firm step, to the poor crushed forms lying there. As he strode across the room, one Frenchman, looking at him with sad eyes of envy at that health and strength, said to me with a sigh, '*Monsieur marche fort;*' adding, 'Shall I ever be able to go home, do you think?' The gift of a few cigars brightened up many a pale face. He had served with the French armies, he could talk to them of their regiments and their old officers, and his presence was like a gleam of sunshine lighting up the weary hours.

After he left the hospital, I took leave of the poor fellows, and then went to the church to summon the ladies there. It was also requisite to find the *curé* to administer the last sacraments to a dying man, and I hoped to meet him, supposing Mass would not be over. I entered the church and found the ladies, but no *curé*. I asked if he had been there. They said No; there had been no service that morning. I was very much surprised, for that of the morning before was a most touching sight. The church was not very large and had no aisles; the wounded were ranged on mattresses in a double row down the sides, leaving the path up the centre clear, except for two or three tables, on which were the necessaries of the surgeons and nurses. The space within the altar rails had been carefully kept free from all intrusion, and Mass had been celebrated every morning at eight.

The greater part of the wounded were Catholics, and the rest lay quiet and listened and looked with interest at the priest. The irreverence of the *infirmiers*, who were German, and the surgeons and their attendants, even at the most holy moment of the service, could not destroy the solemn effect; and when the priest raised the Host, in which the humble, undoubting faith of the poor soldiers saw their uplifted Saviour present amongst them, and turned painfully on their bloodstained beds to worship and adore, it must have been a cold and stony Protestant heart that did not feel how glorious was the faith that could thus realise amidst such agony the Redeemer close at hand, to forgive and bless and receive the freed spirit to a home where 'there is no complaining and no leading into captivity in the streets.'! I regretted the omission of the daily service, and having announced our departure for noon precisely, I went to the *curé's* house.

I found him just returned from a village about two miles off, where he had walked to celebrate his daily Mass. I asked why he had gone so far with his own church close at hand, and the answer was, '*Madame*, I had not a drop of wine to consecrate.'

'Why did you not go to the stores?'

'I *Madame*, I did but they refused me. I asked only for this little quantity (showing me a medicine phial), but they would not give it me.'

I thought of the half-dozen emptied bottles I had seen on the Knights' dining table, and I did not envy the frame of mind that could thus deprive the sufferers of their greatest and holiest consolation. The contents of a couple of flasks supplied immediate wants for a day or two, and I tried my powers of persuasion on Frau Seeman for a bottle of even *vin ordinaire*; but I shared the fate of the *curé*, and retreated upstairs, metaphorically speaking, shaking the dust off my feet as I went, and wondering what good the Knights of St. John and their stores were to anybody or anything.

I found Louise and the surgeon packing up all the stores and nailing them down, in expectation of a visit from a number of army surgeons, coming to get all they could, not for ambulance, but regimental use. A sudden exclamation of Louise's from the inner room showed she had discovered the reason of the angular points and hard knobs in the straw, from out of which she was digging all sorts of small boxes and packages, finishing by the discovery of a roll of waterproof sheeting, fifty yards long, under her pillow, and acting as a bolster, upon which she remarked, in a reproachful tone, 'Now, how could we be expected to sleep with a roll like that under one's head?' to which there was one unanswerable rejoinder: 'But we did!'

A clatter of swords and spurs up the rickety stairs announced the arrival of the German surgeons, and in they came. From all the villages, from the camp, every brigade had sent by deputation for everything there was and was not, and at that very time three waggons were taking away stores belonging to the Knights back to Pont-a-Mousson, they evidently expecting ours would remain. With the greatest good temper, under great provocation, Mr. Parker treated the demands as impossible to grant in their full extent, declining to re-open boxes in the absence of the General, and giving as little as possible, knowing how very far the use that would be made of them would differ from that intended by those who had so nobly subscribed their money, not to supplement the military chest of the German Army, but to help where help was really wanted.

It is to be hoped that, warned by the past, in any future National effort of this sort, the subscribers will insist on having some voice in the distribution of their money and goods, and not leave all blindly to the caprice and personal feelings of any small executive committee with irresponsible power, however well adapted individuals may be for the office of control over hundreds of thousands of pounds sterling. Our stores were worth about 500*l.*, and many were most expensive and comparatively useless. Had they been selected by an army surgeon accustomed to the rough work of field ambulances, he would never have chosen costly articles only fit for a London or Paris hospital, and many things which were sent were utterly useless; for instance, the *spongio piline* and the oiled silk; *gutta percha* tissue, at a third of the price, answering the same purpose, while the *spongio piline* only served to line splints, for which tow was equally good. But the frightful waste of money will be more clearly seen as we go on.

This affair being settled, the surgeon went off to an operation and Louise to her stables, leaving me with strict injunctions not to leave the garret, nor to part with a single article, in case of further demands being made. I finished putting up my little baggages, and was leaning out of the window, looking into the street, wondering where our waggons were, when I heard steps behind me, and, turning sharply, saw two Knights of St. John entering the inner room. I called out, but they did not hear me, and, going in after them, I found them trying to read the label on a case of *gutta percha* tissue. I said it was the ladies' bedroom, and begged them to come out. The senior then said that he understood we were going, but of course our stores would be left for their use. I said No! certainly not; the stores would go with us. Such were the General's orders, and we should report ourselves to Prince Pless. They muttered and grumbled all in vain. I persisted, and finding it was no use, they departed.

I was very glad, however, to see the waggons drawn up on the other side of the road. They had been obtained by requisition, and, as this word will often have to be used, it may be as well here to explain what it really means. In most cases licensed robbery. Everything in the shape of horses, waggons, drivers, provisions, fuel, and bedding, the commune: or parish is bound to furnish at their own cost on warrants signed by any German official; the cost to be repaid by the *mairie*, or, as we might say, corporation of the place, after the war.

Carriages, waggons, and horses, however, are invariably seized for the conveyance of military stores and the convenience of the officers of the invading army, and no money will procure them; but a warrant from the official in charge of the train service to some other official in possession of the desired vehicles generally has the right effect.

The carriages and horses rarely, if ever, come back to their owners; the waggons and their drivers are taken from the farms to wander in the track of the army, receiving only scanty food and forage; but, after all, it is the requisitions in large towns which offer such a sure means of getting anything required and paying nothing for it. The working of this system, however, will be better seen when we relate our residence in Orléans. Yet even this taking of waggons and horses shows what the misery of an invaded country is, for it must be remembered that not only the invaders but the defenders must avail themselves of every mode of transport for troops and munitions of war, and the seat of war is often as unhappy under one as tine other.

Think, too, of the entire stand-still of all farming operations—no ploughing, and consequently no sowing, no carrying the produce to the nearest market, no communication between town and village, no means of going to see friends or transact the commonest business fifteen or twenty miles off, and the railways either unused or taken up solely for the military movements. The loneliness of the roads, the hush of all the noises caused by the daily occupations of village life, the corn left ungarnered and rotting in shocks on the fields, some reaped and lying where it fell, the absence of all men except the very old and the very young, mark what are the hourly deprivations of war, not to speak of the terrible scenes which the neighbourhood of a battle or the passing of a great army brings about. We fully intended to send back our waggons; but as the drivers afterwards took it into their own hands and escaped, we are certainly not responsible for their fate, whatever it might be.

Louise soon returned, followed by Mr. Parker and one of the Swiss surgeons, and we were nailing up the last of the chests when the door suddenly opened and in came the secretary, breathless with haste, and in an evident state of excitement. We stared with astonishment, he having told us he was off direct to England. He began by saying he had been to Ars-sur-Moselle, and brought us lanterns, blankets, tea, sugar, and bread. We assured him that we regretted he had taken the trouble, as we were off to Pont-à-Mousson. His anger was excessive. He disputed the right of the General to give us orders, and Louise and I declared, however that might be, we would not be under his orders again.

We had been told before we left England by Colonel Loyd Lindsay to report ourselves to Prince Pless at the king's headquarters; this we should certainly do, and end the uncertainty, and it was simply to the headquarters that the General was about to take us. He then said of course we left the stores behind us, and to this we replied that the orders of the General were imperative—the stores were to go with us, not another article was to be given at Ste. Marie, and we declined to accept any orders from him, now or at any future time, and for so doing we would be answerable to the committee at home. He grew so angry that the surgeon took him out into the street to try and cool him down, and here he commenced giving away a quantity of cigars he had brought with him in a light waggon to all the soldiers standing about.

A German officer interfered, said there were plenty of cigars in store there, and he had better take them back with him. On this a most violent scene ensued. Now, he had in hand 200*l.* of the committee's money, and with some of this he had bought the various stores he brought up, and which he afterwards gave away recklessly on the journey to Pont-à-Mousson. In reckless giving, however, he was not worse than many others, and it was often a source of bitter regret to us, when we thought of the hardly earned shilling of the workman, and the widow's mite, and the school children's pennies that had gone with the princely donations of the wealthy to make up the enormous sum that has made England famous for ill-regulated charity through the length and breadth of Europe.

We were very sorry that no one gave a helping hand to Mr. Parker. He and the Swiss had to move down every box, and lift them into the waggons, whilst the Knights of St. John and their orderlies stood and looked on. Determination, however, carried the day; but, in consequence of all these delays, it was one o'clock before we started. We were not offered any dinner before we left, but we were now anxious to get fairly off. The work at Ste. Marie was so far done that things had been got into order, the wounded were being rapidly evacuated by death or removal, and it was evident that in a couple of days more only those cases would be left which would probably have to remain there weeks, whilst the imminence of fresh battles rendered it necessary for us to push forward to our original destination.

The secretary, having no further business in Ste. Marie, accompanied us in his waggon, and with three others of our own we left Ste. Marie and the Knights of St. John, turned up a little lane which led from the main street to the back of the village, and emerged on the battlefield, which lay between Ste. Marie and Gorst, on the road through Vionville and Ars-sur-Moselle, and past Cormy to Pont-à-Mousson.

CHAPTER 7

The Burning of the Red-Cross Banner

Our cortege made its way slowly up the muddy lane and came out on the wide-open bend of the battlefield. It was a huge plateau, the distance bounded by low woods, and as the afternoon sunshine came out bright and clear it looked sadder, than ever. Our road crossed it, and we were very glad when it took a slight dip and brought us to the entrance of St. Privat, a ruined village, and up to the door of a house of the better class, occupied as an ambulance and also as quarters for soldiers, many of whom were lounging about, idle and dirty. We halted, and the secretary, calling to some Germans to assist him, commenced a distribution of goods, principally those which he had brought with him; but one box of English stores was so hastily broken open that next day the Swiss surgeon brought to me half-a-dozen valuable lancets and knives which he had found in the straw of the waggon.

How many were lost on the way no one could tell. The bread was given to the soldiers, who, as the secretary said, had not very large rations and must be hungry; probably they were. The German soldiery have an immense capacity for eating, but the poor miserable peasants who came around, and begged even for the broken bits of biscuit we had, were rather more hungry still; but the argument used then and afterwards, when good port wine sent from England was given to the troops, was, some might think, unanswerable: 'Poor fellows! they have hard work before them, and require strength.'

It seemed ages before we moved on. The secretary was evidently in no hurry to get to Pont-à-Mousson. At last I ordered our driver to push on, and he had to follow; we came out again on the wide, barren plain, and we overlooked a valley in which stood a large village, Gorst, we were told; but just where the road descended, yet still on the bend, was a lonely building. It looked as if it had been a barrack, and was surrounded by a wall enclosing the yard, which extended about fifty yards in width, between the building and the wall. It was a mere shed, the roof had fallen in, and the iron rails of the staircase hung, broken and twisted, from the side wall of the top storey. It had evidently been burned, how we knew not, and the intention was evidently to hurry past it; but the Swiss surgeon and our English friend stopped the waggons and begged us to get out and see the ruin, and as a waggon behind broke down at this instant and had to be repacked, the secretary had no excuse for urging us forward.

We entered within the ruined enclosure. A fearful smell met us; it was the first time we had ever experienced it. We knew it afterwards too well at Bazeilles. And what were we walking upon? Not cinders; the charred morsels were too soft for that? We turned sick with horror; human beings had perished here by fire. We went out directly, and saw the blackened skeletons of horses and pigs in the stables. Why, with the open country all around, had no effort at escape been made, and what were the charred morsels of wood, like the remains of a flagstaff, that had crushed in with the roof, and those remains of iron bedsteads? Standing in the court-yard, we heard the story. From that flagstaff the Red-Cross flag had floated. It was a deserted barrack, occupied as an ambulance on the evening of the battle, and in it were three hundred French, wounded.

The Germans passed on, Gorst was occupied, and two or three days after the battle they commenced firing on the barrack. They saw the flag, but persisted that it was occupied by soldiers. It caught fire, and as the wretched occupants, those who could rise from their beds at least, tried to escape, they were met by a fire of musketry, and all perished together; and there was the ruined, roofless barrack, standing alone, its blackened outlines, cut clear against the blue sky, sad witnesses of a sad event. It was a miserable mistake is the only excuse; but the flag should, at all events, have induced some enquiry, before cannon and rifle did their murderous work on those sheltered under it.

Saddened and oppressed by such a fearful scene, we remounted our waggon and drove on. Gorst was as dreary and deserted as all the other villages. A few scared women appeared, and one or two old men. We asked for a little water, and a woman ran for a glass and got us some from a pump close by. She seemed half-frightened, but our assurance that we were not Prussians encouraged her, and she told us all the boys and men in the village were gone to the war, and there was nothing left to eat. They had not even bread; all had been taken from them, even the potatoes in their little patches of garden, and their clothes, such as were useless being cut to pieces before their eyes. But revenge would come someday. From first to last that was the cry; and it will come, if not in our day, in that of the children who from childhood are being trained all over France for the great day of triumph—the entry into Berlin. It may be a dream, but it is a widespread one, and those who live to a good old age may see if it is realised or not.

After an hour or so we entered Vionville, a very pretty place, with a wide central street, and here we came to another stop. The secretary ran off after sundry friends, and, whilst we were waiting, an English gentleman with a knapsack on his back came up and introduced himself as Mr. Herbert of the British Society. I told him our troubles with the secretary. Nothing could be more kind and considerate than he was, and he begged us to write to him, giving us an address, and he would come to our help at any time. He was on a walking tour round the battlefield and the villages. I am sure he must have seen the greatest misery and distress, and if he knew as well as we did of the large stores of the Knights at Ste. Marie, he must have wondered why they did not ride round the neighbourhood and afford relief to the ambulances where the wounded were starving, and to the peasantry who were also dying of hunger.

The peasantry were French, and the Knights never professed to relieve them; but the ambulances were, to say the least of it, neutral, and the sick and wounded have no nationality. And why, with all this pressure of want, stores were sent back to the huge central depot at Pont-à-Mousson, no one could tell. It was, perhaps, the utter ignorance of the Knights as to its existence. We can safely say they never entered an ambulance at Ste. Marie, never rode out to enquire into the condition of those established not two miles from that place, and what they did, or why they were there at all, is beyond comprehension. They ate and drank the best of everything, they occupied the best houses as quarters, and enjoyed a perpetual picnic safely out of danger, but sufficiently near to say they had gone through a campaign. They were indeed carpet Knights, and have their spurs yet to win.

We got tired of waiting, sitting, as we were, in an August sun, and when the secretary brought a gentleman, whom he introduced as Mr. Appia of the Geneva Society, I told him plainly we were being detained here, I knew not why, and it would be dark before we got to Pont-a-Mousson, and did he not think he had better move on. He said most assuredly, and instantly asked the secretary to go on, and we started, having been one hour in the main street of Vionville; and here more stores were given to the soldiers, some bacon, I particularly remember, for a piece was reserved, which we were told was for our dinner. We got fairly out of Vionville at last, and as far as some trees; here we came to another halt, and the Swiss surgeon came up and told me the secretary was proposing to light fires and cook the bacon, and have a kind of gipsy party, and he was very uneasy. He had promised the General to see us safe to Pont-à-Mousson by seven o'clock, and really, if we were to light fires and cook bacon, we should not be there before midnight.

We remonstrated violently against this new detention, and the idea was given up. The bacon was served round raw with a slice of bread, and we were so hungry we ate it, and having very soon finished, we insisted on going on. The surgeons mounted the first waggon, and by dint of keeping up its boy driver to his work we jogged along faster. Our driver was a stupid-looking peasant, speaking only German, and his horses were harnessed with the loosest traces that ever were seen, which had at intervals to be disentangled. He looked like an utter idiot, and for such we took him. It would have been better for him had he been only an idiot, as we shall see.

After leaving Vionville, we descended from what may be called the upper level by a most lovely gorge, the sides clothed with rich foliage down to the little stream which runs through it. We came across many a beautiful bit of scenery in these parts, so rarely visited by travellers, no railroad being within several miles, and we came to the decided conclusion that a waggon is the only way of travelling by which you really see the country. There is a remark in *Eothen* that we Europeans do not understand the true enjoyment of travelling. We go from place to place, that is all. We found the truth of the idea. We lived our day as if this quiet state of passing over the ground was our normal condition, arriving at a decided resting-place, a break in our usual course of life, and we saw more of the country and the people than years of railroad travelling would have enabled us to do.

We gradually descended to Ars-sur-Moselle, and once more saw the Roman aqueduct. We had passed through it on our way to Ste. Marie, but had missed the beauties of the gorge in the darkness of the night, and after leaving it must have lost our way, for we certainly did not go through Vionville. The long, narrow street was crowded with troops; a Red-Cross flag hung from almost every house.

The shops were all open and a brisk trade was going on, but more in what are called fancy articles than food or clothing. There was but little of those to be seen. We drove through the town, and after another hour or so found ourselves by the bridge of Cormy. We did not cross it or enter the town, but went steadily on. It was quite dark when we reached Pont-à-Mousson at half-past nine instead of seven.

We halted in a large square, surrounded by arcades like Bologna, and were very glad to hear English voices calling to us. There were our friends. Of course, they had finished dinner, and it was so late that we were glad to go to the quarters they had found us. The ladies all occupied a third-storey room in the second-best hotel. The little *salle-à-manger* was crowded with soldiers smoking and drinking, and it was impossible to sup there. The good people of the house declared it was impossible to serve us upstairs, but I caught a small boy, who was running about with clay pipes for the Germans, and the offer of a *franc* enlisted him.

We got some knives and forks, plates and glasses, and I went into the kitchen and saw a pair of chickens in the oven. They were for the German officers' supper, but a little private arrangement transferred them to my share, and my *aide-de-camp* mounted the stairs in triumph with our spoils. What a supper we made! We really had had so little since we left Brussels, that even the moderate quantity we eat was more than we could well bear. Our gentlemen had gone to quarters somewhere else, and the General told us he would let us know before noon if we started for headquarters that day; he must first ascertain where they were, or not.

Our waggons were left in the centre of the 'Grande Place,' under a Prussian guard. I had proposed bringing in, besides our little baggages, the one small portmanteau we each of us possessed, and Louise quite agreed it would be safer. However, the General declared that no one could run off with the things with two sentinels watching the waggons, and we bowed to his superior judgment, particularly as he had a very valuable tin box there himself. The hotel seemed dirtier than ever when we went down next day. It probably was, in times of peace, a very fair one; but what could be expected with every room full of soldiers.

Many of them brought in their own rations and cooked them themselves over the kitchen fire. The officers required suppers up to two in the morning, and there was no refusing the imperious conquerors. A blow with the sheathed sword, or the smashing all the glass in the room, would have been the mildest form of punishment. There was no help, and no redress, and no pay. The poor people told us their sorrows, and gave us coffee. The Red-Cross badge was too often the pretext for demanding lodging and food by requisition, but we always gave it clearly to be understood we came to help and not to oppress, and that we should pay honestly, as in peace time, for what we had.

After coffee we went out. I remarked to Louise how insecure two of the portmanteaus were, the General's box and the leather trunk of one of our ladies. Louise pointed out that her trunk was fastened by a chain, and mine buried under a heavy chest that required two men to move, but she thought we had better tell the others. We went back to do so, but they were out, and we waited a little while in the *salle-à-manger*. The Swiss surgeon came up to the window, and handed in the instruments he had found scattered in the straw. He had had his orders to go direct to Nancy, and with much regret we took leave of him and his friend. They told us of some very good hot baths, and we went to them. They were far superior to any I ever had in England, and we only paid a *franc* for each, including a plentiful supply of hot towels and a special room, which, we were assured, no 'dirty German officers' had ever used.

On our return we passed the waggons. The two trunks were gone! We instantly gave the alarm. The General came up, and a search was commenced. Mr. W— declared directly he distrusted the driver (our supposed idiot), for he had found him selling the forage given out for the horses, and Mr. A— said he had always disliked the downcast look of his face, whilst Louise and I persisted we had always thought him more knave than fool. All these complimentary opinions, however, did not find the lost baggage, and the only thing to be done was to replace, as far as possible, the contents of the portmanteau of our lady companion.

I told the secretary that clearly the society ought to pay the damage. Had the baggage been brought in, as we requested, this would not have happened. I begged her to make an estimate of the value. She made one, far too moderate, not even valuing the things at a fair price. Part of the sum claimed the secretary paid, saying he could spare no more. I trust the rest may be paid. When I named it to the committee they hesitated. With all the thousands they flung recklessly away they need not have scrupled at giving a five-pound note to replace necessary clothing, lost on actual service by one who was certainly a most active, faithful, and unpaid servant. The General gave notice to the German authorities. His box contained his uniform, and was therefore very valuable, and also his medals. The driver was instantly arrested, and the provost-marshal offered to shoot him then and there;

but it was considered advisable to try and screw the truth out of him. Either he had not taken the things, or was not alarmed at the provost marshal's threat, for he confessed nothing.

The day passed on, and no orders were given. Finally, we were told to be ready at six a.m. precisely the next morning, and a fresh waggon was found to replace that of the driver, consigned to prison for further examination. We walked a little about the town. It was very dull, the shops mostly shut, and, like all towns occupied by troops during war, very dirty; the central square littered with straw, broken bottles, and all the debris of a bivouac. German troopers have a peculiar habit of riding on the footpaths and pavements, and it does not add to the cleanliness of a place, and is peculiarly inconvenient. Probably they do not do it in Berlin, and it reminds one of the arrangements in Damascus before the massacres of 1860, when the terrible punishment inflicted on the Mussulmans compelled them to change their insolent order, that no Christians should walk on the side-paths, but run their risks in the midst of the confusion of an Oriental street.

Did the Prussian generals take a hint from this, and try to force the unhappy people of the occupied cities into the dirt and danger of their own streets? It really seems so. I have often wondered, if the French had invaded Germany, would they have been as arrogant and contemptuous and unfeeling as the German soldiery. Would they have forgotten as completely that their turn might come someday, and as they had sowed so they should reap? Perhaps so. Military success is a hard trial of character. Few pass it unscathed, and the hardheartedness it engenders is only one of the many forms of the demoralisation which are the result of even one campaign.

We were glad to shut ourselves up in our own room, from which, later in the evening, we descended to the *salle-à-manger*, and finding a small table, we took possession of it. Amidst all the noise and smoke we were rejoiced to find that the soldiers had not yet come into dinner, and the room was filled with Frenchmen, whose kindness and courtesy made us quite at home. Dinner was a difficulty. Some German officers were dining in a small room which opened off ours, and demanding everything there was to eat and the attention of every waiter. My pipe boy of the night before gave us a hint what to do, and the next dish that he brought past us I quietly took out of his hand, and so on till we had got enough, and the officers dare not storm at us; but we very soon adjourned upstairs, resolved to have a good and long night's rest before our march of the ensuing day.

CHAPTER 8

The Chase After the King

It was a bright, sunshiny morning when, on the 27th of August, we all assembled booted and spurred at 6 a.m., ready to start on our first day's pilgrimage in chase of the king's headquarters. The aged Knight of St. John, it seems, had declared that it was too dangerous for the ladies to go on further, and that the stores had far better be left at the depot of the Knights of St. John. It was not wise to contradict the venerable Baron H——. So he was implored to go to bed and to sleep, and the General, knowing his usual habits, arranged that ourselves and the baggage were to start at an early hour, the greatest care being taken not to awaken the baron, and when later in the day Mr. W——'s light carriage, which conveyed the General, Mr. A——, and Baron H——, should overtake us several leagues away from Pont-à-Mousson, it would be too late for the Knight to object.

Fortunately, his morning sleep was a prolonged one, for several delays occurred. The gentlemen were obliged to go to the provost-marshal and give evidence as regarded the robbery, and evidently the provost-marshal had not had his breakfast and begun his daily official career, for we had the pleasure of sitting waiting in the waggon and watching our friends sunning themselves in the balcony of the provost's house for at least an hour. The lost baggage was not discovered, I believe it never was; but I suppose that ultimately the driver was convicted of being the thief, as we heard afterwards that a few days after we left, he was shot.

At last we started and went slowly on over very pretty country, a splendid Route *Impériale*, and not a trace of war to be seen anywhere. We read, and worked, and chatted, admired the view, wondered where we should sleep at night, and met with no adventures of any sort. We passed through one small village, and just beyond it a peasant boy overtook us, and told us that over that very road, not many days before. Napoleon III and his son had ridden, on their way back from Saarbruck, and the great French Army had turned off to the right, pointing to a road which diverged and crossed the plain in a lower level than the one we were on.

We asked him how it happened that at his age, eighteen or nineteen, he had not been summoned to join the army, and he answered, with a bright smile coming all over his face, 'The luck I had, *Madame (la bonne chance)*! I was drawn in the conscription. Ah! see now, what for! to be shot dead, or wounded, or prisoner. Only a few days were left me, but the Prussians came; they ordered, on pain of death, no one should leave the village who was of age to fight. Did I wish to go? No, madam; a thousand times no. I said a very good day *(bien bon jour)*, and thank you. I shall stay with the plough and the cows and sheep, and here I am, two arms and two legs and my head on my shoulders, and the rest of the boys may fight if they like. What matters it to me? King or emperor, it is all one to Baptiste. Thank you, *Madame*, good luck to you (this in return for two ten *centime* pieces); you go to nurse the wounded. Ah! I will never trouble you; a very good day.'

And off went our heroic friend, his dog at his heels, whistling some gay French airs. Quietly and steadily we drove on, and at last we came where two roads parted; one turning to the right, round a rising hill, was evidently our onward way, the other wound up the hill to a village on the height. Just at this time we saw the carriage of our friends rapidly coming up the long straight road behind us, the baron still sleeping. They told us to take the road up the hill. It was three o'clock, and we could lunch at the little *auberge*, and up it accordingly we went. We found that the village was called Gironville, and its situation was certainly lovely. It stands on the wooded height, which seems suddenly to block the road, overlooking an expanse of cultivated country, with here and there a distant group of white houses and a church tower to mark the scattered villages.

The church of Gironville and the graveyard round it rose directly behind the little street of the village, and was approached by rough stone steps placed on the hillside. The inn itself was rude enough, but very clean, and with an abundance of eggs and butter which was astounding under the circumstances; but the merry old landlady explained it by telling us the village stood off the main road, the great armies marched past down below, and had no time to stop and mount the steep road to the village.

Besides, it was too poor a place to tempt even the *Uhlans* to turn aside to make requisitions. The arrival of so large a party as ours utterly broke down the good old *dame's* resources, and Louise and the General took possession of the great kitchen fire, and cooked eggs and bacon, while Mr. W— and myself found plates, and knives, and glasses in corner cupboards, and the baron discovered a large, cold, brick floored room, not invaded by the peasantry, which he considered more adapted to our dignity, and where he insisted on our lunching. I am sorry to say that we should all have preferred the kitchen, for it was not a very warm day, and the fire was very pleasant; besides, eggs and bacon are much better transferred instantly from the frying-pan to the table. However, not choosing to leave our escort to lunch by himself in solitary grandeur, we submitted, and the result was a series of fatiguing journeys to fetch fresh supplies.

After lunch Louise and I wandered up to the little church. It was closed, a very unusual thing in France, but a woman came to open it. It had no architectural beauties, and was very old and simple. Returning to the inn, we saw a little crowd in the street; conspicuous in it were a fat baker in his white apron and our friend the Admiral, who was delivering a lecture on the politics of France to the admiring villagers. Whenever he was missing, his tall form and merry Saxon face were sure to be descried in some such a situation, and the natives listened and looked in wonder at his size and his eloquence. It was just five when, as he would have said, we got under weigh once more, and we humbly suggested 'where were we going?'

'To the camp near Châlons,' was the answer, 'by way of Commercy. Before we overtook you, we were afraid you might have turned off to the left, and gone by way of St. Dizier, which you would have found occupied by the French.'

As we never had the slightest intention of going anywhere except slowly along the straight road till our friends came up, they need not have alarmed themselves on that account.

The General urged on the drivers, the horses actually broke into a trot, and in an hour, we entered Commercy. Going a trot in the waggons is not a pleasant process; the store chests bumped about, and we were considerably shaken. Those vehicles are never designed to go beyond a dignified walk. In the light and brightness of an August afternoon Commercy looked a very pretty town, with no edifice of any peculiar size or beauty in it, except an old *château*, modernised into a barrack, and a very comfortable inn.

The German Army had passed quietly through it, leaving only about thirty troopers in the place, which, though containing some 4,000 inhabitants, was not of sufficient importance to require a garrison, and so escaped the scourge of a military occupation and the heavy requisitions which accompany it. At this time the Germans had not committed the excesses they afterwards did when success had blinded them to all considerations, except that they were victors living amongst the vanquished, where might makes right, and much was done that caused even their own officers to say, 'This is not war; it is pillage.' So Commercy looked even cheerful in the evening sunlight.

When next morning we descended early to breakfast, Louise and myself strolled into the kitchen. We always found amusement and information in chatting with the people, and heard and saw many things that otherwise would have escaped us. One thing that morning surprised us, the enormous quantity of butter.

Certainly, the fair and fertile plains in the neighbourhood were admirably suited for pasturage, but we had seen so little of late that it was a novelty to us. It was neatly made into half kilogrammes, about an English pound, and wrapped up in cool green leaves. It had evidently been brought in from the neighbouring farms, and was sufficient evidence that the invaders had spared the cows at all events. We assembled round the fire, and listened to the tales of the passing of the two grand armies.

At last we were properly packed into our waggons, and provided with pillows of hay, Louise and myself voyaging together. Again, a lovely day, and no signs of war and devastation on the country we passed through. About noon we arrived at a small village called Ligny, and halted for lunch. We had, besides the Knight and his cross, a bodyguard of two Prussian soldiers, who, as it turned out, were solely and wholly for the safety and protection of the said Knight.

At Ligny these soldiers and our drivers entered a barn in which was a good deal of hay, and not only took enough for their horses at the time, but laid in a stock sufficient for several days, and also in so doing quite spoiled our comfortable couch in the waggon, by piling it up too high. This afforded us a good opportunity of indignantly tossing it out, and thereby pacifying the unfortunate farmer, who justly remonstrated that he was bound, he knew, to furnish the forage for one meal, but not to supply it for two or three days. The Prussian soldiers would listen to nothing; but we made our coachmen disgorge their surplus hay.

At this time, though we were about to leave, the Admiral was missing, nor did we see the usual crowd. He emerged in triumph from somewhere with two geese and a rabbit, which he declared he had stolen, and on being remonstrated with on the style of his proceedings, as being highly objectionable, modified the statement by declaring he had paid for them in German coin of little value, and resembling dirty silver, which the deluded owners of the geese accepted as *francs* and half-*francs*. Probably he got them cheap, we'll hope it was no worse; but ever after that, the legend ran that he announced us everywhere in the following terms:—

We are the English column. We have five ladies; we have a great many stores. I have stolen a goose; will you have it?

Not knowing where we should get our next meal, but evidently feeling bound to make restitution somewhere. Everybody was so astonished that nobody ever accepted the offer, and the geese in their feathers travelled on with us.

We pursued our way, thinking of our own quiet England, and almost fancying we could hear the ringing of the church bells for the afternoon service. There was little distinction between Saturday and Sunday through all the occupied departments, and the soldiers of the 'Pious King' seemed to put it aside as a sort of luxury these people had no right to indulge in, and from whose observance they themselves were specially absolved in right of conquest. Requisitions must be made, troops moved, and the routine of war go on, just as on any other day; but as we came into Bar-le-Duc, everyone was walking about in Sunday costume.

The town was full of Bavarian soldiers, and Mr. W— and the General thought it better to push on to a quiet village called Ruvigny, just beyond. The only difficulty was the baron. He had started with the object of going to Bar-le-Duc, and had enquired at intervals all the way along how far it was still to that place; but he was soundly sleeping, and it was thought better not to wake him, but to bring him along to headquarters. He was going to meet a son, whose corps was with the advanced guard, and therefore it was useless his staying in Bar-le-Duc; besides, he saved a great deal of trouble with outposts and sentries, and therefore, on all accounts, he was allowed to sleep.

What a gay, pretty town Bar-le-Duc looked as we drove slowly through it. It was here the Young Pretender, Bonnie Prince Charlie, passed three years of his exile; and here, too, in the Church of St.

Pierre, are the remains of several princes of the House of Lorraine. It is a thoroughly French-looking town, and we were told many Parisians had country houses here, where they passed the autumn. A group of Bavarian officers in their light blue uniforms were standing in front of the hotel, and it was certainly a wise decision to go on the four miles that still lay between us and Ruvigny.

We soon arrived at our destination for the night, and found the little hotel unoccupied. Twenty-four hours before the headquarters had passed through; and here we heard the news of the flank march from Châlons to intercept MacMahon's army on their way to relieve Bazaine and Metz. It was therefore, clear that we must turn away from the Châlons road, and follow the advance of the army by St. Menehould and Grand Pré.

The great battle of the campaign was evidently close at hand, and an early start next day was resolved upon. The baron was assured we were close to Bar-le-Duc, and sat down to dinner with that comfortable conviction. His notions of geography had got more confused than ever since we left Ste. Marie-aux-Chênes, and he was quite resigned to be carried about in a comfortable carriage and allowed his undisturbed repose, assured in his own mind that someday or other he should find himself at Bar-le-Duc.

As usual, our early start ended in breakfast at nine, and getting off at ten. We may be permitted to observe here that the ladies were always ready. It was the gentlemen whose *toilette* seemed such a prolonged occupation, for we used to hear them beginning to stir about at a very early hour, but it was certainly not a very early one when they made their appearance.

Another quiet march brought us to a small village, through which the German Army had passed only the day before. We were close on the track now. We halted to rest the horses, and walked to the house of the *curé* to get the keys of the church. He was absent, but his old housekeeper received us most cordially, and showed us her once neat kitchen, now in the dirty and disorderly state always the result of a room having been occupied as sleeping quarters for soldiers. They had demanded dinner and supper, and in no inconsiderable quantity; but though many empty bottles showed the ravages made in her master's cellar, she insisted on our drinking some of the wine, made, she told us, from the produce of a vineyard close by.

The church looked quite new. It had been lately restored, and the stones and debris had not been removed from around it. It was airy, clean, and spacious, but nothing worthy of remark in it. It was an unusually large church for so small a village; that was all. In it we met a young man, by his dress a farmer or small proprietor of a better class. He had just ridden in from the neighbourhood, and told us the French picquets were close at hand. As he then ascended the tower, he probably went to look for them. We were rather diverted at the idea of what a waking the German baron would have from his dreams if they did pounce upon us. It was all one to us. Indeed, we began to think that the exceeding unpopularity of the German Armies rendered it by no means agreeable serving with them, and if the French lancers had caught us, we should not have regretted it very much. At least, I can answer for Louise and myself.

The country about us was hilly and well wooded. We could not help remarking, as we went along, the utter solitude of the roads. We never met even a peasant's cart, nor did we see a living being in the fields by the roadside. The corn was standing in shocks; there was no one to garner it in. The scattered cottages were deserted. We were indeed coming close to the seat of war.

Late in the afternoon we came near St. Menehould, and the General proposed to drive on in the carriage and see the state of affairs—if we were really and truly on the right track, and what prospect there was of obtaining a night's lodging. It seemed an age that we waited, St. Menehould being hidden by the rising ground up which our road took its way. It was, in reality, an hour before we caught sight of the returning carriage.

St. Menehould was full of troops, but the king had gone on. There was a hope of a lodging in some private house, and we were, at all events, to rest there for the night, even if we had to sleep in the waggons. The entrance to the town was excessively pretty: across a bridge, with an old *château* on a high rock overhanging the stream. A vast number of troops were encamped for the night on the meadows which bordered the river, the Aisne, and the long street in front of us was blocked with provision and ammunition waggons.

It was at St. Menehould that poor Louis XVI was detected by the postmaster Drouet, from his likeness to the head on a coin he gave, when the post-horses were changed; and it was at Varennes, some sixteen miles farther on, that he was arrested by the same over-energetic official, who had ridden on horseback to overtake the king's carriage and intercept his flight to the frontier.

We had plenty of time to indulge in historical reminiscences, for just over the bridge we came to another stop. Night was closing in, chilly and damp, and we were very glad when the General, who had gone on into the town, sent the Amiral back to show us where to go. The waggons and horses were left in a large open square with trees on one side of it, and we ourselves, with our little baggages, walked with our guide round the corner and into the main street. The town seemed much larger from the crowd and confusion in the streets. The hotel, Mr. A— told us, was impossible; but three rooms had been found in three different houses, besides one for the gentlemen, and the hospitable owners had refused all remuneration, and only expressed their anxiety to make us welcome.

Giving them all due credit for kindly feeling towards those who had come on an errand of charity, we learned afterwards that we conferred quite as great a favour as we received by accepting lodgings in a private house. It was far better to have English ladies than German soldiers clamouring for wine and brandy and supper, and too often pocketing the little ornaments about the room, if they happened to strike their fancy.

However, we were most warmly welcomed by our hostess, a pretty young married woman, showed into the very best bedroom, which was thoroughly comfortable and even luxurious, and, very cold and tired, we refused all the offers of our kind hostess to find us something of what was left (for they had had Prussians in the house all day, and some were even still quartered there), and would only accept a cup of coffee and a morsel of bread, and were beginning to take off our boots, when a knock at the door was followed by the entrance of Mr. W—, to tell us they were all very hungry, and had resolved to have a good supper in their rooms. The other ladies were there, and they were to cook the Admiral's rabbit and a chicken they had found somewhere, and he begged us to come over the way with him.

A mental calculation how long a rabbit and a chicken would take to cook under evidently unfavourable circumstances determined us to decline the supper party, and we discovered next day we had had at least two hours more sleep than the rest; so very long did it take to get ready the table, prepare the eatables, and find bread, knives, forks, &c. All night long, however, the rumble of heavy artillery and the marching past of troops never ceased. Now and then the shrill call of a trumpet rang out in the still air.

The army was in full advance, and when we rose in the morning few soldiers were left in St. Menehould. Our start was deferred, for the roads in front were so blocked that it was better to wait awhile, and we should reach Grand Pré just as soon. The king was there, and we should there receive our final orders.

We left the town about half-past ten, and escaped the crush on the roads. We halted, as usual, about one o'clock in a little village. This was now the 30th of August, and already vague rumours of French defeats were flying about. A drunken man reeled past our waggon calling out, '*Perdue est la France!*' and snatched at my railroad rug, which I snatched back again, remarking, 'If France is lost, that is no reason I should lose my *couverture*.' The General was very anxious to press on. Great events were occurring, or about to occur, ahead of us. Our halt was cut short, and we took the rest of the road to Grand Pré at a lively pace.

Along a straight route *Impériale*, through a fragrant pine wood, over a flat country plain where the distant road dipped down to reach a village, the tower of whose church we saw rising suddenly before us; then slowly through a blocked-up street, and we were in Grand Pré. There was a sudden stop to let a carriage and four go by, preceded by outriders in old-fashioned cocked hats. It was the king himself! There was fighting in front, about six miles off, the people said, and he had gone out to the battlefield.

Chapter 9

England to the Rescue

The General, who had preceded us into Grand Pré, ordered our drivers to turn up a street to the right off the central market-place, and we found ourselves opposite a handsome red brick house, the contents of one window by the side of the hall-door showing the master was a chemist. He, with his wife and son, were waiting to receive us, thankful it was no worse—that is, Prussian troops—and welcomed us into the rooms vacated only an hour before by the king and his immediate staff. A piece of white chalk was produced, and 'Ten officers of the Medical Department' was written on the door. This included the ladies, of course, and looked very absurd, but was very useful. We deposited our baggage, and while the gentlemen went into the market-place for news, we saw the horses and servants all placed together in the stable, and from the little garden in front watched the confusion going on just at the end of the street.

For two days, our host told us, the great army had been passing day and night. Every house had been turned into quarters for troops, and every scrap of provision carried off. All day they had heard distant firing, and no one knew what the next twenty-four hours might bring forth. It was seven o'clock before the gentlemen returned. They had heard of two horses to be bought at only twenty pounds each, and having brought their saddles had invested their money on the purchase of them. That is, the General and Mr. A——, Mr. Parker and Mr. W—— had arranged to take on a small selectin of stores in the carriage. The baron, who had a bad cold, was to be left for the night in charge of us, and they would send back for us directly they had ascertained the exact locality of the battlefield, and where our services would be of most use.

We all sat down to supper, and had the honour of finishing the king's leg of mutton; and whilst we were still laughing over the absurdity of our so immediately succeeding him as to eat up the supper intended for him, we heard loud lamentations outside, and Mr. W— went to see what had happened. He found a lady who was in such a state of fear at the arrival of so many Prussians, and so perfectly convinced that they were about to burn down the town, that she was imploring our hostess, a friend of hers, to allow her to hide herself and her daughter, a pretty girl of thirteen or fourteen, in the first convenient cellar.

Mr. W— tried to pacify her and induce her to return home, but she wept on and refused. He then suggested having a guard in the house in the shape of a couple of the English ladies, and, with a vague and indefinite trust in their power to hold the entire Prussian Army at bay, she consented. Mr. W— most good-naturedly pleaded with us on her behalf, and Louise and myself volunteered for the service. We finished our suppers, got our hand-bags, and prepared for our expedition. Our host and his son said they would go with us as far as the house, and having received our final orders to be in readiness at an hour's notice we went off in procession. We found the house was in the market-place, and a very nice one. Mr. G—, the husband, was there, safely locked up with a servant and a poor old lady of ninety, bedridden and literally paralysed with terror.

We were shown into a very nice room, and Madame G—assured us, after nine o'clock at night, when the retreat sounded, she should be better if the town was not burned down, as she fully expected. We declared that we did not see why the Prussians should burn their sleeping quarters over their own heads, but she only shook hers, and said, 'That was nothing; they were used to it.' We resolved at once to go to bed, and were just dropping off to sleep when, after a tap at the door, *Madame* entered with her daughter and a mattress, and implored us to allow her treasure to sleep on the floor under the shadow of our protection, and would we promise, promise on all we held most sacred, to defend her with our lives. We sat bolt upright, to make the affirmation more energetic, and said, 'Certainly.'

The poor child being laid down in her clothes on the very hard mattress, and requested to compose herself, exit *Madame*, after taking an affecting farewell of her daughter. Five minutes afterwards in she came again, to beg us to put on our brassards over the sleeves of our nightdresses and keep our left arms out of bed, that the Red Cross might be visible directly any marauding Prussian entered the room. As the idea seemed to afford her great comfort, we consented, only remarking that 'we did not allow Prussians in our bedroom;' and off we went to sleep again. Ten minutes afterwards in she came again, and informed us that the enemy were just about to set fire to the other corner of the town. We begged her to let us know when the flames reached the market-place; but after that she came in at intervals of certainly not more than five minutes each, to tell us that she heard dreadful shrieks, or smelt smoke, or was sure that the flames would reach us very soon. And so, the weary night went on, till at half-past three a.m. she rushed in again to say her mother was dying.

This was something real and tangible, and Louise directly got up and went downstairs, and came back to tell me she thought it was true, and the family was most anxious the old lady should receive the last sacraments; but not one dare venture out of the house to fetch the priest, and she herself had volunteered to do so. Of course, I said if she went I should go too, and dressed myself in haste. Madame G— persuaded the old servant to take the biggest of lanterns and show us the way, and off we went. It was a lonely night, or rather morning, with the intense darkness that precedes dawn; not a sound was to be heard, not a living being to be seen. I objected to the lantern as unnecessary and likely to attract attention; but it appeared to be 'the proper thing' in Grand Pré, if anyone went out after dark, to have a lantern; that is, anyone who was somebody, and as Mrs. Nickleby says, 'Let us be genteel or die.'

We blundered on, feeling very sleepy and tired, till the old woman and her lantern stopped before a house in a side street, and I gave a gentle ring at the bell, so as to avoid waking up any Prussians who might be quartered there. It was answered by the priest himself, an elderly man with grey hair, who said he would come directly. The dying woman was one of his oldest parishioners, and he did not wonder that the excitement and fear of the present time should prove fatal to her.

Having thus given the message, we suggested going back directly, and leaving him to follow when more fully dressed, but he begged us to wait and go with him to the church. It would be better; for himself he had no fear, but he had to bring the Host, and he dreaded insult from some foreign soldiers to his precious charge. We willingly consented. His old housekeeper came down and took us into the kitchen, and told us of the wreck and ruin in their poor household from the passing troops. At last the *curé* appeared, and we walked up a dark lane or two, till we emerged on a platform shaded with huge elm trees, and overlooking the country below. The moon was setting, and the watch-fires glimmering here and there marked the bivouac of a division of the German Army. The old church threw a heavy shadow on the platform, bounded by its low wall, and so perfectly calm and peaceful was the scene, that it was impossible to realise the fact that the rising sun might shine on two mighty armies meeting in a death-struggle.

The scent of autumn roses was strong on the quiet air, so quiet that the flame of a candle would not have flickered in it. We could willingly have leaned over the low wall for hours and looked on the fair scene below us, the dark woods, the open fields, and the dying watch-fires, but the turning of the key in the church door recalled us to present duties, and we followed the priest in. How strange it all looked by the dim light of the lantern: double rows of beds, neatly fitted up with mattresses and blankets, extended down each side of the nave and in the aisles, but no one yet occupied them.

They were so white and clean that they stared out at us in the darkness with a singular effect, the pillars of the aisle throwing weird shadows as we passed, on the beds below. The priest turned off into the sacristy, for there the Host was kept in these troublous times, and requested us to follow him close, and let the old woman and the lantern bring up the rear; and so we emerged from the church, the priest first, bearing the Host, and a little bell to ring if he met any of the faithful, and Louise and I well up behind, and slightly keeping on his right and left, to answer any questions that Prussian patrols might ask. The lantern behind threw a long streak of light down the black street, and the only sound was our steady tread and the clank of the old woman's *sabots*.

But we did not meet a soul. The Germans were too weary and the natives too frightened to prowl about at four in the morning. Only once a door opened and a baker looked out, the reflection of his oven fires showing our little party distinctly. The priest rang his bell, the baker knelt on his knee for an instant, and we passed on into the darkness, like a phantom train. I ventured to suggest that the little bell was likely to attract attention, but the brave old man said he was not afraid, and of course we were not, or we should not have been there. Finally, we arrived at the house, and leaving the priest in the room of the dying woman, we went upstairs, fairly worn out. Just as our eyes were closing in sleep, up rushed *Madame* again—the Prussians, the Prussians, they were in the house!

It was not a false alarm this time; and hastily putting on our dresses, not forgetting the brassards, down we went, and found one soldier in the little hall and two or three grouped round the door. The soldier inside did not look at all ferocious, and the others were evidently waiting patiently for something, so the best thing was to be indignant, and ask what they wanted. The enemy saluted politely, and said they had fallen behind their regiment and had missed it. They could find no one to give them intelligence, and seeing a light in the house, they had knocked to ask it a regiment, describing their dress and facings, had gone through the town. Strangely enough, just as we entered Grand Pré, we had met it, and been told they had marched far and fast, and left many '*trainards*' behind.

We were able, therefore, to give them the desired information, and we asked if they were tired and hungry. They said 'very.' I observed that they could not sleep in the house, but I could procure them some bread and wine. They said how grateful they should be, and turning to *Madame*, who, not understanding a word, thought I was pleading for their lives, I said, 'If you'll give them a bottle of wine and a loaf of bread, they will go quietly away!' 'Give them only bread and wine,' shrieked *Madame*, echoed by *Monsieur*; 'they shall have all they require, only let our lives be spared;' and *Monsieur* ran off to his hidden store (of whose existence I was aware), produced a couple of bottles of good wine and two large loaves of bread. The poor corporal's eyes brightened, as he took them. 'Tell *Madame*,' he said, 'we have not eaten since daybreak yesterday. Goodnight, and many thanks. *Schlafen Sie wohl* (may you sleep well)!' and he bowed himself out and closed the door. *Madame* gave a groan of relief, and observed, 'What do we not owe you! We should all have been murdered and pillaged had it not been for you!'

The story the soldiers told us was a strange one. It was not probable they could hear news of their lost regiment in a French house at four in the morning. I think they wanted lodging and supper, but finding that without trouble and offending English ladies they could not obtain them, they gladly accepted the peace-offering I suggested, and slept in the market-place. However, all parties were mutually satisfied with the arrangement, and at last we were allowed to rest in quiet. Day was beginning to dawn, and we slept soundly, till at eight *Madame* came to awake her daughter and bring us coffee. We then went back to our original quarters, and found them all in despair. There was no bread! The army that had passed the day before had carried off all that had been baked, and all that the flour in Grand Pré could make. Carts with flour had come in and bread was being made, but a sentinel was placed in every baker's shop, and every loaf was to be kept for the troops as they passed through on their way to the front. All that long day (August 31) they were pressed on, regardless of fatigue and heat, regiment after regiment passing through at intervals, and it was evident no bread could be had.

One of the Prussian soldiers of our escort told me that if I could get an order from the general in command, I could get some bread, so I started off with him to find that official. Just over a bridge that crossed a very small stream and up a road to the left we met three officers, one of whom, my soldier said, was the general himself. It was no time to hesitate or wait for an introduction. I stopped the great man and requested an order for bread. He was most kind and much amused. He asked, 'Did I know a good baker?' Fortunately, I had tried in vain at the family baker of the chemist, and found him a very respectable man, with two sacks of good flour, and a Prussian sentinel watching him. I therefore said I did know a very worthy baker. The general offered to accompany me, and we turned back together. We had to pass our headquarters, and great was the astonishment of some of the party who were lounging in the garden to see me parading with an illustrious general and two or three *aides-de-camp* behind.

We arrived at the baker's, and a knot of women, congregated about the door, took to flight. The neighbourhood expected the instant execution of the baker, and the poor man himself shivered with fright as the general, stooping his tall form, just kept his spiked helmet clear of the doorway, and requested the baker in very good French to tell him how long it would be before the bread was baked. The baker said, 'As fast as he could;' and the general turning to me asked for how many persons I claimed bread. I said boldly 'twenty.' I knew anybody would be glad to have it, and it would, according to the system of 'requisitions,' cost nothing. The general then quietly turning to the sentinel said, 'When this soldier comes (pointing to my orderly) let him have twenty large loaves of bread.'

Of course I thanked my friend, and he bowed himself out, his spurs and boots creating fresh consternation in the minds of the inhabitants of the neighbourhood, and my baker looking aghast. Requisitions meant payment by a ruined town after the war, and I hastened to disperse the cloud on his rosy face, which shone brightly through the flour, by dismissing the orderly with orders to return when the bread was ready, and then paying my friend beforehand for his bread, assuring him England came to help, not to oppress.

After telling our host at the headquarters house that bread would be shortly forthcoming, Louise and myself went back to our quarters, where we were obliged to make our appearance at intervals, and console Madame G——. Here we found some people lamenting over the distresses caused by a Prussian invasion in a large and solitary house just across the bridge and out of the main street, and begging us to go and see the lady who lived there. We went off accordingly, and soon arrived. The house was a very good one, belonging to a large brewery, and certainly it was a scene of the utmost desolation.

The stables were empty, the horses had been taken by the Germans, the plants in the garden torn up and trampled down, and inside it was worse. Not a piece of furniture remained unbroken, except in the room of the unfortunate mistress, who lived there with her son. The poor servants showed us the kitchen. Every utensil that could be useful—pots, pans, gridirons and frying-pans, knives and forks—had been carried off; chairs and tables cut to pieces in mere wantonness. Some of the officials—for over 180 officers and men had slept there— had taken possession of the bedrooms upstairs, and in the morning had cut the mattresses and sheets to pieces and carried off the blankets.

The son begged us to go in and see his mother. The poor woman was in bed, but welcomed us as friends. All her 'household goods' lay broken and strewn about the room, and she herself, always an invalid from heart attacks, was in a pitiable condition. The son was half broken-hearted, half indignant; he had applied in vain to the mayor to represent to the *commandants de place* the unnecessary ravages committed by the German soldiers. We gave all we could of the sincerest sympathy, and begged him to indulge us with a glass of beer.

He took it as we meant it, as a high compliment, and from a hidden cellar produced a bottle of beer of his own brewing, and of excellent quality. He offered to give us as much as we liked to carry away with us, and only regretted we had not passed the preceding night there, to be a help and comfort to his poor mother. All things considered, perhaps we were as well with Madame G——. However, disturbed our repose was, it could not have been as bad as with 180 reckless soldiery wrecking and ruining the quiet home of the poor brewer.

We returned to Madame G——for our dinner-breakfast, and on our way, we strolled on to the platform by the church. The view was lovely, though it wanted the quiet, dreamy charm of the night before, and coming back down the very same street we had descended with the priest, we passed a group of women gossiping together, and were amused by seeing one of them turn suddenly, silence her companions, and point to us, when she thought she was unobserved, saying, 'Look, look! the English ladies who saved the house of Madame G—' After breakfast, we went to headquarters; no message had come for us, yet a low, dull sound like distant thunder was heard, and many said it was the firing of heavy artillery.

Our host and his son offered to accompany us to what seemed to be the public promenade of Grand Pré. There was an old castle, now used as stables and farmhouses, and through the central court-yard we emerged on a raised platform overlooking the country for miles. This platform was simply the higher ground on the north side of the castle, but on the east, where it overlooked the plain below, was bounded by a low wall, and the steep bank sloped sharply down to the route *Impériale* which led through Beaumont and Douzy to Sedan.

The platform and the fields on the same level, extending westwards, were cultivated as cornfields. The corn was quite ripe, had been cut, and lay in shocks about the field. It was a glorious autumn day. The open country below was bathed in a flood of sunlight. The tall poplars, in a double row, marked where the road went, and as far as the eye could see it was blocked by the long, long train of waggons and columns of soldiers.

As they passed below us, we could hear the talking of the drivers to each other, and their German oaths as they urged on their tired beasts. We loitered on the platform for an hour, conversing with our host, the mayor, and several other citizens, doubtless of 'honour and renown.' Everyone had a different story to tell of what was passing beyond the low grass-covered hills that, in the distance, bounded the view; but no sound of war could be heard, just then no rising smoke clouded the deep blue of the sky. The view was exquisitely sunny and dreamy, and softened down in a golden mist, like some lovely Claudet unspoiled by the fading of the long years since it came, in all its freshness, from the great master's easel. The mayor was an individual of some forty years of age; he looked robust enough to endure the hardships of the present times, but he was quite broken down by billets for lodging, requisitions for forage, and the difficulty of procuring flour.

He at present was cheerful. The Prussians had all gone on to the front, the flour carts had come in, and His Worship, in a buff alpaca coat, white trousers, and a straw hat, was enjoying his cigar in well-earned repose. He expressed himself graciously delighted to have such worthy assistants as ourselves (Louise and myself) in keeping the peace of the town, and assured us he was of opinion that all the soldiers had gone forward, and we should have a quiet night. We returned to headquarters, and promised our host that we would only go and see Madame G—and come back.

We went down the street, and were just entering the market-place when a scared maidservant met us and implored us to go down and get the Prussians out of the brewery. They were there again, and her mistress had sent for us; but as we looked round the market-place we found it crowded with Prussians and Bavarians. Two regiments over 1,000 strong had come in, and there was nothing to eat in the town! The situation was difficult. We knew the soldiers would search every hole and corner for bread and wine and meat, and finding none would grow violent. To add to the excitement, a messenger came hurrying in to say the Prussians had entered a little village about two miles off, and finding nothing to eat or drink had set fire to it. Our host's son, with a very white face, came up to us and told us it was all true; the smoke and flames were already visible. We crossed the market place as quietly as possible: Madame G— had double-locked the door and put up the shutters, but on our knocking and calling out who we were let us in.

Things were looking black, and Louise and I went upstairs to watch the scene below, and saw the two officers in charge sitting on their horses, as bewildered as anyone what to do. An idea struck us how, at all events, to secure the safety of Madame G—'s house, and we ran down and proposed to Madame G—to invite the two officers to supper and a bedroom. I said there was bread and wine and soup in the house, and we had a goose they could roast (one of the Admiral's). *Madame* was weeping, and said, 'How could they roast a goose?'

I replied, 'The baker next door will bake it,' and *Madame* saw the difficulty overcome, and implored me to go and get the officers and the goose. Louise volunteered to keep the door against all comers, and off I went, and with the politest air possible presented the compliments of M. and Mde. G—, very worthy citizens, and would the noble commanders accept a very good bedroom and such a supper as the reduced state of Grand Pré enabled M. and Mde. G—to offer? The Bavarian officer instantly dismounted, and in very pretty French begged his best thanks for so much kindness and hospitality. 'Might his friend accompany him?'

'Most certainly.'

'Might he immediately offer his thanks to *Monsieur and Madame* also?'

'Most certainly. Would he follow me?' He did so, and I presented him to Mde. G——, who was uncertain what her fate was to be, shooting or hanging. He thanked her most courteously, and said as soon as he had attended to the wants of his men, he would present himself for supper. *Madame* brightened up, and I asked if he would kindly write on the door that the house was taken up as *commandants'* quarters so that no one might occupy their bedroom. A piece of white chalk was procured, certain cabalistic signs scribbled on the door, and our friend bowed himself off, saying, '*Au revoir*,' whilst *Madame*, exclaiming 'We are saved,' became on hospitable cares intent, and recovered all her cheerfulness. Louise stayed to assist her, and I went off to headquarters to fetch the goose.

The rest of our party, by the way, were living sumptuously on the remains of the king's provisions. The worthy chemist suggested, if I took the goose through the streets, the hungry Prussians would seize it; so, I threw a blanket over my arm, hid the goose in it, and sallied out again. As I crossed the market-place I was stopped by some thirty or forty Prussian soldiers. One of them advanced as spokesman for the rest. He was a stern little man, in spectacles, with a very decided manner. He said in very good French, '*Madame*, you are English. Have the goodness to explain to the deluded people of this town that we must have bread.'

His manner was studiously courteous, but I hugged my goose close as I answered with equal courtesy, '*Monsieur*, I regret it, but there is no flour in the town.'

'*Madame*, look around you. It is not a thing to be believed, that in a town with so many good houses there is no bread. Tell me not so!'

'*Monsieur*, it is unbelievable, but true. The army this morning took all the bread with them.'

'*Madame*, I regret to say it, but we have not eaten for twenty-four hours; we are very ferocious. If there is no bread in half an hour, you will be all hanged upon the lampposts.'

'*Monsieur*, I shall regret it very much; but that even will not bake bread without flour.'

The little man burst out laughing, and then sighed and said, 'I am very hungry. Oh, that I were back in London with my dear violin.'

A memory of his face dawned upon me. 'Is it possible,' I said; 'are you from London?'

'Yes, *Madame*; do you not remember me? I am E. P——.'

What visions of concerts and concertos floated before me. How I wished I could ask him to supper; but the goose was a small one, and he had hungry friends. We took an affectionate leave, and I earnestly hope he found some bread.

On I went, when a breathless man stopped me, one of the officials I had seen on the platform of the castle. 'Oh, *Madame*, we are lost; there are a thousand more troops arrived, and the mayor is perfectly disorganised.'

'Then, *Monsieur*,' I said, 'let him go and organise himself as fast as possible.'

'*Très bien, Madame*! but there are no quarters left. Where is he to lodge the men? they will not sleep in the street.'

'*Eh bien, Monsieur*, there are two or three hundred beds in the church; put some of them there.'

'*Madame*, it is a magnificent idea, only they cannot cook their suppers in the church!'

'Then, *Monsieur*, light a great fire outside and lend them the corporation kettle' (*le marmiton de la Mairie*).

'That goes well, *Madame*. A thousand thanks. I will go to the mayor.'

And he ran off. The effect of the advice was seen in the arrival of the mayor in the market-place, in a black velvet coat, black waistcoat and trowsers, and black wide-awake, imploring his fellow citizens to be brave, and above all, as he said, '*Soyez tranquilles, mes enfants*,' evidences of imperfect re-organisation. At last I arrived safely with my burden. We were all courageous and cheerful now, our shutters were down, our front door open. *Monsieur* was lounging on the door-step. We were the *commandants'* headquarters, and no soldier dare invade those sacred precincts. *Madame*, leaving Louise to see that all went well with the goose, and assured that I would remain at the front door, departed herself to visit various friends in the neighbourhood, and relate her good fortune and the safety of the house.

Long before she returned, sundry maidservants arrived, bringing messages from their mistresses. Could the English ladies find them an officer? It would be such a comfort. We were obliged to remonstrate that officers were not plentiful, and we could not find any more; but one persevering maiden returned to the charge, saying, 'If not possible, *Madame*, to find an officer, could we not have an officer's servant?' whilst another withdrew, murmuring, with upraised hands and eyes, against the injustice of fate. 'Think, then, of two whole colonels for Madame G——, and not even a corporal for us!' I must confess it was a monopoly; but what was to be done? The friends would not be parted.

There were only two officers in charge of all the men, '*trainards*' from the main body, probably, and we could not afford to part with them. About seven o'clock they came in. Supper was ready, the soup was good, and so was the wine, the *bouillon*, and vegetables, and above all, the goose, was a great success. With the light-heartedness of the French, *Monsieur*, *Madame*, and their pretty little daughter, finding the officers most pleasant, entered into the spirit of the scene. We all drank wine together and touched glasses, and how the poor fellows, ate, and then laughingly apologised, by saying that, except a few raw vegetables, they had had nothing for twenty-four hours. They were most grateful for a good supper and a kindly welcome, and we all passed two or three very merry hours; the last for many days. At last we wished each other goodnight. The Bavarian, as spokesman, begged his warmest thanks, not only to good M. and Madame G——, but to ourselves, who had procured him so charming an evening. I really hope and believe Madame G——slept that night, secure in the presence of the two Germans.

Nor must I forget to add, that before the supper ended the commanders' servant arrived with the leg of mutton he had received as rations, which was left behind for the use of the house; and furthermore, the servant was induced to accept a bed next door, where he acted as guard to a frightened family. At five next morning they were off. They just knocked at our door and called out a kind goodbye, and before we were fairly awake for the day, they were miles away from their night's quarters.

Chapter 10

Alone on the Hills

There never was a brighter summer morning than that 1st of September, a day that will not be forgotten in the history of the world. From that miserable day may be dated the unbroken cloud of misfortune and treason that crushed the hopes of France, and left her alone and despairing to struggle against a resistless foe. Yet only twenty miles from that great battlefield around Sedan all was as quiet and sleepy as if it had been in some out-of-the-way provincial town of England. The troops had gone on. The provision difficulties were ended, and Grand Pré was just the sort of sunny, idle town at seeing which one would have wondered how the inhabitants kept themselves awake, not to say amused.

There was a low, distant grumble in the air, but no cloud in the blue sky. 'They are fighting in front,' we said, as we sipped our morning coffee; but we did not dream how an empire was being lost, still less of the awful misery that day would entail on the fairest provinces of France. And only twenty miles away! Only the distance of Richmond from London, not half an hour by express train. What a contrast between the strife and agony in front and the calm repose of twenty miles behind.

After breakfast we walked round the town, and seeing a lovely creeper in a courtyard, ventured to enter and look at it. A lady, perceiving us, came forward to welcome us, and asked us to come in and see the view. Like many others, her beautiful house and garden had suffered from foreign occupation. She begged us to go and stay with her as long as we liked; indeed, we had so many invitations at Grand Pré that we might have lived there at free quarters during the war. About noon I went to see the lady at the brewery. The Prussians had left, and, thanks to everything having been wrecked and ruined the day before, they had not suffered much additional damage.

As I was returning, I met Louise, coming to tell me the General had sent a Bavarian officer to order us to go on directly to Beaumont. He had asked me, before he left Grand Pré, how long we should take, after receiving an order, before we could start. I replied, I thought, with no packing to do, one hour ought to be enough, and of this I had duly warned the rest. Louise and myself instantly gave the news at headquarters. It was half-past twelve; I ordered the start for half-past one. The drivers and German escort had had their noon-day meal. I paid off all scores, bought some forage, and they promised us everything should be ready at the time appointed.

Louise and I returned, and our kind hostess, heartbroken at our departure, yet contrived to give us a charming little breakfast, and at a quarter past one we arrived at headquarters. The waggons were packed, the horses harnessed, the drivers ready, and the Prussian soldiers in their light carriage, prepared to go off instantly; but that was all! The rest of the party were invisible, and, to my horror, I found them only just beginning an elaborate dinner. I spoke of the necessity of obeying the orders we had received, and enunciated the magnificent sentiment, 'Duty before dinner,' and then went out to see to the packing of our little baggages.

I was followed by the Knight of St. John, who had passed his time in bed, except at the hours of dinner. He asked me if we really were going forward. I said, 'Yes, directly, by order from our commander, the general.' He said we should not go forward; it was dangerous, it was useless, and the stores must remain behind. I said I was not under his orders, and the stores were in charge of the general, who had left them in my care, and both ourselves and them should go on. Just then out came Louise. I hastily explained, and implored her to get the rest of the party to leave their dinner and come away. She saw the necessity, and hurried back. Meantime the baron grew violent, and declared all the waggons were his. I denied it. He then claimed the soldiers' cart as his, and ordered the soldiers to turn out our light baggage and take the stores; they must go back to the depot at Pont-à-Mousson. And then he went back to his dinner.

Louise came out. Her efforts had been vain, and she gallantly said, 'Let us go on with the stores, and let the others follow;' and so it was settled the Prussian soldiers declared they would go. It was a lonely, dangerous road, and they would not leave us, and I promised them ten *francs* each when we arrived at Beaumont, where the General was quartered for the day. Then I went back with Louise and told the rest what had happened, that there was opposition made to our leaving, and implored them to come away. There was not a Prussian soldier in the town except our two guards and the old baron, and the Bavarian officer. We two could manage them; but troops might come in at any moment, and the baron would seize the stores, and they would be sent back to swell the collection of goods in the depot at Pont-à-Mousson for Prussian use alone.

All in vain; so, I left a paper with the route, and ordered a rendezvous at Sommeurthe, six miles short of Beaumont, knowing that with no baggage they might possibly get there first, and then went out. The baron rushed after me, perfectly furious. He ordered the soldiers to stay behind, and, doubling his fist at me, threatened vague punishments, if I dared to take away the baggage. I said I was resolved, and he turned into the house, not believing we could go alone with five hundred pounds worth of stores over twenty miles of lonely road. The soldiers were very grieved, but they could but obey orders, and they helped us to transfer the light baggage to our waggons. We ordered one to remain to bring on the rest of the party, under escort of the Bavarian officer and a troop of dragoons, whom he was instantly expecting; and then, taking a cordial farewell of all who had been so kind to us, we told the first two waggons to move on, and, mounting on the third, took the road to Buzancy, the first village between Grand Pré and Beaumont.

It was just two o'clock when we got off—two English ladies and three Alsace drivers speaking only German. The country we had to traverse was on the outskirts of the great battlefields. Camp-followers and *trainards*, or, as we call them, lingerers, infesting it. And the chance of getting somewhere between the contending parties, or finding ourselves in the line of fire of some battery of artillery, was also not a remote one. If, as we wound slowly up the road leading out of Grand Pré, our hearts half failed us, it was not fear, but a sense of the heavy responsibility thus laid upon us. It was our duty to obey orders; it was our duty to save the stores for those who might so sadly need them.

But in fulfilling that duty we never for one moment doubted that, in the hour of anxiety and danger, we should not be 'Alone upon the hills.' So on we went till Louise, seeing we were going due east, remembered that we ought to go due north, and we had no map with us. We stopped a peasant boy and found we were going straight to Verdun, and must retrace our road almost to Grand Pré. Having been nearly an hour coming thus far, we were not inclined to do this if we could avoid it, and he suggested a cross-road which would bring us to Buzancy, where we could rejoin the main road. At a farmhouse on the rising ground beyond we should probably find a man to direct us. We turned off accordingly, and as we traversed the high ground, and looked back on the little town where we had passed those long two days, we congratulated ourselves that there we had protected and comforted four poor, frightened, oppressed people; but no foreshadowing came to us on that autumn afternoon with its golden sunshine of the dreary winter days when it should be given to us alone again, with only God and our own English courage, to keep, to protect, and comfort four hundred helpless beings committed by Him to our care.

So, on we went, so slowly that we had perpetually to get down and urge our driver on. Travelling in times like these is not very safe, and it was better to keep together. The utter loneliness was something appalling; not a bird flew across our path, no sound of life except the slow grating of our broad wheels on the dusty road and our continual cry, 'Forward!' It was very hot, a blinding sunshine, no shade of trees, only low hedges and scattered orchards. In the distance a few cottages but no living being visible, yet what sound of war and tumult might suddenly break that strange silence no one could predict.

On we went up a long white road, and then we came to the highest level of the rising ground, and looked to our left over a vast expanse of champaign country, with blue hills and woods in the distance. The meadows were fresh and green, the trees just stirred their branches to the slight summer breeze, but down below were long lines of dark figures; they changed places every now and then, and here and there were little tiny black dots, that seemed to explode in a puff of white smoke that went up slowly, to linger against the blue sky before it dispersed.

Beyond were heavier white clouds of smoke and a dull echo on the air. The little black dots were skirmishers, and the long lines troops in order of battle; the smoke came from cannon and rifle, but the golden sunshine threw a halo over all and softened down the distant outlines, and that was our view of the great battle around Sedan. 'They are fighting down there,' we said, and we turned off the hill road and descended to the valley, and became intensely interested in the finding of some intelligent peasant to guide us to Buzancy, for to us the battle was ended.

A battle is very pretty ten miles off, very exciting on the spot, very dreadful when it is ended, and all that is left of the strife and the defeat and the victory is the agony on the battlefield of those lying there, moaning for help, and, even worse still, the cottages crowded with sufferers, the stables and barns full of groaning men, no beds, no light through the night; too often no bread, no water, no wine, and all help insufficient for the time. How they listen for the ambulance carts coming to take them to some house where assistance and nursing can be found. How many crawl away into some low shrubbery or wood or amongst the long, cool grass, and days after are found dead, not from wounds, but weakness and starvation.

With all our improved means of helping the wounded, this is too often the case. But the summer is so merciful compared to winter, when the snow buries dead and dying alike, and a white heap, a little higher than the white field around, is all the guide to find some poor fellow gone beyond all human help.

This had not been realised to us as we halted in the village and looked for someone to guide us in vain. We were half inclined to laugh at our predicament. I started off and thundered at several doors; still in vain. At last I spied an individual peeping round a corner, and dashed at him. Finding it was not an *Uhlan*, he ventured forth, and, on being offered a consideration, consented to guide us to Buzancy. He mounted by our driver, and we tried to get some information from him; but if he ever had possessed any wits they had been all frightened out of his head, for beyond saying everybody in the village had run away and he was alone there, and shrieking 'right' and 'left' to our drivers (the German for which we taught him), nothing could we get out of him. He was evidently bent on escaping at the first possible moment, and as soon as we had ascended another hill, and he caught sight of a church spire, he gave a sigh of relief, said '*Voilà Buzancy!*' jumped off, hardly waiting for his fee, and became invisible.

Our drivers were not inclined to stop at Buzancy, even to rest their horses. Our private opinion was they were terribly frightened, and inclined to keep as far from the scene of action as possible. But as we insisted on going on and as every mile we went we were coming nearer, it became a great point with them to go as slowly as possible, whilst with us it was to get to our journey's end before dark. This unfortunate difference of opinion caused a great deal of trouble, and we bitterly regretted not having a little revolver. We had no intention of shooting ourselves by firing it off; but it has always an effective appearance, and they would not have known it was not loaded. Evening began to close in and not one of us had the least idea of where we were. The horse in our waggon began to go on in an eccentric way, stopping suddenly and pulling all to the right, and we speculated how much further he would go, and what we should do if he dropped dead; but the solution of the difficulty being too much for us, we left it alone, and contented ourselves with hoping he would not drop dead. And so, hours passed away.

At last we saw a group of dirty-looking soldiers assembled round a broken waggon. They were camp-followers, and we feared that they would seize one of our waggons to go on their way with. I spoke of this to our drivers, and implored them to get on. They would hear nothing. A desperate remedy was needed, and looking suddenly to the left, and pointing to a clump of trees, I cried out, 'The French, the French; we shall be all made prisoners.' Louise aided in the outcry, our driver got frightened, the others caught the alarm, and they actually lashed their horses into a gallop past the suspicious party. It was so quickly done that they had no time to stop us, even had they been so inclined. At all events we avoided troublesome questions and demands, and we rushed on down a long hill and fairly out of their sight. Below us in a valley lay the village of Sommeurthe.

How glad we were to see the lights that showed the place was in military occupation! Anything was better than the darkness of night on those lonely hills. The road was a sharp descent cut in a hill-side and going round a corner, a low bank on the right hand, and a very steep slope down to the little stream that ran through the valley on the left.

Just as we began to descend, our horse made a dead stop, and then staggered. It was all over with him, for the time at least, and the driver was compelled to unharness him, and tie him up behind. The waggon was thus left with one horse only attached to the pole. The driver walked and fell behind to speak to one of the other drivers, who had lingered, and our horse naturally pulled to the left. I called to the driver. He was lighting his pipe, and before he could reach the horse's head to turn it round the waggon was over the side, and going slanting down the slope.

How we escaped I know not, except that the wheel caught against a large stone, and the earth being soft, the downward progress of the waggon was checked, and it came to a standstill. The heavy chests would have overbalanced it in another moment, and I saw them swerving over. I was on the right-hand side, and sprung out, Louise followed instantly; but the escape was a miracle, and so we felt it. Half-way down an angle of forty-five, with a stream below, and heavy boxes bringing the vehicle head over heels, is a most unpleasant position. We recovered our coolness sooner than the drivers, who yelled and chattered like monkeys, and at last the horse and waggon were turned up the bank, and what to do was the question. We could have gone on in either of the other two waggons, but to leave the one we were in behind was impossible. Very valuable stores were in it, so we decided it should go at a foot pace (all it could) ahead of us, and one of us mounted each of the other two waggons as guard, for darkness was closing in.

Our progress was slow, but happily downhill, and most thankful were we to enter the village street. I saw a gentleman in a white cap run out into the centre of the street, and call to several others to come and meet us, and I cried out to Louise in delight, 'Here is Mr. W—' (he, too, had always worn a white cap). One of the gentlemen stopped the waggon, and the supposed Mr. W—in the white cap came up and held out his arms to catch me as I jumped off my throne of hay, saying, 'I am so glad to see you. I had just sent out a patrol of *carbineers* to look for you. It is so dangerous on those hills.' The tone was foreign, the gentleman spoke in French, and looking up I saw it was not Mr. W—. We did not explain our mistake, but we did our misfortunes.

Another of the party was speaking to Louise, and asked, 'Were you not afraid?'

'Not at all,' she said; 'we are English.'

He laughed and said he had lived many years in England, and had been a merchant at Liverpool. He added, 'That gentleman with your friend is the Prince of Tours and Taxis. We heard from some of your party, who passed through an hour or two ago, that you were on your way, and His Highness was so anxious that he ordered out a guard to search for you.'

The prince then told us the rest had gone on, hearing the General was at Beaumont. Of course, we were vexed. They had been ordered to wait at Sommeurthe for us, and had they done so we too could have gone on; as it was, it was impossible. There was not a horse to be had, and the prince suggested it was so dark and late we should lose nothing by waiting till the morning, and making an early start of it. By that time, he would find us a horse, and he would also try for quarters for us. I believe he gave us up his own room in a small house, and slept in his carriage. Nothing could exceed his kindness. He came up with us, to show us the way, apologised for the rough accommodation, and explained that he and all his friends had had no meat that day, which must plead his excuse for not asking us to supper. Little could be spared from the wounded, who were coming in fast; but a loaf of bread and a bottle of wine he could give us, and would we give back what we did not require?

We deposited our hand-bags, and went out to see our stores safe, the Englishman, as we called him, with us. Whilst returning we were stopped by the prince. He pointed to the church close by, saying, 'That church is full of wounded, and we have *nothing*, literally nothing. Can you not give us something? Lint, medicines, extract of meat, anything.' Now, we had been ordered to bring on the stores untouched, but in a case like this to refuse would have been heartless. I said if the prince and some of his men would help me to open and afterwards nail down some of the store chests, I would give all I dared. He gladly consented, and we mounted the waggons; the prince going hard to work himself. We got out lint, cotton wool, and a quantity of Liebig. They were most gratefully accepted. The village was utterly destitute, and no help at hand; our arrival was most timely.

The prince bade us a kind goodnight, saying he had ordered the Englishman to escort us to Beaumont at 6 a.m. next morning, and we promised that more stores should be sent back by him the instant we could communicate with our chief. We went off to our little room, had our supper of bread and wine, and slept soundly till some of the people of the house awoke us at daybreak. They were very sorry they had no coffee or milk to give us, so we took a piece of bread each and a little wine, gave back the rest, and with many thanks departed. Our escort was waiting for us, the waggons ready, and at half-past five we drove slowly out of Sommeurthe on our way to Beaumont.

One painful scene we had witnessed at Sommeurthe was still present to our minds. As we were unpacking the chests the night before, we saw led through the village street as prisoners a man and woman, their hands tied behind them. They had been found on the battlefield that afternoon cutting off the finger of a dead officer to get his ring, and we knew their doom was certain. That bright morning a grave, hurriedly dug by the roadside and hastily filled in, was all that was left of two who, the night before, had been human beings in full health and strength. Such scenes were too common.

At Conny we had seen a man with his clothes half torn off his back led struggling and shrieking down the street. He was a spy, and his fate was sure. In both cases it was deserved; but in all such sudden and terrible punishments there is something revolting to our feelings of mercy and the gentle doctrine of pity and forbearance which we profess to believe in and practise. War puts aside, and perhaps by necessity, all such considerations, but it is not the less sad and deplorable.

CHAPTER 11

The Last Hours of the Empire

The morning air was fresh and cool as we drove out of Sommeurthe to reach Beaumont. The sun had hardly risen, and the dew was still hanging on the branches of the trees. The road was utterly lonely, and as we went slowly along, we saw a dark object on it. The driver of the first waggon dismounted and picked it up. I looked at it in utter astonishment. It was my waterproof cloak, which had been left in the waggon that conveyed the rest of the party, had fallen out, and remained ever since seven o'clock the evening before just where it fell. Can anything give a clearer idea of the desertion of a high road by all ordinary traffic? I reclaimed my property, not much damaged by the muddy road and the night dews, and we drove on. Our kind escort knew nothing of the battle said to have been fought the day before, nor where the French were.

A crushing defeat of MacMahon's army was spoken of, and wounded had come in in large numbers; but the state of ignorance and confusion of mind prevailing in all who are near a battle is a singular fact. Every man knows isolated incidents of his own corps or brigade; but no one can give a general idea of the affair. I doubt if even the general in command knows much about it. Perhaps he pieces together the reports of his officers; but it must be as impossible for him as for anyone else to have the battlefield and every manoeuvre upon it spread before his eyes like a map. A white mist hid the distance, and so we journeyed quietly on, speaking of England, till we entered Beaumont, passed down a road with orchards each side, enclosed by walls, crossed a little stream by an old stone bridge, turned into the main street of the town, and almost directly afterwards into the central square, Grande Place, or whatever it was called.

What a scene of confusion was there! Provision and ammunition waggons. Ambulance carts, mixed up, together with troopers, some on horseback, some dismounted, men of all regiments pushing here and there, and heaps of straw round the church in the centre of the Place, on which lay men in every stage of suffering from wounds—German and French side by side. The church was full, and even the side streets had wounded lying on the doorsteps. Where to find our friends was the question. A Prussian officer who rode up was accosted by our friend, and informed us they had found quarters in the mayor's house, just down a by-street, and there we accordingly went. A Frenchwoman came out to receive us, exclaiming how anxiously we had been looked for. Her husband ran upstairs, and in another moment Mr. A— came down with a hearty welcome. They had been very uneasy about us, and sent out a patrol to look for us; but the General had consoled the party by observing he should have been dreadfully alarmed in any other case, but as it was Miss Pearson and Miss M'Laughlin he was quite sure they could take care of themselves; and the baggage and they would be at Beaumont early in the morning.

And there we were by half-past six, with the stores all safe, feeling very proud of our successful effort to save them. God helps those who help themselves, and in times like these personal considerations must be put aside. The duty imposed on those who have any charge committed to them must be done, and to fail in doing it is better than not to try under every difficulty to carry it out. Besides, dangers and hindrances that look so vast at a distance vanish into nothing as they approach. A little more fatigue, a little more suspense, a few more anxious throbbings of the heart, and a stern resolution that come what may the duty shall be done, and difficulties vanish like frost in sunshine, and the struggle is over, the battle won.

We dismounted—for getting out of a carriage it could not be called, to get off a heap of hay—and entered the house. There was a general effect of confusion and wounded men. Almost directly afterwards the General came down, congratulated us most enthusiastically on our success and pointed out its result—that we had brought on help where it was most terribly needed, and where, owing to the difficulties of the way, none had yet come. That word 'difficulty!' It is too often an excuse for leaving undone a tiresome task. Perhaps we were unconscious then, as we certainly were afterwards, of the danger we had incurred.

The General, the Prince of Tours and Taxis, our escort, the Englishman, all seemed to know it. But except heat, weariness, and nearly being tumbled over a precipice, we had seen none. I believe both of us had a singular unconsciousness of peril, which blinded us to it, and certainly saved us many painful hours. We got what breakfast we could—some bread and coffee; whilst Mr. A— and the General occupied themselves in finding fresh horses for us, for they said we must press on to the front.

Whilst trying to boil some water for our coffee a priest entered, and begged us to dress the wounds of some men lying in a house hard by, whom no one had yet attended to. We went with him, and entering a small room found it full of wounded. We did what we could for them, and first got some water. We unfastened their stocks, and washed the blood and dust from their faces and throats. They were lying on straw; and therefore, to undress them was useless; but we took off their coats laid them over them, and dressed their wounds. One poor fellow was in such a state that I saw he was beyond our help, and begged the poor woman of the house to fetch a surgeon. She returned with one belonging to a French Ambulance; he examined the poor man's leg. It was shot through by a ball, the bone broken, and the wound already gangrened. The surgeon spoke most kindly to him of the necessity of immediate amputation; he refused to have his leg cut off, and the surgeon said very quietly and gravely, 'Then, my poor lad, you have but twenty-four hours to live. I leave you for half an hour, and I shall return for your answer.' We dressed them all and went back to the house.

There were so many wounded in Beaumont, and such urgent need of help, that, had we not been bound to get to headquarters as fast as possible, we should have stayed there. Whilst we were all discussing matters two or three French surgeons arrived, one an elderly man, much decorated. The General received them most kindly. They told us that they had two ambulances there, and that the Germans had taken away everything they had—instruments, medicines, all were gone— and they earnestly begged for help. Just at this instant in came several German surgeons to ask for everything, possible and impossible, and I pleaded the cause of the prince and the promise I had made to send him back some stores. A large collection was put aside for him, and then we turned our attention to the wants of our present friends. Nothing could exceed the jealousy of the Germans at the idea of anything more being given to the French than to them, whilst we felt how badly the French ambulances had been used, and how necessary it was to give them the largest assistance.

The General said to me in a whisper, 'Tell me to put aside for your immediate use on the battlefield a large quantity of things,' Louise and myself instantly began to claim our proportion, and considerably more. The General said, as there were two German ambulances and two French ambulances, four equal parcels must be made, and then one for us, and one reserved for the use of Mr. Parker, when he rejoined us. This was done, and the Germans were requested to give receipts for the various articles handed over to them. The French did the same. The General whispered to me, 'Tell the old French surgeon to stay behind the Germans, and to be very slow writing his receipts.' As I spoke to him he burst into tears as he told me of his wounded, without a single thing with which to nurse or dress them, and the nice stock of instruments and medicines which had been so carefully got together, and which were all taken away from his assistants and himself. A small cart came for the German lots, but the head surgeon was evidently suspicious and discontented.

Just after they left, we called to some French orderlies attending on their surgeon to add to their store the heaps nominally laid aside for us, and at that very instant the head German surgeon came back again, saying, 'I have only two parcels; I ought to have three.'

'Not at all,' said Mr. A——, who was trying to stand before the remaining piles; 'you have had three that is more than your share.'

'How so?' asked the surgeon; 'I saw but two I was to have one lot of things for myself.'

'So, you had,' said Mr. A—— 'there were three lots put aside for you, only *Mademoiselle* here was so stupid she mixed up the three lots into two.' *Mademoiselle* tried to look guilty, and the German took himself off, evidently not at all satisfied as regards the two or three heaps. The gratitude of the poor French surgeon was beyond all bounds, and he took instant precautions to hide up his treasures where the Germans would not be likely to discover them.

All this business having been transacted, and the new horses for the waggons having been harnessed, we prepared to start. The poor horse whose failure the night before had nearly caused our topple over the high bank was shot, it being discovered he had glanders, and one other was tied behind our waggon, and so annoyed us by munching the hay which formed our seat, and thereby bumping us perpetually in the back, that we begged he might be transferred to some other waggon, where there were only store-chests to interfere with his amusements. The rest of the old lot of horses were left behind, and as the new horses were powerful French artillery ones, used to dragging heavy guns over open country, it was possible to go forward at a great pace, but where no one knew. To Sedan, the General said, for doubtless the French had retreated beyond it. Who could dream of the surrender of that splendid army, which was only the next morning to become a sad reality and an everlasting stain on the page of French history?

The sun was still shining bright as we rattled out of Beaumont, the General and Mr. A— on horseback, armed with long hunting-whips, which were afterwards very useful. As we went on the sky seemed to become clouded, a lurid haze to hang all about, and the brightness and beauty of a summer day to be gone. We were on a long, straight road, overlooking many miles of country. To the left, bodies of troops were moving about in the distance, and a thick cloud of smoke arose from a village some miles off, which we could just see; but our road was as lonely as usual. Presently, however, a cloud of dust rose before us, a gleam of red was visible in the midst, and the General, who was in front, rode back to us and said, 'Look out for the saddest sight you ever saw—French prisoners in thousands.'

On they came, Prussian dragoons on either side, four or five abreast. Every corps in the service was represented there—Artillery, Dragoons, *Chasseurs*, *Zouaves*, the Line, all unarmed, of course, and unwounded, tramping heavily to the rear, where the railroad waggons waited to take them away far from La Belle France to the Northern land, amongst strangers and enemies. They walked with a quiet and subdued air, but with a firm and steady step. They were not beaten men, as we knew afterwards. Conquered and betrayed, but still hopeful of some victory that should retrieve the loss of yesterday, they came on and on, till the heart was sick to see them.

Twenty thousand passed us by as we halted, not to break the lines. Even their guards, soldiers themselves, seemed to feel for them, and allowed them to halt for rest, and spoke in softened tones to them. It was before the days of *Gardes Mobiles* and *francs-tireurs*; these were the flower of the armies of France—Crimean, Italian, and Chinese medals on almost every man of that sad throng. It was a relief when they had passed and the cloud of dust hid their red *kepis* and trousers from sight. The General spoke to one of the officers in charge of them, who afterwards talked to us and told us we could not get into Sedan.

The emperor was still there, and the place had not surrendered; but he thought we could get into the suburb of Balan, only we should have to pass through the burning village of Bazeilles, which was somewhat dangerous and very dreadful to see; but as there was no cross road, we could not avoid it, and so we went on our way to Douzy, the first village on our road to Sedan.

Just before we entered the village, we had to cross a small stream by a wooden bridge. A party of cavalry were in the level water meadows below, guarding more prisoners, who were huddled together in long lines, trying to keep each other warm; for a cold wind was blowing, and everything looked dreary and desolate. Just as we were crossing, a cry was heard, and we beheld the hindmost driver lamenting over the loss of the horse which had been tied up behind his waggon. He had been staring at the prisoners in the field, and some sharp Prussian soldiers had cut the cord and walked off with the beast. Now, as it had been 'required' by the Prussian Knights of St. John at Pont-à-Mousson a few days before, there was no occasion for his loud lamentations over his ruin and evil fortune.

Douzy looked utterly deserted; not a woman or child to be seen, only German soldiers and some French prisoners wandering idly about. As we halted in the main street a cry was raised; a number of chickens and ducks had been unearthed from a barn close by and were running wildly out. Captors and captives joined in a hunt, and picked up sticks to knock the poor birds down with. The scene was most absurd, but nothing could relieve the oppressive weariness of Douzy. The grey sky, the dusty streets, the closely shut houses, the absence of all light or warmth of colouring, were most depressing. The Admiral had, as usual, collected a small crowd of German officers round him, but there were no civilians, male or female, to listen to his eloquence.

The General spoke kindly to one or two French officers and took their addresses, that he might send news of them home to their friends. We did not then appreciate what a blessing such a trifling kindness might prove; but afterwards, when we saw the piteous appeals in the Belgian papers from dear friends and relations longing for news of those they hoped might be prisoners (not in the sad lists of the killed and missing), we realised how many a weary month of agonising suspense was spared by that thoughtful act.

We were sitting in our waggons, watching the scene, when a German general came up and begged us to have some wine. An *aide-de-camp* brought a bottle and some glasses, and when we had taken the wine, we naturally gave back the glasses. 'Pray keep them;' said the *aide-de-camp*; 'they may be useful. Take anything you like; it is nobody's now, and may as well be yours.'

It was a delightfully lawless sensation to go shopping with nothing to pay to select whatever pleased us, with no consideration of the bill, to be sent in next Christmas. One felt like a comfortable high-way robber, sanctioned by the highest authority, and no forebodings of Newgate in the distance to cloud our perfect enjoyment of everybody's property except our own. Under the circumstances it was Spartan forbearance not to take a beautiful *barouche* (quite new) and a pair of splendid horses which the Prussian general pressed on our acceptance. He had found them, he said, in the *château* he had taken possession of (a large house close by). He really had no use for them, somebody would run off with them that evening, he was sure, and really, we must be so tired of our very uncomfortable waggon, he must insist on our having a better conveyance; and he began to call to Fritz, and Wilhelm, and Johann to bring out the carriage and harness the horses. We were young campaigners then, and had a shred of conscience left, and we declined, but we were tempted to regret it many a day afterwards.

The Prussian general's theory was right: somebody, no doubt, took the carriage and horses, and they probably are being driven '*Unter den Linden*': now; whilst I trust that we should have had sufficient strength of mind and rectitude of principle to restore our '*voiture de luxe*' after the war. Carriages and horses were great temptations where there were none, and we met a wandering omnibus the other day which had been 'required' in Mantes, had passed the winter in Orléans, and was going on to Paris. It may find its way back some day; but as it has been all repainted in white, with a Red Cross on the side, I fear it will cost some trouble and expense to restore it to its pristine yellow. They were lawless times; I trust we shall never know such in England.

The General told us we must get on as fast as possible. Sedan had not surrendered, and there was an idea that a sortie on a huge scale would be tried. The suburb of Balan was occupied by the Bavarians, and there, he thought, we could find some sort of shelter for the night. He feared we should find getting through Bazeilles difficult, but not impossible, and that we must be prepared for sad scenes, for hardship, and even danger, such as we had not encountered; for we should have to go quite close to the walls of Sedan, and the guns might open fire at any time. All these possibilities had also struck us; but it was no time to turn back. We had no wish to do so, and only begged him to take us to the front as fast as possible, where our services would be most useful and our stores most needed. We bade *adieu* to the German officers and the dreary village of Douzy, and at 2 p.m. clattered out upon the long, straight, and poplar bordered road that led direct to Bazeilles.

CHAPTER 12

The Saddest Scene of All

We left Douzy at 3 p.m. at a rapid pace, and went along the road, as regular and straight as is usual with all routes *Impériales*, that led to Bazeilles. Look in Murray, and you will find at page 648, route 180, the simple statement:

'Bazeilles, four miles' (from Sedan). 'At this village is or was the *château* where Turenne was nursed, and an avenue planted by him. Near here the Count de Soissons defeated the army of Richelieu, 1641, but perished on the field of battle.'

That is all! But Murray must add a longer and sadder record now to his next edition. We may simply say that before the war it was a neat and pretty town, with broad streets and white stone houses, very many standing apart in their gardens—the country residences of the wealthy shopkeepers and merchants of Sedan. It might be described as a 'very select town' of 1,200 inhabitants. It had its *mairie* in the central place, a handsome building with a large entrance-door and many windows, and a balcony from which His Worship (if French mayors are so designated) had proclaimed the latest bulletins of 'His Imperial Majesty.'

It had its neat little hotel, and many good shops, and residences of weavers, very few cottages; in fact, it was 'a genteel suburb' of Sedan. On this quiet little town the scourge of war fell heaviest, and we saw it only a heap of blazing and blackened ruins. Even as we drove along, a heavy, thick smoke arose in the distance, a lurid mist seemed to hang over the open fields on either side, where small parties were busy digging shallow trenches here and there—the graves of the fallen soldiers.

We went on, the General and Mr. A— lashing the horses with their long hunting-whips. Scattered bodies of troopers passed us every now and then, and waggons full of knapsacks and other equipments; but every moment was of importance, and we did not stay the full gallop of our horses for troopers or waggons. The great cases bumped as if they would break loose from their lashings. The drivers stared and muttered at the unusual pace. We held on by the sides till the gallop slackened, and the General, riding up to us, said, 'Don't look out; it is too bad for you to see.'

We said, "Better face the worst at once,' and he replied, 'Yes, you are right; look out, and nothing you'll ever see in hospital will alarm you afterwards.'

We did look out. Shall we ever forget the horror of that scene? A long street, every house burning, some smouldering, some blazing still; no human being there, but dreadful forms lying about the streets in attitudes of pain and agony, their clothes still smoking, with clenched hands and upturned faces, the blood issuing from their mouths, showing how fearful their deaths must have been. All were Germans, and there were deep gashes on the throats of some that told a tale of revenge, and possibly murder, that had been done by no soldier's hand. The church and *mairie* were only wrecks. The *mairie* had been made into an ambulance, but the flames had caught it. There was no one to help or save, and the floors had crashed in with their helpless occupants. Not one single house was left. Death and destruction reigned there, and the smell of burnt flesh lingered for many a long day with us, turning us sick at everything that bore the slightest resemblance to it.

On every side of us the fire had extended up the main street, down the cross ones, smoke and flame, crashing ruins, and burning bodies. We feared the hay in our waggon would catch, and tried to cover it up with rugs and our waterproof sheet. Sick, and faint, and smothered, we longed to be out of that terrible place; but the horses winced perpetually. With the noble instinct of their natures, they would not trample on the dead, and we were obliged to go slowly.

It seemed hours before we reached the central Place, where there were ruin and death still around us; hours before we got out of that fearful town, and breathed a long, deep breath of pure air on the road beyond. But as we left the town one sad, touching thing we saw. A small cottage on the outskirts had escaped the flames, and there were wounded there, for a Red-Cross flag was hung out of its lattice window—only a coarse white handkerchief, the cross traced on it in blood. Over all hung a deep cloud of sulphurous smoke, that in mercy hid from the country round the awful fate of Bazeilles.

How it all came about will, perhaps, be never truly known. It was held by the Marine Infantry against the enemy, who, in this case, were aided by their own countrymen; for, mistaking their blue jackets and caps for Prussian uniforms, they were fired at by both sides, and lost as many by the balls of the French as they did by those of their foes. The village was twice taken and retaken by the Bavarians, and it is said that when the Germans were driven out the first time by the French the peasantry cut the throats of their wounded who had been left there, and that when it was retaken by the Germans they, in revenge, set fire to the town.

Certainly, it had been burned by hand. The houses stood separately, yet everyone was destroyed, even where it was impossible flames could catch from one to the other. Whether or not the popular tale is true no one will ever know. Others say a Bavarian trooper entered the place just after it was taken, asked an innkeeper for water for his horse, and was told in no courteous terms to fetch it himself. That he seized a burning brand from the hearth and set fire to the house, and the mania of destruction spread like wildfire.

Why the *mairie* should have been fired, with all the wounded in it, German as well as French, is a difficult question to solve. Military reports and popular rumours always differ, and both I believe to be equally worthy of credit. At least, we have found them so, and in this instance various accounts were given. There is some truth in all, but often mistakes; and certainly, both French and German telegrams and reports were singular flights of fancy. Everyone said the only reliable news came from England, and the newspaper correspondents we met deserve every credit for their endeavours to be exact. They all had their own predilections, French or German, but all honestly endeavoured to give the best account of passing events, and the slight colouring of personal feeling maybe easily forgiven.

We were too ill from the scene we had witnessed to care much about looking at the road we were travelling upon, and it was only when we came near a village, we were told was Balan that we could rouse from the half-sick stupor which oppressed us. Here we encountered a number of Bavarian troops. As we entered the place, we saw that we were indeed in the heart of the battlefield. Though the destruction had not been as complete, as at Bazeilles, yet many houses hard been demolished by shot and shell, and were only smoking ruins. Dead bodies lay about the street, and in one place were a carriage and pair of horses. A shell had struck them, and driver and horses lay dead; their blood splashed upon the wall, against which they had dashed in their last agony.

The carriage, though overturned, was unharmed; of its occupant, if it ever had one, there was no trace. The road was strewed with articles from the houses around which had been pillaged; books, china, and wearing apparel were thrown about. We saw a very pretty hood of white cashmere, trimmed with black velvet, lying on the ground beside where our carriage halted, and, as we admired it, a soldier picked it up and presented it to us. A great number of leaves of music books were also lying there. They were separate leaves, or rather cards, such as wind instruments have placed upon them when playing on the march. We had time to look at it all, as our chief was consulting with the Bavarian colonel what to do.

To go on into Sedan was impossible. It had not surrendered, and the only alternative was to take possession of one of the many sacked and deserted houses around us. There was one with a perfect roof, which was something, and with two or three loftier houses between it and the guns of Sedan, which was something more, and on this we decided; and the colonel ordered the Bavarian soldiers who were occupying it to clear out. It was an original style, certainly, of 'taking a house.' Furnished lodgings it could not be called, for nothing was left except a mahogany bedstead, too cumbrous to carry off, some tables, and chairs. There were stables, still smouldering, but the drivers extinguished the last remnant of fire, and our horses and waggons were housed for the night.

We tried to discover what sleeping accommodation we could find. The bedrooms were in a dreadful state; the floors littered a foot deep with the contents of all the closets and drawers, torn and cut up into pieces, linen, books, bonnets, dresses, papers, chimney ornaments, mixed up, so to speak, into one heterogeneous mass. The kitchen was worse; the dirt was inconceivable, and every utensil seemed to have been used for something it was never intended for.

To clear up and clean out was our first endeavour, and whilst doing so some of the party discovered a way through the garden to a *château*, next door, where the pillage had not been quite so complete, and where we should have removed our whole establishment, except for two objections. First, it was too high, more exposed, if the guns on the ramparts had opened fire; and next, and most important of all, the poor master lay shot dead in the kitchen. He was a merchant of Sedan, it appeared. His wife and daughter had taken refuge there, but he remained to guard his property.

The Bavarians arrived, loudly calling for wine; and, with the idea of saving his cellar, he gave them sour cider. They resented the insult by shooting him dead, and there he lay amidst the wrecks of all the kitchen had ever contained, with the fatal crimson marks on his breast that showed where the balls had entered. No burying party was at hand; nothing could be done but to cover decently his white upturned face, and leave him literally with his '*household gods shattered around him.*'

Here, in this *château*, however, beds, blankets, and a huge box of wax candles were found, some candelabra, and some cups and glasses. They were borrowed for the occasion, and transferred to our humbler residence next door, and we arranged our bedrooms. Supper was now the question. The kitchen had been cleaned out and a fire lighted, but all our researches did not enable us to discover anything to eat. Liebig, however, supplied deficiencies, and some vegetables from the garden; but it was sad work to search for them. Amidst the lovely flowers near the house, and beyond in the kitchen garden, dead men lay, seeming asleep in the evening light. We got, however, a few potatoes, carrots, and salad, and I remarked particularly one patch of very fine green potato plants, promising a good crop, and we resolved next morning to begin there.

Night was closing in as we re-entered the house. Every door had been broken open by forcing in the panels, and the shutters of one of the lower rooms had also been broken away. In the one we selected, though the windows were gone, the shutters remained. We closed them, lighted the candles, and began our soup with a few pieces of bread left from our breakfast. Every moment we expected the much-talked-of sortie, and listened for the opening roar of the cannon planted on the walls so near us; but all was silent, except the challenge of the Bavarian sentinels, whose grand guard was next door, and tired and worn out, we were glad to lie down on the mattresses we had found, and slept as profoundly as if all the horrors around us were but a dream.

We were roused at some unearthly hour in the morning by a loud shout proceeding, as it appeared, from the Bavarian colonel, who was informing our General that the sortie was coming and that he was going, having received orders to retreat to Douzy. His information must have been of the worst description, as it afterwards appeared the emperor had surrendered himself and his army at 11 p.m. the night before.

The colonel was resolved, perhaps, to leave us in an unsettled frame of mind, as he trotted away, leaving the village totally undefended;

for he added the pleasant suggestion that probably on his leaving the peasantry would become excessively troublesome, and darkly hinted at robbery and murder. This combination of anticipated horrors induced us to get up and dress, whilst Mr. A— saw to the harnessing of the horses to the waggons; but two or three hours passed away, and nothing happened.

Louise and myself sallied into the garden with a distant view to roast potatoes for breakfast from that especial plot we had seen. But as we got up to it, past some shrubs that hid it, we stared and rubbed our eyes. Were we dreaming still! Instead of the green plants was a tomb, a cross of iron placed on a square block of stone, a fresh wreath of flowers hanging upon it, and a lovely cross of chrysanthemums lying on the newly-dug grave! We forgot all about our breakfast, and tried to find some clue to the mystery. We went into the street, and found one solitary Frenchman, who, seeing we were not 'Prussians,' told us he supposed it was done in the night.

The Bavarian guard had drunk hard and slept soundly, and doubtless it was then that the body of some general officer had been interred there. That probably, also, the fact of seeing an ambulance flag had been the inducement to bury it there, in the hope the grave would be undisturbed; that the iron cross had been taken from a stonemason's yard close by, as we might see for ourselves; and that perhaps after the war we should hear who it was.

He did not know; how should he? these were no times for meddling in other people's business; but would we let the wreath and cross of flowers remain? It was nothing to him; why should it be? But, doubtless, it was some brave soldier, and the flowers did no harm. He certainly knew more than he chose to tell us; but we assured him that whilst we remained no one should profane the last resting place of the man, whoever he might be, on whose tomb might truly be engraven the grand old words that answered the challenge when the name of Latour d'Auvergne was called in the ranks of his grenadiers, '*Mort sur le champ d'honneur!*'

As we were finishing our breakfast (so called by courtesy), we heard in the distance strains of martial music. The distant fields were half hidden by a golden mist, the Meuse was flashing in the sunlight, and the raindrops of the night before were glistening on the leaves and hedges. If we could have avoided the sad foreground, and only looked across the green meadows to the hills beyond, we might have fancied it the gay music that preluded some great festival. The air was so like 'God save the Queen' that for a minute we listened, believing it to be so.

At that moment the late emperor was passing as a prisoner through the ranks of the victorious army. It was evident that something important was going on. The General mounted his horse, and said he would ride into Sedan and go to the headquarters to report our arrival, and ask for orders as to our destination. He begged us to remain in the house to await his return, as the village was so close to Sedan that it was in a disturbed state. He took a Red-Cross flag in his hand, and rode off.

He had hardly been gone before a trooper galloped furiously down the road towards Bazeilles; and some peasants going past, to try to re-enter their desolated homes and save what they could, told us that the French were about to break out of Sedan and force their way to the Belgian frontier. About half an hour afterwards we saw a vast mob of French soldiers coming up from the town. At that instant a regiment of Prussian cavalry rode by and formed four deep, completely blocking the road, whilst picquets were sent into the gardens and lanes on either side to prevent the French getting past.

It looked as if things were likely to get exciting, and we placed ourselves well behind our courtyard wall, where we could see all in comparative safety. The officer in command went forward alone and met two or three of the French. Apparently, he convinced them of the hopelessness of the attempt, for after a short parley they retreated, and the cavalry withdrew into the park of the *château* we had inspected with a view to a possible ambulance.

The roadway had been clear and all quiet about half an hour, when a small maid-servant came timidly stealing up to the front door, and asked leave to enter. We asked her her business, and she said she was the servant of the house. Her master and mistress were in Sedan. They had left several days before, and had carried off the greater part of their furniture. She had remained in the house till the bombs were falling round it and the French were finally driven back, and a sergeant of the marine infantry had entered suddenly and begged her to retreat into Sedan, as the battle was lost and the enemy close behind. On this she fled, but in her haste she had left behind her the cat and two kittens, and she had come back to search for them, and to see who occupied the house or if it had been burned down, and to ask if she might take away a few vegetables and some salad, as there was very little to eat in Sedan.

We graciously accorded her permission to take her master and mistress some of the contents of their own garden, and showed her that the house had not received serious damage. We took her upstairs, and she wept over the ruin of her crinoline, which was indeed but a shapeless mass, and the utter destruction of her best cap; but we consoled her by remembering we had seen the kittens, indeed we had given them something of the little we had the night before. She grew quite cheerful, but the sight of the kitchen again overwhelmed her, and she sat down on the remains of a chair and lamented for all her pots and pans, which she assured us were once beautiful to behold; but just as she was growing hysterical with her grief a faint mew was heard.

She started up, and the next instant the two kittens came racing in. They had heard her voice, and emerged from the hole where they were hidden to greet their mistress. She caught them up in her arms in a state of frantic delight. 'Oh, my little ones, my heroes! have you stayed here to guard your master's property? And the bomb shells have spared you. Ah! what courage you have! You ought to have the Cross of Honour! Oh, what happiness, my loves, to see you again!' The battle was lost, the house was wrecked, the emperor a prisoner, and the Germans in their quiet homes; but all faded into nothing before the joy of finding the kittens, though it was damped by sorrow for the still missing mother cat. The poor girl expressed her delight that we were in the house, and she knew we would not steal the things.

This we might safely have promised, under any temptation, for, as she said, everything had been carried off. She begged me to escort her back into Sedan, as the peasant who had brought her out was gone on to Bazeilles; so, we started together. It was well to look straight forward at the green bastions of the town, for the sights by the way were not good to see, and, as we got close to the first gate, I met a burying party, and begged them to go to several places I pointed out to inter the dead. I saw the poor girl safe into the town, but it would have taken me too long to go to her master's house with her.

The streets were a mass of soldiery. The Germans had not entered, and guns, swords, and belts were being flung about in every direction, and broken, to prevent their falling into the enemy's hands. Old officers stood about, some crying like children, and the frightened inhabitants were peeping out of their windows to watch the scene of confusion below. I returned, and found two or three of the marine infantry begging for five minutes' rest and a little soup. They had got past the guards, and were making their way over the wooded hills behind our house to the frontier, only about thirty miles off. It was no business of ours to detain them, so we gave them water to bathe their feet and a little soup, and they went out through the garden, to avoid the high road. Poor fellows, they gave us a sad account of the destruction of their battalion from the double fire of friend and foe, and we hoped that they might get safe away, and avoid that long captivity in Germany which we too truly apprehended would follow.

Then came a gentleman of the place, who begged us to go to a house two miles away, where many wounded were needing help. This we could not do, as we were ordered to remain till the General's return in the house, nor could we leave the stores. We, however, gave him various things for the wounded, and we proposed to him to send us all the wounded he met who could walk, and we would dress their wounds and give them some soup.

This was accordingly done, and we were kept busy till the General came back. He had been to headquarters, seen Prince Pless, and received orders to go on to the little village of Donchery, three miles beyond Sedan, and close by the *château* of Bellevue, where the emperor passed his last night of freedom. He went to order the waggons to be ready at four o'clock, the streets of the town being still so crowded that it would be useless to attempt to drive through them; and as it would be too late that night to commence any work at Donchery, it was as well to remain quietly, and get what dinner we could in Balan.

A carriage drove past. We caught sight of its inmate. It was Mr. Parker! We rushed out and I 'hailed' him. Sundry dreadful ideas had been started that he had been burnt in Bazeilles. Why no one knew; but we were all delighted to see him. It seemed after leaving Grand Pré Mr. W— and he had gone on to Beaumont, and finding the battle further ahead, had pushed on, missing the General and Mr. A—, who were quietly sleeping as Mr. W— and Mr. Parker passed through. They had been on the battlefield close by Bazeilles, and narrowly escaped being shot by getting behind a wall. They had gone into Sedan that morning, and Mr. Parker was just setting out on an expedition to find us and bring us up. He was, of course, enchanted to find us so close to the scene of action. The General, finding he was with us, said he should like to ride over the field, and he would meet us at Donchery, and off he went accordingly.

I proposed to Mr. Parker to show him the ruined *château*, and as there was also a very fine one opposite, he said he thought we had better look at that too, in case we wanted a good house for an ambulance. It was an enormous place, but as rent was no consideration, we agreed it would be wise to do so, and leaving Louise and the paid nurse in the house, we started off. Her statement is, that she immediately told the nurse to lock the doors, which was done; for the General having unfortunately said we were going, the Bavarian Guard began to take possession of the house. Louise then, being, as the old ballad says, 'of a frugal mind,' resolved to devote herself to the washing-tub, one of which had been, discovered in the back premises. We had not had the chance of 'a wash' since we left Brussels. Water was very scarce, for here at Balan and round Sedan every stream was choked with corpses, dead bodies of men and horses were floating in the Meuse, and very few wells and cisterns were uncontaminated by blood.

But a pump had also been found in an outhouse, and these advantages, combined with the total impossibility of finding a washerwoman, induced her to tuck up her sleeves and go to work herself upon our mutual garments. The suds were flying about in all directions, as often happens with amateur efforts of this description, when the kitchen door opened suddenly, and she saw the captain of the Bavarian Guard. It flashed upon her directly that he had entered by the shutterless window and crept through the broken panel of the drawing-room door, and that he meant mischief.

He was very small, very ugly, and very sandy, something like an ill-bred Skye terrier, and Louise prepared to frown him down. What he said she did not comprehend, but she felt it was something very impertinent, and in a select mixture of French and German she ordered his instant 'evacuation,' and showed him the door. It is to be presumed that she looked sufficiently ferocious to impress him with a sensation of fear, or the polyglot language in which he was addressed had a weird and awful sound, for he took to instant flight and retreated by the way he came.

It must be remarked he had watched all of us out before he tried this game; but then and ever afterwards we found that the Germans are easily subdued, if only anyone has the courage to turn upon them. We soon afterwards returned, and resolved not again to leave the house, for a party of officers were drinking and smoking in the court-yard, and our stores were not nailed down.

One of them, a captain of *carabineers*, had paid its three or four visits, and on each occasion had graciously accepted Liebig, melon, coffee, and potatoes, till we really thought we should have to nurse him in a horrible fit of indigestion; and now they came to borrow the last half of our last melon and all the sugar, a loan still accumulating at compound interest. But what was worst of all, as showing the black ingratitude of human nature, when late that evening his comrades arrived with rations and wine and sundry good things, he never offered us any, and became loftily unconscious of our existence as we passed and repassed the table where he was sitting.

Mr. Parker was busy re-packing the boxes, which had been opened to give out stores in the village, and all being ready he and I sallied out to the stables to find our waggons and drivers, anticipating an early arrival at Donchery; but imagine our consternation when we found all were gone! We could hear nothing of them, except that they had been seen going back to Douzy an hour before, and had told some man who was lounging about his ruined cottage that they were afraid to go any further.

What to do was the question. Omnibuses and waggons were standing idle in every stable-yard of Balan, but horses there were none; and whilst Mr. Parker and I were arranging to try and send some Bavarian troopers after our runaways, I was summoned into the house to see a strange sight in those days—an English gentleman, and not of our party. I hastened back to see who it was, and if by chance he had brought any news from home.

CHAPTER 13

A Miserable Village

I found Louise talking with a very pleasant Englishman, who told us he had met with the General as he was riding out of Sedan, homeless and hungry, and who had suggested his coming on, where at all events he could get some soup and a rest. He was the correspondent of the '*Standard*,' and no one could be more kind than he was. Forgetting his fatigue, he started off with me to seek for horses, and as we went down the road an officer galloped past us and, reining in his horse, claimed acquaintance with me. It was our Bavarian commandant of Grand Pré, but I did not recognise him in his shining helmet and long white cloak. I explained our position, and begged him if he overtook our culprits on the road to arrest them and send them back, which he promised to do, and rode off at a rapid pace.

We prowled about the village street and into every stable and yard; no horses were there. The dead bodies were yet unburied, and the place was deserted. My friend offered to take on three of the ladies in his waggon, with only their hand-bags, as he was going to Donchery, and so it was arranged; Miss McLaughlin and myself remaining behind with Mr. Parker, to see what the morrow would bring forth. Their journey, we heard later, had been tedious and difficult, owing to the crowded state of the streets of Sedan. They arrived very late at Donchery, and could only find miserable accommodation.

The unfortunate French Army, 80,000 strong, had not yet been consigned to that miserable island on the Meuse where so many perished of cold and hunger. They were throwing their arms and accoutrements into the ditches which surrounded the town, and into the river itself, and were still lingering about the streets. Hundreds escaped, though the Prussian lines had closed all round the town, and hundreds more might have done so, the frontier was so near. But many still believed that had not MacMahon been lying desperately wounded, unable to move, and almost unconscious of what was going on, that he, at the head of 80,000 well-armed and unwounded veteran troops, would and could have cut a passage through the lines, even if half had perished in the attempt.

But the emperor had signed the capitulation, he was a prisoner on his way to Germany, and the army of his conquerors were preparing for their march on Paris. Sad tales are told of the ball given at Sedan, which delayed the advance of MacMahon's army by twenty-four hours, when, had the troops been pushed forward, it is said Metz might been relieved; and legends are still current of the more than sardanapalian luxury of the emperor's travelling suite; of his thirty carriages, which, whilst crossing the bridge over the Meuse on the afternoon of that fatal 1st of September, prevented the French batteries from playing on the Prussian troops beyond; of generals declining to leave their breakfasts that they might hurry on their men to check the enemy; and never will the French think otherwise than that utter incapacity and, worse still, treason of the blackest description consigned their best army to death and imprisonment.

But the full extent of the defeat and misfortune was unknown to us, when, after seeing our companions off, in charge of their kind escort, Louise and myself returned into the house to see what dinner we could prepare, and whilst she endeavoured to find some of the cooking utensils I went off into the garden to look for vegetables. I saw in the distance a piece of very young-looking carrots, and remembering how very hard those I had brought on the preceding evening had been, I went to it to try for some better ones. But lying amongst them, crushing down the pale green leaves, was a dead Prussian, shot through the head. Poor fellow, he was a young man, with fair hair, and except for the wound and the bloodstain on one side of his face, he might have been sleeping. I covered up his face with a handkerchief I found in the breast of his coat, and left him lying there, in the quiet garden.

Mr. Parker had made another excursion to see if our absconding drivers had been found, but of course they had made the best of their way in a homeward direction. The Bavarians had taken possession of all the bedrooms, so we resolved to make up a bed in the dining-room, on the heavy bedstead, and Mr. Parker, with his usual good-nature and cheerfulness, declared he preferred a mattress and blanket in a corner of the kitchen to any other more luxurious arrangement. We were very cheerful over Liebig and coffee, and whilst sitting round the kitchen stove we heard the clatter of a horse's hoofs and the firm step and clear voice of the General. He had been benighted on the field of battle, and, instead of going on to Donchery, had ridden into Balan, knowing he should find a stable for his horse and a shelter for himself, for it was now raining heavily.

We welcomed him as best we could on our scanty means, but some boiled haricots, which had been too hard for our dinner, were by this time arrived at a softer stage, and he made a supper off them. He arranged with Mr. Parker that both would like an early ride round by Floing, where the cavalry had perished *en masse*, and return to us about eight or nine o'clock, and the General would then go into Sedan, and request from the Prussian *commandant* the use of some train-waggons and horses, as so many, captured from the French, were standing idle.

He was very indignant at the impertinence of the Bavarian captain, and the continued annoyance they had been to us by trying to come into the kitchen to cook their rations, when they had a large fire and every convenience in a sort of wash and bakehouse at the back—a system carried to such an extent that, when a good-natured soldier was chopping some wood for Louise to cook by, an officer forbade him to do so, and ordered him only to chop the wood for their cooking.

However, being indignant was utterly useless, and we all went to bed, or rather mattress. The first part of the night passed off in profound tranquillity; but at early dawn, or rather before it, Louise, hearing the gentlemen moving about, was seized with an idea how comfortless it would be for them to have no breakfast, and that she would get up and make it. I remonstrated, first on the ground that the male sex always looked after themselves, and secondly, that there was no breakfast to make. To which she rejoined she had found some cold bacon she could fry, and had a little chocolate she could warm, that the male sex, were not capable of taking care of themselves, and that, as they were going over the battlefields, they must have food first.

This difference of opinion resulted in my staying in bed and her getting up, but, truth to tell, I had had no solid food for three days, not a drop of wine, hardly any bread, and I could not eat the so-called bacon, which was nothing but a piece of some horrible fat. I was weak and tired from actual want of nourishment. It was two hours before our friends got off and Louise came back. We resolved to sleep till eight o'clock, when we expected them again. But we had hardly tried to close our eyes before we heard the lock of the door being tried. We thought it was fancy, but presently the other door was attempted. Louise called out to know who was there, and the answer was a burst of insulting laughter. Fortunately, we had barricaded one door the night before, and the window shutters fastened inside. We dragged a heavy box against the remaining door, and felt pretty sure that the Bavarian officers, whom we knew were prowling in the hall, could not enter; but there we lay. Bright daylight came on, and we could not open the shutters, for the windows were broken, and we felt utterly helpless, alone in the house with this set of ruffians round us.

The annoyance of attempting to get in continued, as it seemed, for hours. At last we heard the bugles for parade and a clatter out of the house. We got up and dressed, and ventured to peep out. Our persecutors were gone, for the time at least, but they had carried off all that was left of our bread, though that very little and very old, the small remains of the bacon, and most of the cooking utensils. We had no water to wash with, for they had thrown all kinds of dirt into the open cistern, the pump would hardly work, and we felt very dirty and dispirited. We began a search, and found a little flour in a jar in an out-of-the-way corner, and Louise made a few flour cakes. How we longed for the return of the gentlemen! and to get away from this detestable neighbourhood.

Presently the small maid-servant arrived from Sedan. She feared we were gone, and had come to see what was the fate of the house. She, on being closely questioned, said she knew a neighbour who had returned, bringing out of the town some mutton, and she thought, if she was entrusted with a five *franc* piece, she could get us some mutton cutlets. The very idea was encouraging, and we sent her on the errand. She actually found the neighbour who had the mutton, and for three *francs* and a half brought us what we should call in England the worst half of a neck of mutton. To cook our chops was a great struggle, but we succeeded; we had still some coffee, though no milk, and with the flour cakes began what we considered a delicious breakfast, when horses' hoofs rang on the pavement of the yard, and we ran out to welcome the General and Mr. Parker. How hungry they were, how astonished they were to see hot mutton, and how they enjoyed it. They had ridden far and wide over the battlefields and been to Floing.

We had no curiosity to walk over the hill behind the house to see the other parts of the field. The battle had been all around us, even in our own garden, where forty-five dead bodies were found, hidden amongst the shrubs, and in the private lane leading to the coach-house. We had no desire to see more horrors than fell to our share in the way of duty, and we gladly began to prepare for our departure.

The General rode into Sedan, and in about an hour returned with a train of waggons, horses, and soldiers, sufficient to convey the baggage of a regiment. They were French artillery, prisoners of course, and the Prussian commander had ordered out some vague number to assist us. Our chests, much reduced in number and weight, were distributed at the rate of what Louise declared was one a-piece in the great ammunition waggons, and the soldiers formed an imposing array in the road. Poor fellows, how sad they looked! unarmed, and servants to anyone who claimed them from their masters the Prussians. They brightened up under the influence of kindly words and real sympathy—who could help feeling it?—and they said that, after all, serving English ladies was very different from being at the beck and call of German officers. The *sous-officier* in command was a most intelligent, bright, well-educated young man named Louis Bobard.

His sister was a governess in an English family in London, and before we had made acquaintance ten minutes he had given us his name and a short greeting written to her on a piece of paper, which he had found an opportunity of slipping into our hands, to be delivered as soon as we could. What amused us most of all was the spare horses led behind the waggons, it looked so excessively formidable and was so truly ludicrous, considering the feather weight in each waggon and the three miles we had to go.

Finally, the horses were ordered to be harnessed to the carriage which had brought Mr. Parker. Louis, and Hippolyte, his second in command, being detailed to ride by our side, we expected to start directly, when a hue and cry commenced. The pole of the carriage was gone, nowhere could it be found; and that was not surprising, for we ascertained that the Bavarians had burnt it for their bivouac fire. Now, as there were trees all round, to say nothing of firewood ready chopped in the yard, it was a wasteful proceeding. An appeal was made to the Prussian officer in command, for by this time the new guard which had replaced our tormentors had arrived, and he remembered he had seen a carriage with a pole in a neighbouring coach-house, and ordered one of his men to fetch the pole. This was done, and at last we started, thankful to be out of that miserable village; but one thing upset all our gravity just as we were going off.

The little maid-servant had prowled about, jealously watching lest we should carry off any of the shreds of property remaining, and filially she discovered being hoisted into a waggon a small rough deal box, value in material about sixpence. It had been lying about, and taking it for one of ours, some lint and other parcels which had been turned out of a nearly empty large chest, which was left behind, had been packed into it. She began a series of lamentations over our thievish propensities and the loss of the box. It was the dog's box, her master had made it himself, and did we intend to be so wicked as to carry it off? Considering the state of things, it was too ludicrous. We declined to unpack the box, and shewed her the much better one we had left. All in vain; she refused to be consoled, and we left her locking up what was left of the doors, in spite of all assurances that the next body of troops who passed would insist on finding quarters there.

We drove at a rapid pace into Sedan. The streets were pretty clear now, the prisoners all on the island of the Meuse, but the usual train of military waggons blocked the gate on the other side of the town. At last we got through, and on to the road leading past the Château Bellevue, where the emperor had slept the night after the battle, and past the little cottage in front of which, as legends say, he and Bismarck sat and settled the fate of an empire. As we were driving along with our imposing cortege we overtook a pedestrian so evidently English that we stared, and he bowed, and, coming up, told us he had seen our friends in Donchery, that morning. It was Mr. Landle, of the *Illustrated London News*. He got on the box and drove with us to Donchery.

Sedan is a very small town, built in a valley through which runs the Meuse, and surrounded on all sides by hills. It is walled around with deep ditches and drawbridges, so that the gates once shut, getting out was impossible. It is as pretty a specimen of a trap as could well be imagined, and I was assured afterwards that, had the gates been shut when the French Army were retreating, the battle would not have been lost. They could not have got in, and must have fought it out. That is the opinion of the townspeople; but it could not alter the fact of the German batteries, being allowed to be planted on those hills, firing shot and shell at leisure into the crowded town below.

It was just six o'clock as we passed over a wooden bridge and up the narrow street of Donchery, deep in mud, wondering where our friends might be, when we caught sight of them looking out of the window of a small cottage. They greeted us with delight. The General, who was riding by our side, proposed that Louise and myself in the carriage should go with him to report our arrival to the head physician. We enquired for the residence of the general in command, and drove on to the little central Place. Here a lovely band was playing gay waltzes—what a mockery it seemed of the wretchedness around—and the

Prussian general and a group of officers were standing listening to it.

Our General introduced himself and us, and the head physician, who was there, gave us a hearty welcome. He took us off directly to see a house that was being fitted up as a hospital, showed us where the stores would be placed, and suggested our sleeping in some rooms there; but the Prussian general opposed this. He thought it would be far pleasanter for us to have quarters elsewhere, and sent an orderly down a side street to a house vacated that morning by some staff officers to find us quarters. We followed, and found ourselves in a charming little house, with most respectable people, who, though we were unpaid lodgers, were only too glad to escape quarters of soldiers, and begged us piteously to pitch our tent there. This we did by leaving our baggage. A stable next door was found for the horses, and the little army soon deposited the store-chests in the new hospital. Before dark we were safely housed, and the poor people, finding we were too late to get our rations, kindly cooked for us what they had.

We held a long consultation that night. The little money we had was all but exhausted and the stores nearly used up. We had tried to communicate with England and failed, and Mr. Parker and the General strongly urged my going home for a few days to report our progress and bring out stores. The General was going on with the headquarters, and Mr. Parker would not leave the ladies again; so, I consented to go, if I found I was not actually wanted. The next morning, we went to the hospital. We were most graciously received, and entered the wards. There were no wounded, only fever cases, and plenty of German orderlies. So little was there to do that I was glad to see some of us employed in sewing up sheets in a peculiar German fashion. At early dinner Mr. Parker and all of us decided that this state of things would never do.

In the afternoon the correspondent of the '*Illustrated London News*' came in and quite agreed that we were wasted there. He mentioned the Anglo-American Ambulance in the great Caserne Asfeld, Sedan, how they were crowded with wounded, and no help, and begged us to go to them. We resolved to wait a day and see before we decidedly left the service we had been attached to. We wanted orders, and to get them seemed more imperative than ever; and it was settled I should start the next day and return as soon as possible. That evening, too, my knee, which I had hurt falling on a stone at Grand Pré during the struggle to change the baggage to our own waggons, became very swelled and stiff, and kneeling beside the low beds—only mattresses laid on the floor—was impossible. Thus, I was temporarily useless and so my departure was finally arranged.

The next day no further work offered. We looked round the Hospital. The German orderlies did not care about our assisting them, and it was too evident our stores, not ourselves, were the attraction. But I deferred my start, hoping to the last we might have orders. That afternoon Mr. Landle, of the '*Illustrated London News*,' and Dr. B——, an Englishman in Her Majesty's service, but of German extraction, tempted Louise and myself to go on an expedition to the railway station to see if any fast trains were available. It poured with rain. But we persevered; we found a train starting with French wounded, who were allowed to go to Mézières, about ten miles further on in the French lines. At Mézières they would find trains for Lille and the north-west of France. There were so many prisoners in health and strength that the Prussians did not then care to take to the rear a number of helpless men.

We found that it was very uncertain when the next would go, if at all, and the only way was to drive to Pois St.-Hubert, the nearest station on the Luxemburg line, and thence take train to Brussels. We returned wet, and miserable. But what must have been the fearful sufferings of the poor prisoners on the marshy island of the Meuse? The sad tale has been already told most truthfully and graphically by Mr. Seymour, M.P., in a letter to the '*Daily Telegraph*,' published about the second week of September. He visited the island on the day following this miserable afternoon of rain, September 6, and his account has been fully confirmed by the statements of various soldiers whom we afterwards met—how they had no bread, and no possibility of buying any, no shelter, no great coats or cloaks; they had been taken from them or lost on the battlefield.

A soldier, afterwards an *infirmier* in our ambulance at Orléans, told us that he himself was one of those who saw starving soldiers eating the entrails of dead horses. Louis Brancard escaped with some 1,400 others, and rejoined his battalion of the marine infantry, to be again wounded and a prisoner on December 4; but fortunately, we obtained for him from the Prussians a commission as *infirmier*, and he remained with us till the peace left him once more free.

No provisions had been sent out with us, such as casks of biscuits, Liebig, or preserved milk, and even had we gone to the island we had no means of affording any relief. Our own rations allowed by the Prussians, and which we accepted because we could buy nothing, were very scanty. I do not think the meat given for six persons was more than we often saw one German soldier carrying home for himself. The prisoners were evacuated at the rate of some thousands a day, but the number that perished by famine on that sad island will never be known. Herded together like sheep, strictly guarded, but no common precaution of humanity taken to feed them, what else could be expected. Their blood is on the head of whoever had the command at Sedan, and who let helpless men die for the want of the bread his soldiers flung away as hard and dry unless fresh from the bakehouse, and sent rations to the guards, who ate the soup and meat and bread and drank their wine in stolid indifference to the starving crowd around them.

We were glad to find shelter in our quarters, and Mr. Parker coming in with a gentleman, a German physician, who would be glad of a "lift' in the carriage to Pois St.-Hubert, and it was therefore settled that he should come in the evening to make final arrangements. Mr. Landle was to come also with letters and sketches for his office in London, which I had promised to convey, and it was suggested that we might as well give them a cup of coffee. So, after dinner we prepared for our evening reception by lighting two more of the Balan candles, and to add to the festive appearance of the scene we placed a black bottle of sherry, which Mr. Parker had bought in Sedan, in the centre of a round table, with a ring of glasses encircling it, and so received our guests, who brought their own cigars. Dr. B— came in also, and it is to be hoped that the pleasure of our society compensated for the muddy walk they had to take to come to the house, for except coffee and dry bread they had nothing else.

We waited for Mr. Parker to propose a glass of sherry round, but he, always thoughtful for our comforts, just as he was meditating where the corkscrew was, was seized with the idea that, perhaps, some of us might be ill where nothing was to be had, and it would be wise to keep it for such an emergency; so he said nothing, and the bottle remained unopened. We were all very cheerful, however; and if it ever was a matter of surprise to any of our guests why that bottle was simply used as an ornament, we hereby beg to explain, and should this narrative of our doings come under their eyes, we also beg to apologise for the inhospitality, and to assure them that, in spite of Mr. Parker's real kindness in thus guarding against future want for us, we should have been happy to have shared the contents of our cellar (one bottle) with them, for, generally and individually, we always received from Mr. Landle, Mr. Austin of the '*Standard*,' and all of their fraternity, the greatest kindness and attention, and found them very pleasant, highly educated, and gentlemanly companions.

CHAPTER 14

To England and Back

The morning of the 7th of September was bright and fine when, at the appointed hour, 5 a.m., I made my appearance, ready for the journey; but with the well-known unpunctuality of the male sex in general, neither my two escorts, Mr. Parker and Dr. M—, were there, nor were the despatches of the General finished. It was past seven before we left, and drove at a rapid pace through Sedan. It was far more empty and quiet now. The French were on their island, and the Germans were at breakfast. We passed through Balan, and, though still ruined and desolate, the dead bodies of men and horses had been buried; but the road beyond was even now strewed with knapsacks, helmets, rifles, and all the litter of a battlefield.

As we neared Bazeilles, we saw a little thin blue smoke slowly curling up into the morning air from the still smouldering ruins. A few peasants were digging in the ground floors of the roofless, windowless, smoke-blackened houses, we thought to search for anything that might have escaped the general ruin. We heard later it was for a far sadder object. Many women and children had hidden in the cellars during the fight, and then when the town was fired by hand, and the Bavarians were rushing from house to house with lighted torches, had not dared to escape, and so perished in the burning ruins.

One man was found, strange to say, with an iron chain, still attached by a belt, also of iron, round his charred form. So local legends say, but I never heard any explanation, probable or improbable, of this wild story. Many walls had fallen and cumbered the street with heaps of brick and stone, but all traces of war had vanished, and the destruction of the pretty town might have been caused by some every-day event.

We drove steadily on till at last, on a very very long road, we became aware that our axletrees were red-hot, and we made all haste to a little house we saw which professed to give, according to English parlance, 'Good accommodation for man and beast,' and there we got down, while water was thrown on the wheels, and they were put into safe order. We were over the Belgian frontier, it seems, but where it began or ended, I know not. I think we passed a couple of Belgian hussars a few miles farther back; but as neither hussars nor travellers seemed to take the slightest interest in each other's proceedings, I cannot really say if they were the frontier guards or not.

As we were waiting in the little sanded parlour of the *auberge*, I suddenly spied a French paper—the only news we had seen since we left Luxemburg. The three of us read it together, and saw that France was once more a republic. It was such a delight to feel restored to a knowledge of the events passing around us. In the midst of conflicts that changed the destiny of a great nation we had been ignorant of the result of them, except that the emperor was a prisoner, which fact had been announced to us by the triumphal music of the Prussian bands.

After a breakfast of eggs and bacon we went on and on over those interminable swells of down land, up and up, till we suddenly began to descend, and there before us, in a picturesque gorge with a stream rushing through it, was the romantic town of Bouillon, with the grand old castle of the great Crusader frowning down from its rocky platform on the houses nestled below. The town was very crowded with refugees from Bazeilles and Balan, and having already rested and refreshed we pushed on to Pois St.-Hubert, over more heights, through a long forest of low trees, till we came down a rapid slope to Pois St.-Hubert, the station, with a few miserable houses, being distant a couple of miles from the town of the same name. We expected just to catch a train; in fact, Mr. Parker did catch one to Arlon, where he was going to try for stores, but this was quite unexpected.

We thought the Brussels train would have gone first, but we had to wait a couple of hours, and when it did come it was on the other side, where there was no platform. My escort and several gentlemen of the neighbourhood, who hearing our business took a great interest in it and most kindly remained to help us, got me safely into a carriage, and we were off for Brussels. We reached it very late at night, and Dr. M— took me to the Hôtel de Suede, where, though there was not a spare bedroom, they took me in and gave me a room somewhere up in the sky, with three or four beds in it, I suppose a servants' room, but very clean and comfortable.

The directress, if such she was, who spoke perfect English, asked me if I would not take something after my long journey. Now, as I had breakfasted at 11 a.m. and it was midnight, the proposal was most acceptable; but it was now so many days since even money could have procured food and wine, that I humbly said, forgetting I was in one of the best hotels of Brussels, if I could have a loaf of bread and a bottle of wine I would gladly pay anything for it.' The kind directress stared and smiled, and as it flashed suddenly upon me that I was where I only had to ask and have if I would pay, I burst out laughing and explained. Bread and wine and something of cold meat were directly brought. Indeed nothing could exceed the kindness and sympathy of all in that hotel with the tired and dirty Red-Cross stranger.

My escort was accommodated with a mattress in the dining-room, and I only hope he slept as soundly as I did, for it was broad daylight before I woke up, dressed, and went downstairs, and found Dr. M— just preparing to go by an early train to Ostend. Now, my experiences of that passage were enough, and finding I could get to London as quickly by Calais *via* Lille, we parted with an agreement to meet at Dover, where both boats were to arrive simultaneously; but I had three or four hours more on land.

I was going for a little walk, when I was requested to speak to some ladies who much wished to see me. They had relations with the French Army at Sedan, and naturally hoped to gain a chance scrap of news of some brigade or regiment in that doomed army; and all the morning the long, sad procession filed into the little public room where I was sitting, with the same anxious question from all, 'What news of such and such a regiment?' and the same prayer to take back to Sedan the few lines of love or sorrow that, if the dear one were in some crowded hospital or ambulance, might come like a voice from home, or the slip of paper with simply the name, to search for it, if possible, in the list (if such existed) of the dead or the wounded and the prisoners at Sedan. Poor breaking hearts, they had come as near to the frontier as possible, where the earliest news might be had, and all was silence.

It was one of the most painful features of the war that fearful suspense as to the fate of the absent, one that neutrals alone could relieve. But surely common humanity might have suggested some relaxation of the strict rule of no communication between the occupied and unoccupied departments, if only it had been permitted for the prisoners to send one open letter to say if they were wounded or only prisoners. Cannot the Geneva Convention take this into consideration, and so heal many a deep wound no surgeon could cure?

I left Brussels in the forenoon, but at Lille I was astonished, when I presented myself at the passport office, where the passports were examined, it being the French frontier, to be told indignantly, as I thought, to go back to my carriage. Seeing my surprise, the official added, pointing to my brassard, 'That is enough, and they say you come from Sedan.' I pleaded guilty, and was surrounded by a crowd, all burning with desire to hear something of the great battle from an actual eye witness. Apparently, I was the first waif and stray that had surged up from the wreck of war, and I was accordingly a great personage for the next half-hour.

At the next station where we stopped there was no buffet, and I was astonished to see the station-master coming up the line, with a tray upon which were wine, fruit, and delicate biscuits. He mounted the step of my carriage, and begged me to take some refreshment, and so kind and graceful was the act, that I accepted it, not as done to myself, but to the badge I wore. Calais was reached at last, I found my expected arrival had been telegraphed, and here a very good dinner was ready, and as I was told that the Paris train was very late, I did not hurry on board.

At last, weary of the station, I took up all my baggage (a hand-bag) and went down to the port. The sun was shining with a blinding glare, but a brisk wind was blowing, and the purple sea was breaking here and there into ridges of foam, 'the wild white horses,': as Arnold calls them, very beautiful to see, but very unpleasant to ride. I went down and took up my place by the companion ladder.

We waited, and waited, but no signs of weighing anchor or loosing cables appeared. The captain said he must wait for the mail-bags from Paris. The tide got lower and lower, the ladder communicating with the shore was a steep descent, when suddenly there came rushing along the pier a wild crowd of men, women, and children, encumbered with more parcels than can be well conceived, and, stranger still, dogs, cats, birds in cages, tied up in pocket-handkerchiefs, and all sorts of odds and ends.

They commenced tumbling down the ladder, arrested by the sailors, who kept them from tumbling into the water, and shrieking to friends and relatives on the pier behind to hasten for their lives, or all was lost. The boat would be gone, and no hope would be left. For one moment, I had a wild notion that the Prussians had taken Calais at bayonet's point, but I discovered directly afterwards they were refugees from Paris. What a motley throng they were!—women and children, and strong men too, who should have stayed behind with the brave hearts fighting for France.

But the cables were loosed, the steam was up, and soon a mile or two of troubled water separated us from that unhappy land. I went down to the cabin, and slept soundly, though my travelling companions did not fare so well, and very wretched they looked when we landed at Dover. It was past 8 p.m. before I reached my home. I had sent a telegram from Brussels to the Secretary of the National Society, and next morning went down there to meet the committee. Captain Burgess gave me a warm welcome, and after waiting some time, Colonel Loyd-Lindsay and Sir Harry Verney came in.

I had been told before I left Donchery to be sure three members of the Executive Committee were there, as not less than a quorum (three) would be likely to make an act legal. Perhaps it might be so; but at that time, they were not disinclined to trust me, nor I them. I presented the despatches; but before they were looked at Colonel Lindsay said, 'First of all, where is Mr. A—'s (the secretary's) ambulance?'

Now this was puzzling. We had never seen him since we left Pont-à-Mousson. Yet he had brought us out from England, so in a state of indecision as to whether we were his ambulance or not, I answered, 'At Donchery, I suppose, if we are his ambulance.' But here I was peremptorily cut short; we were *not* his ambulance. Had I seen his ambulance? Like all women, I felt inclined to be excessively sulky at the dictatorial tone; however, I kept it down, and simply said, in an injured manner, 'I know nothing about it, then.'

The colonel then soothed down, as it seemed to me, and explained that they had 'sent the fellow out' with 800*l*., and had never heard a word of him or his ambulance, which was quite distinct from ours. I said, 'Evidently so, as I have come home with the last money mustered amongst us, and paid my own passage.' A map was then produced, and I was put through my geographical facings, as regarded the neighbourhood of Sedan. I believe I must have answered to their perfect satisfaction, as we all became great friends, and they acted, I must say, most kindly and handsomely.

They gave me everything I asked for, as I tried to explain why such and such things were necessary, especially ready money, to buy on the spot what could not be sent from England, such as fresh bread, butter, eggs, and vegetables, for the sick, and things that did not answer carriage; and I was confided to the care of one of the kindest and most cordial of their officials, with whom I went to buy ready articles not in stock. Those were our palmy days. (I belonged to that great Society then.) We had a regiment of clerks, and another of commissionaires, properly bearded and medalled (three clasps apiece), and hosts of young gentlemen thirsting to assist the good cause at the rate of a pound a day. We went about in cabs, and sent foreign telegrams, two sheets a-piece.

I wonder what they cost. I know one I saw contained nothing that could not have been sent by post; but we had a princely fortune, and what was expense to us? I felt as if I had suddenly become an heiress. I was taken into shops, and chose what I liked, and the bill was to be sent in. It was a trial of virtue. I had a maniac notion of suggesting velvet dressing-gowns and cambric handkerchiefs for the wounded, and astounding Howell and James (close by, too) with a gigantic order, bill, as usual, to be sent in to the committee.

Honesty, however, prevailed. I chose only what I had been requested to get, and took a box of stores of my own (merely actual preventives of the famine we had undergone), mostly presents from private friends, and was told I was a noodle for my pains. Two days of hard work ensued. We had fairly worn out, even in that short time, our only dresses as ordered by the Committee, and I ventured to have four made to replace them.

I paid a very flying visit to my sister, Mrs. Walford Gosnal, at Ipswich, during the hours I was not required by the Committee, and found that I could adhere strictly to the programme laid out for me, that on a certain day and hour I was to be again at Pois St.-Hubert with the stores. I had a most friendly reception at the Prussian Embassy, and it is to the kindness of Count and Countess Bernstorff, and the safe-conduct they sent me, that we owe much of the good we were afterwards enabled to do, and the comfort and safety we enjoyed when all around was troubled; and this was given, to their honour be it spoken, to help us to enter Paris, and later to go into Orléans to help the bishop, himself a Frenchman, with French wounded under his own roof.

Mr. Adams, of Putney, called upon me and offered his escort. He was taking out stores, and our waggons could take them on with his. It was a most acceptable idea, and all arrangements being made, we left Charing Cross on the night of the 13th, for Ostend, *via* Dover. It was a lovely evening, the sea as calm as a lake, and we made a very short passage to Ostend. From thence, *via* Brussels, to Pois St.-Hubert, where I caught sight of our French *maréchal des logis*, waiting with a letter from Louise. Mr. Parker arrived just afterwards at the little wayside hotel where we were to put up for the night. It was too late, he said, to push on to Sedan, where I found our party had gone to aid the Anglo-American Ambulance.

I had arrived over land and sea with all the baggage, and 300*l*. in gold in my little courier bag, to the very day and hour appointed; but the effort was too much. Exertion, anxiety, and the privations of the previous weeks, had done their work, and I was obliged to leave my friends and go to my own room, where, miserable as it was, I could at least lie down and try to rest. That day was the beginning of a severe illness. I was wholly unfit to travel farther; but I was resolved to get on to Sedan, and next morning I got into the ambulance omnibus which was awaiting us, and as we went on our way, I read Louise's letter.

CHAPTER 15

Louise's Letter

Caserne Asfelde, Sedan,
September 11, 1870.

My dearest Emma,—I know you will be anxious to hear how we have fared since you left. You shall be *au fait* of all that has happened before you join us again. I send this by Hippolyte, who comes with Mr. Parker to meet you, and it may serve to amuse you on the dull road from St.-Hubert to Sedan. You have doubtless heard we were here, and you will be very glad, as you thought we were very useless at Donchery. How I wonder if you have brought out the stores? Perhaps not, as Captain Brackenbury has sent over several waggon-loads from Arlon, and young Sims has also arrived with a splendid supply. We have plenty of everything now, and as, doubtless, this is known in England, it will have saved you much trouble and responsibility. Who is young Sims? you will ask. Well, my story will explain that. After you left we went down to the hospital. There was literally nothing they would give us to do, so we took a walk on to the bridge, and there we met Dr. B——. I explained how grieved we were to find ourselves so useless, with such numbers of wounded in the villages all around. He said he had a few men in a convent, if we liked to go and nurse them for him. There was nothing better to be done, so we went. There were sixteen men in all, four wounded, the rest fever and dysentery. We divided this amongst us.

During the afternoon the secretary turned up. He called at our quarters. I was in hospital, and did not see him. He had got an ambulance, as he calls it here, consisting of a train of empty waggons, for conveying the German wounded to the nearest railroad station. Some say he had blankets, but we have not seen them. I wish he would give us some; they would be useful in Sedan. He was as mysterious as usual, and we saw nothing of him. He had a very nice omnibus, which the General required for us, and you will travel in it today. I believe there was some little difficulty about the arrangement; but the secretary had to give in. The Admiral, as you call him, came back in the evening, as jolly as ever, and brought all the London newspapers with him; that is, all the correspondents.

I wish you had been there; they were all so pleasant, I have not had such a merry evening since we left England. We received them at supper! Don't be astonished, when you remember the small rations of tough beef, and the very sour wine, and the soup that was really only hot water. We found the room, and they brought their own provisions—*pâté de foie gras* and champagne! Think of that. And they made us welcome to it all, and we did enjoy ourselves; but the society was the best part of it all. Everyone had his own special tale of adventure to tell us, and we could compare accounts of what we had seen with their experiences. Educated English gentlemen never appeared to better advantage than in contrast with those selfish Knights of St. John, with their long pedigrees and empty heads! They came again next evening. Mr. Parker had returned from escorting you to St.-Hubert, and had met Captain Brackenbury, the English Society's Agent, at Arlon. The day after that was the 9th. The General left with the French troop. I don't know where they are gone; I believe to pursue the chase of the king.

We walked to see the little cottage, just out of the town, where the emperor and Bismarck met. Such a little one, so small and dirty, that they sat outside and transacted their business. I suppose the war will end now. The Germans have no reason for going on with it. The King of Prussia said it was the emperor he was fighting against, not the people. Well, the emperor is a prisoner, with all that splendid army. What more can Bismarck and the king want?

Yesterday Mr. Parker came in and told us he had got work for us at Balan, under Dr. Frank, who had a *château* ready for us, and was anxious we should go. Mr. Parker had arranged that two should go, and two remain to superintend the *infirmiers* here. Of course, there were difficulties as to who should go. You can easily guess them, and I will tell you more when you come back; but it was finally settled I and nurse should go. Fancy our disappointment, after we had packed up and all, to find the head German doctor had put his *veto* on it. We were not to go, and yet he gave us no work at Donchery! Captain Furley called in the evening; he was most kind. A week ago, he suggested our going over to aid the Anglo-American Ambulance at Sedan; perhaps it is through him we are here now. However, that may be, this morning Mr. Parker told us that nurse and myself were to go to Sedan. Dr. Marion Sims had made a most pressing demand for our services. He has 600 badly wounded here, and sadly needed help.

We got here at seven o'clock. The place is miserably uncomfortable, and nothing prepared for us. Dr. Marion Sims says he must have all the rest of us, so the other ladies will come over tomorrow. I do hope to get things a little better before you arrive. We have no sheets, and only one room for the five of us. The whole thing wants setting to rights. I have not been into the wards yet, it is too late tonight, but they seem crowded with sufferers. You remember how anxious Mr. Landle of the "*Illustrated London News*" was we should come here. It was he told Dr. Sims we were at Donchery. He was quite right; we never could be more wanted than we are here. How glad I shall be to have you back again, dear; the week has been an age since you left.

Ever yours lovingly,

Louise.

There was certainly food for reflection in Louise's letter, reflection sadly interrupted by the erratic proceedings of one of our horses, who would persist in turning round to look in at the omnibus windows and declining to go on, except under severe punishment. I was beginning, too, to feel very ill, hardly able to bear the drive, and when we arrived at Bouillon I was only thankful to crawl upstairs in a dirty cabaret and lie down on a filthy bed. Yet thought will not be banished, and I thought on. I was very glad that our party had moved to Sedan, it was so evident the Germans only valued our stores, not our personal assistance. The poor defeated French might be more grateful.

Then I was rejoiced that Captain Brackenbury had taken the command, though how far his power superseded that of the committee I did not know. In London they had never named him to me, except that they had heard from him that some of us were at Sedan. Then about the stores. Young Sims had brought out a great many, and Captain Brackenbury had sent in more; those coming out with me, to follow with the heavy waggon next day, were plainly therefore very superfluous.

Harry Sims had started from London, Captain Brackenbury had telegraphed his proceedings there; why had they sent out such a number of valuable bales by me? However, I was too ill to speculate on the subject, and settled it in my own mind by deciding they had so much money they did not know what to do with it; but my general impression was of a hopeless confusion at headquarters.

Sedan was reached at last, and we crossed the drawbridge and passed into the town. We traversed the narrow streets, crossed the Place Turenne, and stopped short just beyond it, where a steep road turned off to the right, up a hill, crowned by an old keep and a long range of buildings, the Caserne Asfelde, now occupied by the Anglo-American Ambulance, under the charge of Dr. Marion Sims. Here, as our horse positively refused to advance a step further, and seemed hardly able to hold up, I thought it better to walk up the hill and find shelter in our quarters. The road crossed another drawbridge and led on to a green plateau, on which many tents were pitched. The dirt was something frightful; every dressing that had been taken off had been thrown out of the windows, and strewed the ground below. We entered the entrance door at the end of the building; boxes and bales were heaped around it and about the stone staircase. The smell was terrible, and the whole thing seemed to want organising from beginning to end.

I found my way into a barrack-room at the head of the staircase, just outside the swing door leading into the wards, and, unable even to stand, flung myself on the first bed I found there, and asked for Louise. She was attending the operations, I heard; and I had only to lie quiet, half-insensible, till the nurse came in, and, frightened to see the state I was in, ran off to find my friend and beg her to come quickly. When she did arrive, I was undressed and put into her bed, and Dr. Sims was sent for. He ordered me not to stir, and he would see in the morning what could be done.

I tried to give our friends all the information I could, but I deferred asking any questions as to our present position till I was better. I found that we, the lady nurses, dined with Dr. Sims, the chief, an American; Mr. McCormac, an Irishman, taking the second mess, and there being a third downstairs for the juniors. There were some twenty surgeons and dressers in the hospital, besides other assistants, and every bed and tent was crowded with wounded.

Every time the swing door opened the fearful smell came out, and by night I was seriously ill. However, of this I have nothing to say, except that I received the greatest kindness from everybody, a sister's care and nursing from Louise; and next day Dr. Marion Sims ordered me to sleep out of hospital, six in our room being too many. Louise came with me to the Hôtel Croix d'Or, Sedan, from which every day we mounted to hospital, to our different duties.

Ill as I was, the morning after my arrival I went with Louise round the wards, and suggested one or two things to Dr. Sims, which he begged might be carried out. Stores of all kinds were over abundant, and the great thing was to enforce on the *infirmiers* (soldiers permitted by the Prussians to assist) and on the women who had been hired to help, the first principle of order and cleanliness. The other lady nurses were all indefatigable, not only in nursing themselves, but in keeping others up to their duty, and as Dr. Sims remarks, in his '*History of an Ambulance*,' a great change was soon evident.

Louise attended every operation, and her long Hospital training made her most useful on such occasions. It was certainly not conservative surgery that was practised there, and the operations were very numerous. Mr. McCormac was a very skilful operator, and it must have been a splendid school of surgery for all the young men of the ambulance. I preferred our quiet jog-trot way at Orléans, when I saw it afterwards, where we had no secondary haemorrhage and no *pyaemia*, except about a dozen cases out of fourteen hundred, and one of those we cured; where we kept on the legs and arms, even if they were to be useless afterwards, and only lost forty patients out of fourteen hundred. Perhaps it was not so scientific, but it was more satisfying. In both cases I am sure all was done that could be to cure or to alleviate, and if the style differed, it was a mere question. I cannot decide which was really best in a learned point of view.

But what was certainly not best was the system of waste that went on. Imagine three or four hundred sheets being burned because some men with *pyaemia* had been sleeping in some of them, and of course the *infirmiers* had not taken the trouble to put those sheets apart from the rest. Very many more had been sent to the military hospital to be washed, and that institution being in the hands of the Prussians, those universal appropriators had kept them all. A strong remonstrance induced the return of a few. As for shirts and other linen, they shared the same fate; bale after bale was opened and the contents used, but very few ever came from the wash. Indeed, the want of a proper system of laundry was one of the worst features of this great ambulance.

But as there was a storekeeper, whose business it should have been to have seen to the return of the linen, clean and in good order, to the store, no one else had a right to interfere. I had brought out, as I have said, a few private stores, and I was very thankful that among them were half a dozen bottles of sherry; for I distrusted the water very much, especially after Louise's tale, how disagreeable it was when she went there, three days before I arrived, so much so that she avoided touching it. Several of the young men however, were ill, and the water grew worse and worse.

At last they resolved to search the well, and found three dead *Zouaves*. The water after that went by the name of '*Eau de Zouaves*.' And this said sherry, too, was the cause of much refreshment to several weary travellers who came by that way, on business or pleasure bent; for the Caserne Asfelde became the great sight of Sedan. It is not for me to enter into any medical details. Mr. McCormac's book, just published by Churchill, does that.

I will simply give our impressions of the ambulance. Caserne Asfelde was a barrack. A long corridor ran down it, opening on a central staircase, the wards lying on each side; the walls were whitewashed, and the floors, asphalt, very difficult to keep clean, the water settling in the small holes of the asphalt; and no sanitary arrangements whatever. But there was a free current of air through every ward, and plenty of clean linen, and these make up for many deficiencies. The chief, Dr. Marion Sims, was a charming American, with courtly manners, and a certain way about him that impressed one at once with his being a man of talent, and not only that, but a man of strong common sense, and the kindliest and merriest of companions into the bargain. Then came his colleague, Mr. McCormac, a genial Irishman, a splendid surgeon, and a gentle and sympathising man.

Père Bayonne, a Dominican, the Catholic chaplain, must not be forgotten. We often recall his, bright, round, rosy face, his white flannel robe, always spotless in its purity, and leading one to speculate who did his washing, ever ready for duty, equally ready to share in the innocent gaiety of his young friends, his friendly morning greeting, and his loving lament over the lads, 'Good boys! dear boys! if they would only say their prayers, but they never do unless they have got the cholera.' Perhaps the worthy father meant in his own rite; for if ever deeds proved faith it was in the case of the brave and skilful men who formed the Anglo-American Ambulance. Their new chief wronged us much after that; but we have a warm corner still in our hearts for the 'boys' of that ambulance.

Now, Père Bayonne was caterer for the second mess, and M. Monod, the Protestant chaplain, was caterer for the third. It was, indeed, a reunion of Christendom in those days of war. M. Monod was a quiet, well-bred, earnest young man, slight and pale. Two greater contrasts could not be to each other titan the Dominican father and the Protestant pastor, yet they lived together as brothers. Then Turco and Charlie must not be forgotten. Charlie was Dr. Sims' black servant, and cook to the first mess; and Turco was a wounded man, properly a prisoner, but adopted as servant by Dr. Pratt, and new christened John. Both were black and amusing, and had a peculiar way of revenging themselves on any assembled *coterie* they did not like by cooking the dinner most infamously.

While Dr. Sims was there, Charlie dare not play this prank; afterwards he took a dislike to several members of the mess, and thus revenged himself. I should say they suffered severely, but I was, by order of Dr. Sims, dining out of hospital, and so escaped the infliction; besides, I had been warned of it, and specially avoided becoming a victim to Charlie's revenge. I did dine there one day, by accident, and the mutton was raw and blue. I mildly observed, 'Oh, Charlie, Charlie! you could do better than that,' and Charlie replied, as if it were his full justification, 'But, Missus, Charlie did not know you were coming.'

Every bed in the building was occupied by wounded men, mostly French; whilst cases of fever were transferred to the tents. The kitchen arrangements were very poor, no roasting or frying could be done, and the men got tired of perpetual soup and *bouillon*. No regular diet tables could be carried out. They were drawn up and looked very business-like, hanging over the beds, but an attempt to change the hours of the meals and vary the diet was a failure, owing to the fact that the cooks were French prisoners under a military superintendent, and were obliged to return to their quarters by six o'clock, so that the last meal of the day was about four and the first not till 7 a.m. next morning, certainly too long an interval.

The effort to remedy this, by giving eggs and brandy, sago, milk, and other things, was not, I think, a successful one. French soldiers are not accustomed to so full a diet as we English, and I attribute a good deal of the dysentery and diarrhoea which prevailed to this system being sometimes carried out over zealously. Certainly, the laundry and the kitchen were our weak points, and unless the plan had been utterly changed, and we had had sufficient help to organise them in our way, it was unavoidable.

It was fortunate, too, that the weather was lovely and the days long, for there were no means of lighting or warming the wards. The Caserne stood very high, 'exposed to all the winds that blew,' and had the month been as cold as an English September is sometimes, we should have had great trouble in keeping the patients warm. They were all, with one or two exceptions, Roman Catholics; but Père Bayonne, did not institute any religious services in the wards, nor was Mass ever celebrated there.

Every attention was, however, given to the spiritual needs of the dying. On the whole, and considering that it was an ambulance, formed in a barrack under the circumstances of being in the midst of a battle and on a battlefield, it went on as well as possible, and the skill and attention of the surgeons, the ample supply of linen, medicines, and all extras, fully made up for any minor evils.

CHAPTER 16

Caserne Asfelde

To give a detailed account of daily labours in hospitals would be only wearisome. Very few incidents worth recording occur in the quiet monotony of such work, but a few sketches may interest the reader. One ward was occupied by wounded officers, amongst them several who had served with our army in the Crimea. One of them was a gallant old captain, whose faithful companion, a dog, was allowed to range at will in the Hospital and sleep on his master's bed. A legend was extant that this dog had gone through the Crimean campaign; but as the creature was quite young, and the Russian war some sixteen years ago, the story was evidently apocryphal. What was true was, that the dog followed his master into the battle, and was found watching by him when he was picked up, severely wounded, and brought into Sedan.

Another was the colonel of a line regiment. He had been shot through the throat, his case was a most interesting one, and his recovery was a feat in surgery. Every care was bestowed upon him by Dr. Sims and Mr. McCormac. The wound was cured, and he accompanied Mr. McCormac to Brussels when the Caserne was finally evacuated; but there, like so many others, he drooped and pined. His regiment were all dead or prisoners, his career blighted, his country lost, for he was too thorough a soldier to believe in raw levies of *Gardes Mobiles* and *francs-tireurs*, and he died of a broken heart.

Perhaps we saw less of this ward than almost any other, for all the afternoon it was filled with ladies and gentlemen, citizens of Sedan, who came up to visit the officers, bringing with them most unwholesome presents of sweet cakes and bonbons and not very ripe fruit. This was at last put a stop to; but as soon as the officers were all evacuated, by death or removal, the nuisance ceased of itself, for the compassion and interest of the visitors did not extend to the soldiers' wards. I was much surprised on being requested by one lady to take her to a ward farther on, where a soldier was now placed who had been changed from some other room; but the secret came out as we went along, for she explained that the young man was a nobleman in disguise, or rather in the ranks, and therefore was evidently, in her eyes, a fitting object of sympathy, in spite of his soldier's coat and worsted epaulettes.

The wards were divided amongst the English ladies nursing there, and under them were male and female *infirmiers*. The latter were, as, a rule, idle and too fond of gossiping with each other, whilst any extra work, in the way of a thorough wash down of the floors of the wards, required a great exertion of stern decision to enforce the doctor's orders. The night-watch was taken by two Sisters of the Order of the Immaculate Conception, whilst during the day we were assisted by two sisters of the Order of Little Sisters of the Poor.

Some days after our arrival. Dr. Webb requested the services of two of the English ladies with that part of the ambulance serving at Balan, and two accordingly went there. About ten days afterwards arrived a clergyman with two Protestant Sisters. Their dresses were, if possible, more conventual than those of the French Sisters, whose astonishment at hearing that these good ladies were not members of their Church was excessive. The German Protestant Deaconesses they could understand, but not these Sisters, and poor Père Bayonne gave it up in despair. After I had tried for half an hour to elucidate the matter, he only shrugged his shoulders and observed, 'But why do they dress to imitate real Sisters!' Now, these good ladies had not been requested to come to Caserne Asfelde; however, their services were accepted in lieu of those of our ladies who were gone to Balan.

It so happened on the day of their arrival that I had left the hospital about four o'clock, and feeling very ill had gone down to the Croix d'Or, and to bed. Louise came about eight, and related their arrival and the difficulties about their sleeping in hospital. They had wanted a room to themselves, but that was impossible; so, they had to make up a couple of beds in the general sleeping-room, making four in a very small space, and she hoped they would be comfortable. Next morning, she went up to the hospital, as usual, early, and I followed about noon. I found things anything but comfortable. The good Sisters had never undressed, and whether that was a conventual custom, or merely because they would not unrobe in the presence of seculars, no one could decide; but certainly, this could not go on long. To come out of wards full of bad odours in those heavy serge dresses, bringing with them that faint ambulance smell which is so sickening, and not to change them day or night, would be a sure means of infection. Besides, they had breakfasted at the ladies' mess, with Dr. Marion Sims at the head of the table, and though the conversation was purposely kept as quiet and toned down as much as possible, they had requested separate meals, on the ground that it was frivolous, and, to crown all, they had been utterly shocked and horrified at finding a man's cap flung hastily down on one of their beds by Mr. Parker, who, as an old friend, had liberty before breakfast to wash his hands in the general sleeping-room of the ladies (which was used by day as a dining room).

It was so evident that they could not get on there, in such a rough, rambling way of living, that I asked Mr. McCormac to send for our own two ladies to come back, and to send these good Sisters to take their places. He quite agreed, and going into the wards, I was confirmed in my opinion of the wisdom of the change, by finding that one at least spoke little or no French, and in the course of the afternoon the exchange was effected, in spite of a violent opposition on the part of their spiritual director (a clergyman of the Church of England who acted as their chaplain), who could not or would not see how much better it was they should work under their own Mother Superior, who was at Balan herself, and how unsuited they were for campaigning.

They were most valuable nurses there, where all was quiet and the patients were few, and did splendid work; but their wonderful inadaptability to circumstances, their want of pliability, so to speak, and conforming to the actual position, offer a strong contrast to the admirable manner in which, as we afterwards saw, the sisters of St. Aignan at Orléans could put aside their conventual habits, as far as was necessary, and found their rules as rules should be, of leather, not of iron, when Sisters have rough work to do.

Twice all our French *infirmiers* were taken away as prisoners. Throughout the war, the Germans showed a singular disregard of the terms of the Geneva Convention, and when remonstrated with prided themselves upon it, saying, 'Very true, you have the right, but we have the might.' To assert that these *infirmiers* were soldiers simply, after they had been made assistants in hospital, was absurd; they were all unarmed, of course, and might have been left till the ambulance departed. But no; they were marched off at an hour's notice. The wounded, too, were evacuated long before they were in a fit state to travel. At this time, Mézières, about twelve miles off, was still in French possession, and to this little city the poor fellows were sent, and from thence transferred to the towns in the north of France.

I cannot say that much consideration or kindness was shown by the German officials. They were the masters, and they made everyone feel it.

The windows of the Caserne commanded a lovely view. Below us lay the town of Sedan, the blue River Meuse winding through it, crossed by a light iron-railed bridge. In a yard just beyond it were the captured *mitrailleuses* guarded by a couple of sentinels only. In the distance there were the rising hills, covered with trees and verdure, where the Prussian batteries had been planted, and in the valley between, houses and farms scattered here and there, conspicuous among them the Château Bellevue, where Napoleon passed his last night as emperor.

The Meuse looked very fair to see, but the fish were all dead in its poisoned waters, and I was surprised one day to see some men apparently fishing from the bank. 'What can they be fishing for?' I asked my companion a German officer.

'They are fishing for eagles,' he answered. I looked puzzled, and he explained that they were fishing for the brass eagles which had adorned the shakos and helmets thrown into the river, and though the head-gear was ruined, when found, the brass ornaments were valuable. Day after day we saw carts full of rusty *chassepots* come in from the country round, for a strict order had been issued by the Prussians that all weapons found in the fields should be brought to the bureau of the *commandant de place*, under pain of fine and imprisonment. They seemed innumerable, and they must, by their dirty, rusty look, have been abandoned during the retreat into Sedan, for those given up there by the prisoners were bright and clean.

On the same day, I went with this officer to get a pass for a carriage to Carignan, where there was an ambulance we wanted to see, and in the street we met one of the Johanniter Ritters, or Knights of St. John, who asked my friend if he had heard of the arrival of port wine from some 'Merchants of the London Docks.' There was evidently a great deal of it, and the Knight said it had been sent for the sick and wounded, but really as for giving it amongst the ambulances, it was nonsense. It was far more important to keep the soldiers who had to fight in good health, and he was going to distribute it amongst certain regiments who were going forward. I told our storekeeper when we came back, and he agreed that we were fully entitled to a share of the gift; it would be most acceptable. Good wine was very scarce, and he would go and apply for some. Apparently, his application, if made, had no result, for we never saw a bottle in the hospital. It probably went to strengthen King

William's *Uhlans* as they rode forward on their way to Paris.

The stores of linen which Mr. Adams had brought from Putney were of the greatest use. They were good, and mostly new. Very much sent out by various committees was old, and would not bear washing, and much was oddly chosen. We had many a laugh over the singular articles sent out, even including women's apparel. But indeed, we had such a quantity of stores, that I am afraid it tended to waste and extravagance. Good wine was a difficulty. On one occasion Dr. Frank sent in from Balan an urgent request for some. There was none in hospital, and I gave his messenger twenty-three bottles of very good claret, which had been given to me for our own special needs. This was to be paid back to me; but when I left Sedan fifteen bottles were still owing to me by the storekeeper, and I never had one word of thanks for having given all the wine I had to Dr. Frank. Thanks were not needed, it was not given for that; but a little gracious courtesy between fellow-workers is surely a great point at such times. Dr. Frank probably never knew where it came from, and his envoy was by no means what might be called a gentlemanly man.

During the month we were at Sedan we had an almost unbroken series of cloudless weather, only one day of rain. The Prussian bands sometimes played in the Place Turenne, and the French population listened, half sulky, half admiring. 'The Prussians are dogs,' one man remarked to me, 'but the music goes well' (*la musique marche bien*). There were not at this time the acts of cruelty and violence which afterwards disgraced the German name round Orléans. Very heavy impositions had not yet been inflicted. The war was more civilised and humane, and had it ended there the Prussian laurels would have been untarnished; but war has a degrading effect on character, and when we met at Orléans the German troops we had seen near Metz and Sedan the change was a sad and terrible one, and the next generation will feel the effect of their fathers having led a buccaneer life in France, whilst the little children of the vanquished are learning at their mother's knee stern lessons of vengeance and hatred.

Sedan was, however, a melancholy residence. No papers were published, no letters sent or received. All we got came to the nearest frontier town of Bouillon, and were brought on by private hand. That wonderful institution, the Feld-Post, had not yet developed its marvellous capacity for not conveying letters. Confiding souls were not betrayed into trusting to its tender mercies, and we only gained glimpses of the outside world now and then. There was a pause in great military operations. Paris was invested, but no important sorties had taken place, and Metz was still surrounded by the troops of Prince Frederick Charles.

It was the hush before the storm, the end of tine first act of that great drama, and the days went quickly on. Now and then the gates of the city were shut very early. There were flying rumours of some French column, coming by this road or the other, to retake Sedan, but with what object it was impossible to tell. The country was occupied by the German troops, and the place, if taken, not defensible. It was possibly because the towns were useless to the plans of the French generals, or else it was strange that places left with such small garrisons were allowed to remain in the enemy's possession. Being only women, not generals in command of great armies, we saw many things that puzzled us, as not being in accordance with common sense, as we thought; but doubtless they were all right.

All the French prisoners had been sent away by the end of the second week in September, and very few German troops remained. Stray tourists visited the place, but the omnibus service from Bouillon was not yet reorganised. The railway communication was at an end, and there were great difficulties in getting to Sedan from the nearest station. But now and then came some bound on a sad errand, to search for the lost and loved. One was an old army surgeon of the First Empire, still dressed in the blue long-tailed coat, with crimson facings and huge gold epaulettes, and the enormous cocked hat of half a century ago. His only child, he told me, had been dangerously wounded in the knee.

'A captain, *Madame*,' he said, in answer to my enquiries, 'and a *décore*. He has been well nursed here in a private family; but his mother pines to see her boy again, and I have come, *Madame*, yes, all the way from near Marseilles, to take him back to his mother. And they told me these Prussians love uniforms, so behold, I have put on the dress I wore so long ago. It is handsome still, is it not, *Madame*? It will enforce respect.'

Poor old gentleman, it made the tears well up to look at the faded uniform, and the tarnished lace, and the grey head, and think of the dying soldier, for dying he was, and the mother waiting till her husband brought back their 'boy.' I hope he died in his southern home, with his head on that tender mother's breast.

Yet sadder still was the mission of an English officer. His daughter had been betrothed to a Saxon gentleman, who, summoned to rejoin his regiment, left England and his bride-elect at twenty-four hours' notice. He fell in his first battle, shot through the heart, and the poor girl's father had come to search for the body and take it back to Saxony. It was found, and it was a relief to know that death must have been instantaneous. No lingering agony upon the field or in hospital. Death had been more merciful, and this was all the consolation the father could take back to his sorrowing child; yet that was much.

A simple gift of cigars had been sent by her to be given to Saxon soldiers. They were left in my care. I sought out an ambulance where there were wounded Saxons, and the trust was faithfully fulfilled. Such little incidents drifted up like spars from a wreck. Multiply this grief by hundreds and thousands of cases, and you will have one idea of war. For every soldier has a home and parents. Possibly 'a nearer one yet, and a dearer one,' wife or bride. It is a trite remark, but do we realise the force of it when we read of so many thousands 'killed and wounded'? There is one mourner at least for every one of that number—one hearth desolate for ever.

Sedan was at one time encumbered with thirty thousand wounded, that is, including the villages immediately around. Fever and diarrhoea were very prevalent, especially amongst the Bavarian troops, who ate large quantities of unripe grapes and apples. An application was made by a physician of colour. Dr. Davis, of St. Bartholomew's Hospital, who had established a hospital just across the Meuse for the services of Louise and myself in his ambulance, not so much to nurse the sick (he had no wounded), but to see that the German orderlies did their duty, and to prevent the entrance of green fruit. If his German orderlies were as idle and as inefficient, though kind and good-natured, as those we had afterwards at Orléans, he must have had hard times of it. Dr. Davis died of smallpox, about two months afterwards, at Pongy-sur-Meuse, where he had his ambulance, beloved, and mourned by all who had ever come in contact with him.

These *infirmiers* went about with brassards on their arms and weapons by their sides, were drilled and taught as soldiers ready to take their part in any emergency, and expected to be waited upon as if they were generals. In short, the ambulance corps of the German Army was a very large and powerful body, and, as the children would say, 'looked for all the world like soldiers,' and their own surgeons were certainly sometimes in awe of them. We remarked everywhere during the war the vast proportion of German wounded. It was so near Metz, at Sedan, and afterwards at Orléans. Their losses must have been enormous. Will a true statement be ever published? Perhaps not. They do not care to show at what a costly price victory may be purchased.

CHAPTER 17

Under Whose Orders?

Day after day passed on, unvaried by any startling incidents. Death carried off many a poor fellow, in spite of care and nursing, and the hospital became gradually emptied. The tents were taken down, and at last so few patients remained that they were all accommodated on the upper floor, and many of the surgeons and nurses left. Père Bayonne was superseded at last, though the first attempt to replace him by a Jesuit priest resulted in a ludicrous scene. The good father was sitting outside the entrance-door, chatting with some of the 'boys' and smoking his afternoon cigar, when a thin, spare, ascetic-looking priest in black came up the hill, and announced himself to his reverend brother as being sent by the Archbishop of Rheims to take the duty of chaplain there.

Père Bayonne remarked that the said archbishop had nothing to do with him. He did not belong to his diocese. He had been attached to the ambulance as chaplain before it left Paris, and intended to remain with it. The black priest grew excited, and said then he would go himself to the Archbishop of Paris and obtain the order to do duty instead of Père Bayonne. The worthy *père* chuckled, and replied, 'Pray do; go and look for him amongst the Prussian bayonets.' At this defiance the other grew more angry still, and high words ensued.

At last one of the 'boys' suggested an appeal to arms, or rather fists, and Père Bayonne, entering into the spirit of the scene, began to turn up his white flannel sleeves; on seeing which the Jesuit fled down the hill, and declined the combat. Père Bayonne remained till Dr. Marion Sims left, and went to Brussels with him, having arranged to rejoin the ambulance when it took up fresh ground. The service as chaplain was done by two of the priests from the city, but the father's rival never returned again.

About the end of September, I spent one day in going round the villages on the battlefield of Sedan. Balan and Bazeilles were too sadly familiar to me, and both were still desolate and deserted. No attempt had been made in either to repair damages; though in Bazeilles two or three families were living on the ground-floor of their houses, having put up a piece of sail to replace the ceiling and roof. More utter wreck and ruin could not be seen. The little town must be entirely rebuilt before its industrious and once thriving population can return to it. Whatever share the inhabitants may have taken in the battle, surely their punishment was a savage one. It was often called in France the great crime of the war, and certainly nothing equalled it, Châteaudun excepted. La Chapelle, La Moncelle; and all the villages showed traces of the 'work of war.'

Many houses had been destroyed by bombs, the churches occupied by the wounded, and almost every tenable house turned into an ambulance. It is honourable to the people of that neighbourhood, indeed all over the seat of war, that no credible accounts have ever been published of any ill-treatment of German wounded by the poor, miserable villagers. Amidst all their natural feelings of irritation against the invader, they never forgot the sacred duty of kindness to the wounded, and not only refrained from all acts of violence, or even annoyance, but, on the contrary, gave their best efforts to aid the sufferers. Many impoverished themselves in this noble cause, but no pecuniary acknowledgment has ever been made by the German Government of these disinterested services. Perhaps they were included in the 'rights of a conqueror,' as were so many other things.

We passed by the plateau of Floing, where the White Cuirassiers and the Imperial Guard fell *en masse* together. The road beyond dips down towards the Meuse, but on the north side rises abruptly; here and there are gorges, and in one, which opens out towards Sedan, are the villages of Givonne, La Chapelle, La Moncelle, and Illey. In the deep descent of the road the greatest slaughter had occurred; the fire of the batteries had destroyed friend and foe alike. A month had passed since that fatal day, but the traces of the battle were visible still. Men and horses had been too lightly buried, and sad remains of mortality were yet to be seen. In the villages we visited the ambulances, they seemed well supplied with all necessaries.

A few extra comforts were wanting, and a list of these was taken down for Captain Brackenbury, at Arlon, and so perfect were all his arrangements that no doubt the missing articles arrived within a couple of days. Often and often afterwards, amidst the destitution at Orléans, we had to lament that he was not 'Ubiquitous.' His energy, his decision, his clear judgment, would have been invaluable. The National Society had no servant so indefatigable and trustworthy as Captain Henry Brackenbury, R.A.

At Floing we visited an ambulance where many wounded were placed in long wooden sheds. The gift of a few cigars was gratefully accepted. Everywhere ruined houses and half-deserted villages showed the ravages of war, but most of the wounded had been removed. Miss Monod's Ambulance was at this time working at Pouilly-sur-Meuse. All through the war this devoted lady and her companions worked hard during danger and privation such as fell to the lot of few, and though a French International Ambulance, friends and foes met with equal care and kindness. I trust and believe it was so in all places where there were wounded to be cared for.

On the 24th of September Dr. Marion Sims left for Brussels and England, and was succeeded in the joint command with Mr. McCormac of the Anglo-American Ambulance by his son-in-law. Dr. Pratt, to whom he bequeathed his authority and the money he had in store. Shortly before this, Captain Henry Brackenbury had paid the ambulance a visit, and I had had a long conversation with him. When he first ordered our ladies from Donchery to Sedan he had given a written paper into Louise's charge, placing us under the orders of Mr. McCormac (as the English chief), and instructing us, when discharged by him from our duties with his ambulance, to proceed to Arlon (Captain Brackenbury's headquarters), and report ourselves there for further orders.

On the occasion of our interview he reiterated this order, and impressed upon me that no one, not the President of the British Society himself, could give us any orders, except through himself, as their appointed agent on the continent. I told him I was very thankful to know who was our commander, and that all directions he gave should be fully carried out. He expressed himself as perfectly satisfied with all that had been done, and begged me to write to him if anything occurred to require his aid. Thus, our future course was clear.

After Dr. Marion Sims left, the patients were rapidly evacuated. Only two officers remained—the poor colonel, and a cheerful, contented, merry little captain, whose thigh had been fractured, and who, though longing to return to his wife and family near Nice, was the most patient and grateful of men. His delight at, and enjoyment of, any little delicacy added to his dinner were charming to behold. He was all alone in a great ward, and so glad when anyone would go and sit with him and chat over his Crimean experiences and the present campaign, so soon ended for him.

He told us how he was struck by a ball and fell, how he was dragged into some out-of-the-way stable or barn, with nothing to eat or drink and no surgical attendance, till early next morning came some of the doctors of the Anglo-American Ambulance, and dressed all their wounds, and offered to take the worst wounded back to their Hospital. One of these, a superior officer, declined to go, unless he could have special accommodation—a little room to himself, or something of the sort—and as this could not be given in the crowded state of the ambulance, he preferred to wait some other chance.

The poor captain immediately put in his claim—if only a mattress amongst the soldiers, it would be luxury to him—so he was substituted for the colonel and brought away, to be kindly and skilfully tended with all that science and sympathy could do. The colonel was taken to some other ambulance; perhaps was placed in a private house. There were many wounded so cared for; but it rendered the discovery of their fate by their friends more difficult, as the general lists were not very correctly kept, and with such a pressure of business, so many deaths, such countless prisoners, such hosts of wounded, it is not to be wondered at.

In and around Sedan we found a very large proportion of German wounded, and this in spite of their men being transferred to the rear in every case where it was safe to transport them. Dr. Frank's Ambulance at Balan, and near Bazeilles (part of the Anglo-American), is evidence of this. Château Monvilliers, where Mrs. Capel established so well-managed a hospital, had only Bavarians in it; there may have been one or two French, but I think not. It was the same case with Dr. Webb at Balan, also part of our ambulance. He had all Germans. Dr. Davis, at Pongy-sur-Meuse, had 300 sick and wounded, all Bavarians, and instances of this could be multiplied.

At Caserne Asfelde, as I have said, we had almost all French; all French, indeed, after the first few days. The German losses must have been enormous; to judge by these facts, far more than the French. The peasants of the burying parties told us the same, though they added that the Germans buried their dead instantly, and before they buried the French, so that it was impossible accurately to judge of the proportionate loss.

The Caserne was emptying fast by this time (the first week of October), and Dr. Pratt went to Brussels to receive his orders from the French International, to which the ambulance belonged. On his return a meeting was held, and the result was the division of the ambulance into two; one part remaining under the charge of Dr. Pratt, the other under that of Dr. Frank. Louise and myself were selected by Dr. Pratt to accompany his ambulance, with the sanction of the British Society, represented by Captain Brackenbury.

Of the adventures of Dr. Frank and his ambulance we can tell nothing. The All Saints Sisters accompanied it. They went to Brussels, and from thence to Châlons and Epernay, in the German lines; whilst our orders were to go into Paris, if possible, if not into French lines—a very fair division of assistance, as it seems. By the society's accounts. Dr. Frank received some 7,000*l*. from the British Society. Assuredly 700*l*. would more than represent what Dr. Pratt received from them; but then, as his ambulance was also borne on the books of the French Society, he was not entitled to so much. Still, the disparity is enormous.

Mr. McCormac gave Louise and myself our discharge, in compliance with Captain Brackenbury's orders, and we went to Arlon to report ourselves, and obtain the necessary sanction to continue with Dr. Pratt's portion of the Anglo-American Ambulance. I had written to the Chairman of the Executive Committee (Colonel Loyd-Lindsay) to tell him we were leaving Sedan, were asked to accompany Dr. Pratt, and to beg him to speak to Captain Brackenbury about it, who was for a few days in England. At Arlon I received a telegram to say it rested entirely with Captain Brackenbury, who we found was expected that night. Mr. Capel was there in charge, but he preferred our seeing Captain Brackenbury.

Meantime the ambulance had taken a shorter route to Brussels, and we were somewhat anxious for the decision, which we fully intended to abide by. If I relate this in full, it is only because we have, I believe, been accused of 'insubordination.' There was none. We never disobeyed an order; and if there was misunderstanding as to orders, it simply arose from the committee's confused idea as to whose authority was supreme—their own, or Captain Brackenbury's, or the chairman's, or the secretary's, or the executive committee, or everybody in general and nobody in particular—for to this day we have not the slightest idea. We believed Captain Brackenbury, he evidently believed so too; but we were afterwards undeceived. However, on this occasion we waited for his arrival.

Early next day a telegram arrived from Brussels formally requesting our services with the Anglo-American Ambulance. Captain Brackenbury had not been found in Brussels, and Mr. Capel kindly took it upon himself to give the requisite order in the captain's absence, whom we hoped to see at Brussels. We telegraphed this back to Dr. Pratt and started for Brussels. At the station Dr. M'Kellar met us. Captain Brackenbury had been seen, and had sent a note giving his full consent and attaching us for service to the ambulance, not stipulating for any particular place or period of time, and to this hour that order remains uncontradicted.

I annex the two orders:—

Arlon, Oct. 6.

In the absence of Captain Brackenbury, and at the request of Dr. Pratt, as per telegram of today, I authorise Miss Pearson and Miss McLaughlin to join the ambulance now headed by him, and they are at liberty to proceed to Brussels whenever they think proper.

Reginald Capel.

Brussels, Oct. 6.

Dear Miss Pearson,—I have just seen Dr. Pratt, and was in the act of telegraphing to you to come here to join the Anglo-American Ambulance. Dr. M'Kellar now shows me your telegram. Pray go on with the ambulance, as you wish it and Dr. Pratt wishes it. Miss McLaughlin will also be with you. I wish you every success. I remain yours faithfully,

Henry Brackenbury.

Thus, all was done in compliance with orders from the very first.

Brussels looked gay and full, crowded with French refugees. We went to see the stores of the French International Society, and they seemed very scanty compared with the profusion of our own. We had an interview with Captain Brackenbury, who was all that was kind and courteous. He said he did not believe we should obtain permission to pass into Paris, but he thought we should find plenty of work in the immediate neighbourhood. Our departure was deferred some twenty-four hours, owing to the difficulty of getting on the waggons and horses. We much wished to pay Antwerp a visit, but Dr. Pratt requested none of his ambulance to leave the city; so, like good soldiers, we obeyed our chief, as Dr. Pratt was now, and it was only at 7 p.m. on October 8 that we all left by the railroad for Rouen *via* Amiens.

How to get on farther by rail or road remained to be seen, as changes on the route might occur at any moment, bridges be blown up and roads cut, for Normandy was preparing to meet the invader. Amiens was reached at four in the morning, and as the train did not start till 6 a.m. we bivouacked in the station. At ten we reached Rouen, and it was decided that we were not to leave till 6 p.m., and get as far as St.-Pierre-au-Louviers, where the traffic ceased, sleep there, and proceed next morning by road *via* Dreux to Versailles.

CHAPTER 18

'La Belle Normandie'

Our baggage waggons and horses were all duly transferred from the station we arrived at to the station we started from across the river, and here, whilst lounging in the waiting room, we caught sight of a gentleman sitting at a table writing, and he had one of our English brassards on his arms. A courier came in and out, and there was evidently a hitch in their business. Some of our party fell into conversation with him, and his story offered an amusing illustration of the old proverb of sending 'the hook after the hatchet.'

The National Society had become aware of sundry boxes and bales dispersed about the country, and had sent out a courier to find them, get them together, and take them on to Versailles. Why, when so much unpaid service was at their command, they preferred to pay hired servants, I do not know. In this case, certainly not because of superior qualification for the work, for the little man could not carry out his directions, and on telegraphing home to the committee this gentleman was sent out to assist him.

The stray baggage had been got together, but fresh difficulties arose. Fearful tales of the depredations committed by *francs-tireurs* were flying about, and it appeared that to take baggage intended for the German lines through Normandy was a hazardous proceeding. Fortunately for this gentleman, our ambulance was a French one, with French *infirmiers*, and at that time welcomed everywhere as true to France, and Dr. Pratt very kindly offered to throw the shelter of his protection over the captain, the courier, and the baggage, and it was arranged they should go on with us, and at St. Pierre find waggons to take their stores.

We arrived in due time at St. Pierre, found lodging in a small *auberge*, and prepared for a journey next day that we were assured would be full of danger. As we saw it next morning, St. Pierre is a prettily situated village with rising ground behind it, and stands on the banks of the Seine. Opposite are wooded heights, and the country around was green and fertile. An early start had been arranged, but the captain had gone off to Louviers, a town about three miles distant, of which St. Pierre-au-Louviers was the railroad station, to find some waggons, and we had to wait for his return.

The people of Louviers must be a hospitable, kind-hearted race, for the evening before, travelling in the railroad carriage with a lady and gentleman of that place, they had pressed us most earnestly not to remain at St. Pierre, but to go on with them and accept supper, bed, and breakfast, and this simply on the faith of our charitable mission; whilst the captain met with every assistance, and the mayor himself lent him a wagon and a splendid pair of heavy Norman cart-horses, that could drag any weight. This and another wagon and horses he found there were duly returned from Versailles.

Whilst waiting for the packing of the baggage on these waggons, it entered into the fertile brain of one of our party to address the gaping villagers who had assembled round the *auberge* doors in a flowery speech about nothing, which, being delivered in perfect French, with most emphatic action, was irresistibly ludicrous, especially when, pointing to an American banner which was duly displayed out of the window, he declaimed on the reason of there not being a proper number of stars on the blue square in the corner, and being a Southerner, he declared that a great many stars had withdrawn from the assemblage usually displayed on the banner, being ashamed of their company!

On this an elderly and respectable individual, who was listening open mouthed to this flow of eloquence, or rather 'bunkum,' went off into a state of despair, dashed his hat on the ground, began to run his hands wildly through his hair, as if about to tear it off, and lamented over the ruin and disunion of '*la grande Republique*.' It was some time before we could any of us recover our gravity, and by the time we had done so a start was ordered, and the cortege wound slowly up a lane with deep banks on either side, so like an English lane that it was impossible to fancy we were in France, and so near the seat of war.

At Rouen we had seen crowds of men drilling, dressed in their civilian clothes, the black coat of the gentleman side by side with the linen blouse of the artisan; but very little progress seemed to have been made in the arming of them, for old flint-lock muskets abounded. Nor was there a general uprising in the outlying villages. Normandy was hardly awake, and everything looked peaceful and dreamy. We reached at last the level plateau above St. Pierre, and joined the route *Impériale*; and here our light van and store waggons and the gentlemen who were walking came to a standstill, for the heavily-loaded waggons of the captain had stuck in the cross lane we had taken out of St. Pierre, and the horses from the last one were obliged to be attached to the front one and drag it uphill, and then being again unharnessed, all four horses returned to the other waggon and brought it up to the road above. 'Most haste, worse speed,' saith an old proverb. Had we taken the route *Impériale*, a mile longer, but nearly level, we should have avoided the hour's delay which ensued. Thus, we did not make a fair start until 1 p.m. instead of 8 a.m., as originally ordered.

But whilst waiting the arrival of the captain and his baggage we had various sources of amusement to pass away the time. First, we sat on a green bank, though the wind was cold, and looked across the valley, through which ran the Seine, to the grand old ruins of Château Gaillard, the castle of our lion-hearted king, built in proud defiance of his rival, Philippe-Auguste. It is but a ruin now, the 'Saucy Castle,' as Richard called it, when it frowned down on the sunny valley and lorded it over the silver Seine. It has its legends, too, of fair, frail queens who lived in durance there, and one. Marguerite de Bourbon, the faithless wife of Louis X., ended here her sinful life by the executioner's hands, and here the exiled David Bruce found a shelter when banished from his northern home.

Twice the 'Saucy Castle' surrendered to the foeman, on both occasions from famine, once of food, once of water. Roger de Lacy defended it for six months against the French King, Philippe-Auguste, the partisan of Prince Arthur, when that monarch espoused his cause in opposition to that of King John; and later it held out, garrisoned by only 150 men, against the forces of Henry V. There is an old well still in the courtyard, from which in those turbulent times water was drawn for the garrison; but the ropes of the bucket were worn out, there were none to replace them, and the brave little band surrendered from thirst, as Roger de Lacy had done from hunger.

We were looking at the ruin, and wondering what fresh scenes of war and tumult would pass under its old walls, when a cry was raised, 'The *francs-tireurs*!' We sprang up, somewhat curious to see them. Here they were at last, these dreaded brigands; for as such they had been described to us. Would they disregard the Red-Cross banner, the Union Jack, the Stars and Stripes, and fire upon such a combination of neutrality, if could they see them? To obviate this possibility three of the tallest men were mounted on the roof of the store-waggons and waved the standards conspicuously before the advancing forces, whilst an old peasant we had caught was induced to go back down the highroad and explain our pacific character.

It is not to be wondered at that these awful preparations alarmed the *francs-tireurs*, and they began to ascend the slope in most martial order. They had been marching at ease, that is, straggling all about and picking apples, but they suddenly fell into column and levelled their rifles, then halted and held a military council. The result was, skirmishers were thrown out two and two into the fields each side, whilst others came creeping up the road, darting from tree to tree, till they came near us.

It was really very pretty to see, and Louise and myself, feeling all confidence in our female costume, stood in the road watching the advance. Probably our peaceful looks were reassuring. We did not seem ferocious and had no revolvers, the flags were duly visible, so they became reassured, called in their skirmishers by sound of bugle, and marched at ease up the hill. We spoke with several of them. One poor, footsore fellow pleaded hard for 'a lift,' but it was too dangerous. Had we met any German patrol, to have had a *franc-tireur* with us would have been deeply compromising, and we were obliged to refuse.

We soon after started on our way, and at the first village we passed through we over took them. They had got some hot hard-boiled eggs, with which they presented us, and so terminated our first interview with the dreaded *francs-tireurs*. They seemed to us a very superior class of men. In their ranks were several who spoke English very well. Many were landed proprietors, with their servants, gamekeepers, and foresters. They were well dressed and well-armed, and all wore a holly leaf in their caps. We asked the meaning and were told it referred to an old Norman proverb, '*Qui me touche se pique*' (who touches me gets pricked); and assuredly they well maintained the motto of the holly leaf. From no class in the whole army did the Germans suffer so much as from the *francs-tireurs*, the '*Landsturm*' of France.

We slept at Vernon, but here an adventure occurred which might have had serious consequences to two of our party, Mr. Ryan and Mr. Hayden. Mounted on horses as outriders, Dr Pratt sent them forward to order dinner and beds. On coming near the town, a party of overzealous *Gardes Mobiles* met them, arrested them as Prussian spies, and took them to their barrack. In vain Mr. Hayden pleaded he was a medical student from Paris, even saw one of his own friends in the crowd, a young officer, who bore witness to the truth of this; nothing would satisfy the *mobiles*, some of whom were drunk, and all disorderly, and at last they marched their prisoners off, ordering them not to put their hands in their pockets, fearing probably they had revolvers in them, and so took them to the *mairie*.

Here their passports and papers proved their innocence, and they were released after two hours' annoyance. As we drove into Vernon, we were greeted with the news that two of our party were in prison. However, on arriving at the hotel, we found them there, safe and well, superintending supper, not the worse for their detention.

We saw nothing of this Norman town, which gives its name to a good old English family, as we left early next morning. Here we heard that Dreux was burning. We could not possibly pass that way or by Evreux, so we went on to Mantes. The country about here was lovely. The road wound round a projecting bluff, through which the railroad runs to the village of Bonnières, a bright, cheerful-looking place with a broad, steep main street, and past Rosny, the birthplace and home of Sully. The *château* still exists; it was the property of the Duchesse de Berri from 1818 to 1830, but the grounds around it, though well wooded, are very flat, extending down to the river.

We halted for luncheon at a little hamlet, and started about four or five, intending to pass on as far as we could. Mézières would have been our resting-place for the night, but Mézières was a ruin. Nearby some *francs-tireurs* or *Gardes Mobiles* had fired on a body of *Uhlans* with an aim too fatally true, and next day a strong body of Prussians came in and burned the village, and even whilst the few poor, shivering inhabitants who had come back to cower in their roofless dwellings told us the sad tale, the same scene was enacting only fifteen miles away, and the smoke of a burning hamlet was going up on the night air, to protest in the face of Heaven against war and all its terrors, and against the doctrine that an invaded people must neither practise 'defence nor defiance.'

It was very sad to drive in the deepening twilight through the long street of Mézières, to look at the 'comfortable' houses roofless, windowless, floorless, and blackened by smoke, and to think of the household misery entailed by war; the little details of families ruined and gone out into distant provinces to seek a shelter. Sadder still to see those who remained crouching round a fire made of the half-burned beams of their own roof-trees, despairing and hopeless. What was peace or war to them? They had lost all! No peace could give them back their happy homes, recall their dead from some forgotten trench on a lost battlefield; no war could inflict on them bitterer suffering.

And it was the ambition and pride of emperor and king, whose very faces they had, perhaps, never looked on, that caused the war; the rifles of men from some other departments, whose acts they had never sanctioned, that had brought death to the *Uhlans*, and all this misery on themselves. War is very merciless. Soldiers forget they are men, fathers, and sons, and brothers. They lose their individuality, and become one vast machine of evil. We had time enough to think over the 'morality' of war, for in the little village where we halted for the night the beds were not very conducive to sleep.

It was a very little village, named Fling. We occupied all the solitary *auberge*, but there appeared no place for the horses and waggons. Our admirable *avant-courier*, however, informed a sub-official whom he found that he must have places for his horses and *inflrmiers*; if not, the mayor must be hanged early the next morning, and places were found. We knew it was a joke; but the sub-official was frightened, and the mayor, being out of town, was apprised of his danger, and next morning the garrison was called out—two National Guards and a half (that is, a very small youth)—to guard His Worship. We did not see that official, but we left Fling with a splendid reputation for honesty and generosity, for we actually paid our bills—a practice too much neglected by the stronger party in time of war.

We arrived at Mantes about noon, and had time to see the lovely old church of Notre Dame, and after luncheon went on to St. Germain. We drove through the town without a halt, for we were getting very near the German outposts, and came out in the road leading to Versailles. At Mantes our chief had 'required' an omnibus; it was useless there, all traffic being stopped, and his men were all footsore. Our cortege was formed as follows:—Two gentlemen on horseback; four *infirmiers* marching together, one carrying the Red-Cross flag; a light covered cart, containing Louise and myself, driven by one of the gentlemen, a Union Jack and a Stars and Stripes on each side of the cart; the store-waggon, driven by Charlie, with Turco John by his side, and a monkey strapped behind. Then the omnibus with the rest of the folks, the captain's waggon coming last. As we drove out of St. Germain, we emerged on an open road, looking on the left, over flat ground, a valley with trees and houses scattered about it, and a huge rock-mound in the distance, crowned by a fortress.

'There is Mont Valérien,' said one of our friends, and we looked at the far-famed fort with great curiosity. Lines of men were manoeuvring on the green slope which descended from the fort to the valley, and as we looked we heard a dull report, a white puff of smoke broke out from the fort, a shell came slowly, with a graceful curve, soaring in the air, to fall in a green meadow some five hundred feet short of us. The earth flew up in a shower, but no further harm ensued. Our driver thought it better, however, to get on, and the fort was soon hid by a wall and a hedge. Still we heard the boom that showed Mont Valérien was at work. Presently we came out again where the road was open to the country round.

We were jogging quietly on, when one of our outriders galloped up and asked me for the pass which I had procured. We had been sent on first because we had it, but no one had asked for it. We had come at a brisk trot through St. Germain. It was dinner time, and the officials had not descried us; but just as those unlucky waggons of the captains were coming in the rear, some zealous captain of the guard descried them, and demanded what permission they had to go to the front. In vain the captain explained he was an agent of the British National; it was useless, and they had to ride forward for our pass, and we to wait the result—in full view of Mont Valérien.

Presently came another shell, a little nearer, then another nearer still. I requested Louise to emerge from the shelter of the back part of the cart and come and look, but she declared it rained and blew, and Mont Valérien might amuse itself as it liked, and she went on working a red and blue slipper in profound composure. Our driver got nervous, and insisted on driving and getting behind a wall. I declared a little wall was no real protection, and we might as well see what was going on; he preferred the back part of the wall, and there we were placed and had to stay.

I do not for one moment believe Mont Valérien fired at us. There was a sortie from Paris on the side by Bougival. The fort was firing at the Prussians in the fields below, and overshot the mark. As it was, it fell beyond them and short of us, and was very harmless. Shells come comparatively so slowly, that one has time to get over the slight flutter that the first being under fire causes, and, were it not for the danger and destruction they bring about, would be very pretty to watch.

Presently our rear disentangled itself from the outpost guard and we all went on, but five minutes further another stop occurred. Our driver, anxious to hear what was the matter, left me the reins and walked off. Just as he did so a regiment of Bavarian cavalry came tearing down the road, and our horse, having been in the army himself, showed a most decided inclination to dash after the regiment, and probably involve us in a charge, which, with a cart behind him in which were a goodly amount of bags, saddlebags, and other small articles, would have been probably more peculiar than successful. Now, it was an awkward position, for this reason.

At Sedan, two *infirmiers* had been dismissed for dishonesty of the most flagrant description. They had made their way to Versailles, given a false account of their leaving the ambulance, and been enlisted by the agents of the British Society. They accompanied Mr. Thomas, one of the surgeons of the society, to Mantes, and there we had met the party, and Dr. Pratt had identified his old acquaintances. Mr. Thomas had arrested them, with a view of sending them off as soon as he got back to Versailles, and they were being marched along as prisoners in charge of a stalwart Canadian doctor, armed with a blackthorn stick, and competent to manage any two Frenchmen, armed or unarmed.

But necessity knows no law, the prisoners were close by, our escorts were not; and though I had aided at Sedan in dismissing them from the hospital, I was sure they would rescue us, so I swallowed my pride and called out to them. They came instantly to our rescue, and really, we were so grateful that, if we could have escaped them on the spot, I almost think we should; as it was, we obtained their release at Versailles. They held well on to the horse's head, and then came another regiment galloping full speed. They turned off just beyond us, down a lane that led into the fields below, but, as we heard afterwards, the skirmish was then over, and the troops we had seen on the green hillside were retreating into the fort; so our impetuous friends could not have had the chance of charging, and we assuredly preferred keeping on the high road, and not assisting *nolens volens* in such a *mêlée*.

Shortly afterwards we reached Versailles, the only French Ambulance that did so, and were greeted at the door of the Hôtel des Reservoirs by Captain Furley, Mr. Thomas, the Admiral, and many old friends. One word more I must say. To Mr. Thomas's kind care we owed it that we found that we had a most comfortable room in the hotel prepared for us, and the society may well congratulate themselves on the good services done by this gentleman, not only to ourselves—that is a minor matter—but to the wounded of both nations. His bright, cheerful intelligence, his unselfishness, his indefatigable labour, will be, we trust, rewarded by some better recognition than these few lines of a woman's praise.

Chapter 19

The King's Headquarters

We had at last arrived at the termination of our wanderings—the king's headquarters. Here was His Majesty himself, duly installed in the prefecture; here was the crown prince, 'Fritz,' as the French called him, and it may be remarked that he was always spoken of by them almost affectionately, and the name was given in no disrespect, but rather in a kind of strange liking for the man who was said by popular report to pity their nation, to hate the war, and to detest Bismarck. He might possibly be suggested as a ruler for France, and with better chance of success than the distrusted ex-emperor.

'Fritz is kind,' 'Fritz is a brave soldier,' 'Fritz is a good man,' were common phrases even amongst the wildest of the *Zouaves*, and his English wife may be proud of her husband's reputation amongst his foes. We speak feelingly ourselves. The prince may forget an act of kindness shown towards us when we were at Balan; we do not. Our general rode over to his camp to report our arrival, and related how we had nothing to eat or drink. The prince's own luncheon had been but a sparing one, and nothing was left; but he found a stone flask of *Curaçao*, and sent it back to us, regretting he had nothing else to offer. It was invaluable. We were faint and hysterical with fasting, and a morsel of bread and a little *Curaçao* were the most delicious meal we ever partook of.

Besides these great ones of the earth, there was a swarm of little princelings, and amongst them Leopold of Hohenzollern, the innocent cause of this tremendous war. He was a tall, slight, intelligent-looking man, and very popular. His appearance was a great contrast to the heavy look and frame of the Duke of Saxe-Coburg, Prince Albert's elder brother, and the boyish, weak face of the Grand Duke of Wurtemburg. Their lives at Versailles were easy ones. They ate and drank and slept, till reports got abroad that some were sent back to the rear or on to the front, the king wisely thinking them more ornamental than useful in Versailles.

Dr. Pratt occupied himself in trying for the necessary pass to enter Paris, aided by Generals Sheridan and Burnside, and that evening we heard all went well, and we should probably leave for Paris at 3 p.m. next day. We could have no meals in the hotel, and were obliged to go out to the restaurant belonging to it. This was very disagreeable, as it was crowded with German officers, and no other ladies there. However, one of the surgeons escorted us, and the scene was decidedly amusing. How everybody ate and drank! How iced champagne flew about! And how very small the dinner was! We had some soup and some donkey—it was gelatinous, and more like calves-head than anything else—and some sweets, and we paid the full price of a good dinner.

The next morning, the 13th, at 10 o'clock a.m., we were ordered to meet the ambulance, and hear the result of Dr. Pratt's request. We were very grieved to find that the prospect of obtaining permission was a very doubtful one. This was awkward. Fully expecting to get leave to go into Paris, Dr. Pratt had brought away no stores. There were plenty in the city; besides, we should not have been allowed to take them in, and the funds were nearly exhausted. It was a question, if we could not go into Paris, if the ambulance should not be broken up, to be reformed at Tours, within French lines. Dr. Pratt declared that from the neighbourhood of Paris he would not stir, and with the Germans he would not serve, and that we should pitch tents and live close by till we did get in. During this uncertainty he requested none of us to leave the place, so we gave up a visit to an old friend of Louise's at St. Germain—our principle from first to last having been, in great as well as small things, never to disobey orders.

Instead of that we visited the *château*, now turned into a great German ambulance. There were only a few French in it, but French Sisters were the nurses. Of all the terrible places to be ill in, the *Salle des Glaces* must have been the worst, where every pale face, every contortion of pain, every action of the sick or the nurses, was repeated over and over again. It made one feverish only to think of it, and to look at the glare of the light as it struck on the mirrors. The polished floors were as slippery as glass, and the whole place, magnificent as it was, had a comfortless air. The pictures had been carefully preserved by boarding them up, but the unused part of the palace was still exhibited at certain hours, and the Germans wandered through those grand halls, looking with special interest at the pictures of the victories of the Great Napoleon. There was a long ward down below, full of wounded. There almost all the poor fellows had hospital gangrene.

The Sisters showed us the cooking-place prepared for them to heat their *tisanes* and *plaisters*. They were over-worked and badly supplied, and begged us to help them, both personally and with stores; but we told them that Prince Pless had received 20,000*l*. by the hands of Colonel Loyd-Lindsay, from England, only two days before, and surely he could now afford to supply his own great hospitals handsomely. They only shook their heads, and said that no one thought it would make much difference. It would go to the regimental field hospitals, if to any. That would save the government paying for them. I asked if she did not think the 20,000*l*. sent into Paris would do great good. She said, 'In Paris they had plenty of money and stores, and nothing could be bought. The English were very generous; the sum was enormous. She hoped it would do more good than it seemed likely would be done by it.'

That 40,000*l*. represents a great amount of self-denial and charity amongst our English households. They have a right to know how it was spent. Has any account been yet sent in from either government? Will 20,000*l*. be deducted from the war indemnity for all expenses demanded by Germany, or will that sum be given to replace furniture ruined in French colleges, convents, and palaces, in nursing German wounded; or will it be given back to England to form the nucleus of some really practical society for ambulance work amongst our own sick and wounded when next England goes to war? One or the other it ought to be. Let the subscribers look to it.

In the evening several friends paid us a visit. All hope of getting into Paris seemed over, and we heard we were ordered to Orléans by Prince Pless; but Dr. Pratt still lingered, professing his dislike to working in German lines, and consenting to do so only because advised, first, that by coming to Versailles the ambulance had fallen under the orders of Prince Pless, and next that a fortnight's work amongst the German wounded would form a fair plea for permission to go into Paris, or, at all events, leave their lines, and the plan was again discussed of breaking up the ambulance and re-forming it at Tours. Dr. Pratt ordered us to be ready to start with them next day, and ready we accordingly were.

All this time we were constantly meeting the members of the French International, who had a committee-room in the Hôtel des

Reservoirs. All were most kind to us, especially M. De la Roche and the Baron des Bussières. But our mainstay was Mr. Furley, who went, as he told us, by the name of 'the Benevolent Neutral.' If ever we had the right to be proud of a countryman, it was of Dr. Furley. He was a general favourite. Kind, brave, cheerful, unselfish, untiring, peacemaker in general in all little difficulties, Mr. Furley was a sort of patent British Sunshine, quite sufficient to disprove the national French prejudices that we live in a land of fogs, spleen, and suicide.

That evening, as I was hunting for our door-key in the bureau, a very large Prussian officer stopped me, and asked if we belonged to the Anglo-American Ambulance. I said 'Yes.'

'Why are you not off to Orléans?' he said. 'You ought to have gone this afternoon.'

I said he had better find Dr. Pratt, I was simply acting under his orders. He grew furious, and said, 'You are under Prince Pless's orders; you must go at 6 a.m. tomorrow.'

Here Louise called to Mr. Furley to hear how a Prussian officer could speak to an English lady, and Mr. Furley kindly stepped forward and said, 'Really, Dr. Pratt had better be spoken to. These ladies are under his command.' The officer pouted, and marched off to see Dr. Pratt. We heard he was a Prince Piegress, or some such name, and always disagreeable after dinner!

We did not start at six next morning, and things were not pleasant. An *aide-de-camp* brought word that our presence in the town was displeasing to the German authorities, and he requested we would not leave the hotel. This sort of polite imprisonment we quietly declined, and went out to the *château*. In the afternoon Colonel Loyd-Lindsay returned from Paris, accompanied by his valet, who was immediately fallen on by the curious, and closely cross-questioned.

Whether it is to him that sundry extraordinary tales of the interior of Paris are owing I cannot say; but we were irresistibly reminded of Mickey Free, in Lever's *Charles O'Malley* and the unlucky editor who tried to get the true history of the storming of Badajoz out of that mendacious individual. In short, he related such wonderful tales that the most daring war correspondent durst not transmit them to his editors.

The colonel requested to see us, and we humbly waited upon him. He spoke very graciously of our past services, and said he should be sorry to see us connected with a failure; that it was evident the Anglo-American Ambulance must go to pieces, and we had better return to

England 'to end the first act of the drama.' We were utterly astounded and replied nothing, and he continued: 'This is my advice to you—indeed, I may say even more.' At this crisis he pulled his moustache, and subsided into silence. We meekly asked how and why we should go home, as we had been distinctly ordered to keep with the ambulance by Captain Brackenbury, who alone on the Continent had power, according to his own account, to give us orders, and failing him, our commissions ordered us to obey Prince Pless, and his orders were distinctly that we should go to Orléans. He said nothing, only 'You had better leave tomorrow. You are not being treated as English ladies should be. How will you go?'

Now, I knew the colonel was going direct to St. Germain in his carriage, with only his valet, was to sleep there, and go on to Rouen next day. He was going to the very house we should have gone to, the lady being an old friend of Louise's; but I suggested that there was an omnibus went from St. Germain. We had no idea of going in that omnibus, but we wanted to see if he would send two Englishwomen, *alone and unescorted*, a three days' journey through a dangerous country, and through the lines of two armies, when he was going the same road himself. He said he could take us as far as St. Germain, where we should find the omnibus. We bowed ourselves out, determined not to be beholden to him for even a five miles' lift. We saw Dr. Pratt and Captain Furley about it, who procured us a carriage which cost us 4*l*.

Dr. Pratt was terribly cut up at being sent off to Orléans with very little money and still fewer stores. We said we had been attached to their ambulance for service by Captain Brackenbury, that we could not imagine we had been brought from Sedan to Versailles only to be sent back as useless, when so much work lay all around, and we were ready to go on. He said that it was evident, unless money could be obtained, the ambulance must go to pieces.

The English Society's agent, Captain Furley, could only give him 50*l*. Major de Havilland had very few stores in hand, Prince Pless had promised some certainly, and he had procured a waggon and two horses to take them on. But that if we would go to England and try to get the leave to enter Paris, through the interest of Count Bernstorff, Mr. Motley, and Lord Granville, we should do them real service. If we could get it, we could come back direct to Versailles, and send a special messenger on to Orléans to fetch up the ambulance, as we should have to enter by the way of Versailles.

I said, 'But if we cannot get the permission, what then?'

He said, 'That first and most of all; try for nothing till all chance of that has failed. If it is impossible, which I won't believe, get money and stores for us; all you can, from all quarters.' He went on to say, 'Unless we get help, we must break up. Loyd-Lindsay wanted us to do so here, but we would rather go on to Orléans, and if we must breakup do it there.' He added that a fortnight with those Germans would be quite enough, and if the ambulance was not permitted to pass into French lines in a body, that they could break up, get through one by one, and re-form at Tours. He implored us to do all we could, to write them up in the papers, to defend them if they were attacked. He told us how grieved he was that we had to go, even if it were on their service, and never by a single word implied that he dispensed with our services then or in the future.

He also gave us a written list with the names of all those employed in his ambulance, and requested us to apply to the British Society to take upon their staff those men who being Americans were borne at present only on the books of the French International.

We were to go to England to do his business and return when it was done, and of this all his staff were as well aware as we were. That evening we met Prince Pless on the stairs. He told us we were to go to Orléans with the ambulance; that we were sadly needed; that we should be received 'with open arms;' and he sent orders for every attention to be paid to us. It was a sad Sunday next day. We proposed starting at noon to pay a visit to Louise's friend at St. Germain. The ambulance was also preparing to move off to Orléans, and parting in such troubled times with friends is always sad and disheartening; but we were delayed, first by the necessity of getting a safe-conduct for the coachman and horses to come back, and next by the marching down the street of a large body of troops from the army around Metz. We could not break their lines, and had to wait.

All our old friends crowded round. Mr. Furley took charge of us to the last. Loyd-Lindsay was there, but he either overlooked us or thought he had been bored enough with our ambulance and us, for he did not even raise his gold-laced cap. Dr. Pratt asked us to walk aside with him. He reiterated his orders, and said he would write down a list of the stores he required, and we could supplement it with anything else we thought of. He fully authorised us to do that. I said when last in England I had seen the warehouse at the back of St. Martin's crowded with stores. They ought to be able to send any quantity.

There being no paper near, I handed him my passport, which was bound up with many vacant leaves, for visas, &c., and on one of these leaves he wrote what stores he wished for. I did not notice he had not signed it, nor, I dare say, did he think of that formality. When we left Sedan to ask for leave to go with his ambulance, he sent no written request for our services. He did not think, evidently, that the society's agents would distrust us, and when Mr. Capel remarked upon it I was somewhat surprised. As I have said, the request came by telegraph afterwards.

Louise asked him if he had written to his wife. He said, 'No; I am in such a state of worry and depression, I cannot. Go to her directly you get back, tell her so, and tell her all about us, and see if she cannot help you at the American Embassy. She knows some of the attaches; she must work for us, too, in aiding you.' He then wrote down her address, and requested us to telegraph or write any news, and to do all as quickly as possible, for their money was falling short. His last words were: 'Remember, first of all, leave to enter Paris; failing that, money and stores, to get out into French lines, and get our men put on the English staff.'

Thus, it is most clear to all we came back his authorised agents, and we were further assured, not only by himself but by all his staff, that they expected to see us back as soon as we had got one or other of what they required.

We shook hands; neither party could say goodbye. We did not dream how we should meet again. It was fortunate that at that instant, as we re-crossed the street to get into our carriage, a ludicrous circumstance diverted us. There stood the waggon and horses ready for Prince Pless's stores, and up came the messenger bringing them. It was not a princely gift. It did not cost much of the 20,000*l.* given only the day before to buy it. It consisted of two phials, each containing about a couple of ounces, one of opium and one of morphia, and a small box of quinine powders. As an able-bodied child of three would not have been inconvenienced by the weight, it is needless to remark that the waggon was discharged as useless.

At last we were off, the farewell being from all: 'It is not goodbye—*au revoir*,' and the final injunction: 'Write us up in the papers.' We had delayed too late to stay at Miss T——'s at St. Germain, very much to our disappointment, so we drove through to Mantes. Captain Furley had asked us to take back upon our box the coachman of the omnibus our ambulance had 'required' at Mantes, and to give him the advantage of our safe-conduct. Both he and the driver suffered dreadfully from fear of the Prussians, but no one interfered with us till we were far through St. Germain. The coachman had just turned round and exclaimed, 'We are saved;' when up rode a body of *Uhlans*. The officer presented himself at the carriage, and politely asked us whence we came and where we were going. We informed him, from Versailles to England, and produced our pass. He at first declined to look at it, seeing we were only two women; but we insisted upon it. He returned it with the politest of bows, remarked that he wished us a pleasant journey, but he was afraid it-was going to rain, and once more bowing rode off.

We never in any journey experienced the least trouble or delay, except such as was unavoidable from detention of trains and difficulty of finding means of carriage. From everyone, high and low, French and German, we received all the kindness and assistance possible. No disagreeable adventures ever marred those interesting drives through the invaded country. *Uhlan* and *franc-tireur* alike were guards and friends, not savage foes or impertinent enquirers. Whether this was owing to our diplomacy or the absence of the opposite sex, we know not; but the advice we should give, founded on practical experience, is: 'Ladies, when you travel abroad, especially in war, leave the men at home.'

If you have husbands, of course they must go with you, and it will be your bounden duty to look after them; but then domestic duties may probably keep you at home. It is only those who have none who should risk life and health amidst such scenes as it was our duty to go through; and then, with no baggage, a knowledge of the language, good temper and forbearance, energy and determination, there are no difficulties that any woman cannot get easily through. On the whole, we had every reason to congratulate ourselves that our gallant countryman had not offered us seats in his carriage or his valuable escort.

We reached England three days before he did, owing to his being detained at Havre by a storm in the Channel, which began to howl around our steamer as she dashed into Dover harbour, the last mail-boat that crossed for twenty-four hours. But this is somewhat anticipating our progress.

CHAPTER 20

The Battlefield at Home

Between St. Germain and Mantes, we halted at a little village, where the *curé*, whom we had seen on our way to Versailles, greeted us, condoled with us on our disappointment in not entering Paris, and chatted pleasantly whilst the horses were resting. He told us Gambetta had issued a proclamation calling on everybody to fight. Why did he not fight himself? Why did not Trochu fight his way out, instead of waiting for other people to fight their way in? 'But,' he added, 'this is the doctrine which is the ruin of France. This is the doctrine which prevents my writing proudly on my forehead the name of Frenchman; "*la doctrine des autres*," let others do this, let others do that. Why not do it themselves? It is so all through; the doctrine "*des autres*" is our ruin.' It was too true; we had seen it too often, that breaking down under pressure of circumstances, that helpless dependence on others in the hour of difficulty. Always '*les autres.*'

Apropos of this, he related a most amusing anecdote of the ladies of St. Germain. When the entrance of the king into that town was announced, these patriotic ladies held a meeting, and resolved, as they could not prevent his coming in, they would insult him when he did, and it was determined to spit upon him as he passed. The gentlemen, hearing of this, consulted together how to prevent so foolish a proceeding, and arriving at the place of meeting, one deputed by the rest addressed the ladies in a most pathetic speech, declaring that they, the cherished and beloved, should not incur the risk of savage punishment for such a deed, for their husbands, fathers, and brothers, would take upon themselves the act and its consequences, and he, the speaker, would be the first to insult the invader in the proposed manner, even if he perished in the attempt

At this one of the ladies rushed forward, exclaiming, 'Not you, my husband, not you; let some other do it. *C'est pour un autre.*' Out stepped, another volunteer, but again his loving wife forbade him: 'Not you, my cherished, not you; *un autre!*' till the plan was given up by universal consent, and the king made his entry without meeting with any insult from '*les autres.*'

We slept at Mantes. Our host was inconsolable for the loss of his omnibus, and would not believe in its possible restoration after the war. One of our surgeons had left his watch there, and we claimed it. Mine host refused to part with it, alleging that three sacks, which had contained forage, had not been returned with the rest. We remonstrated that the sacks were worthless and the watch valuable; all in vain. We therefore walked off to find the *maire*, who was sitting in council as to the means of defending the place. Things were changed since we had passed; it was now full of *francs-tireurs* and *Gardes Mobiles*. The *maire* most politely left the Committee of Defence and came with us to the innkeeper. A long discussion ensued; the value of the sacks was declared to be six *francs* and a half.

The *maire* justly represented that, if the Prussians came by that way, three *francs* and a half would by no means represent his probable losses. At last, failing to convince the good man that he had no reason to complain in such times of the loss of three old sacks, and no right to detain Dr. May's watch for a debt of Captain F——'s, he gave it up, and said, 'Well, *Monsieur*, your conduct is inexplicable and unjustifiable towards strangers, who have done so much for our wounded; but it shall not be the cause of detention to these amiable ladies. They shall have the watch, and the commune will pay you the three *francs* and a half.' Thus all was pacifically settled, and we left Mantes bearing off the missing property. We earnestly hope that when the Prussians did come—for come they did, in spite of the mayor and the Committee of Defence—and when the heavy requisitions were made on the town, and the officers ate and drank of mine host's best, and ignored his bill, that he was struck with a sense of remorse for the little sum so unjustly and pertinaciously claimed, and felt it a righteous retribution.

We lunched at Vernon, and mourned over the destruction of the splendid railway-bridge. It took three years to build, three hours to destroy, and it was such useless destruction, for the Prussians walked over Normandy and into Rouen in utter disregard of broken bridges and cut-up roads. Just beyond Vernon we came to a specimen of this fact.

Across the broad road was a large barricade, with a deep trench in front; only one small passage was left at the side for traffic, and that was blocked up by an overturned cart. *Francs-tireurs* were ambushed in the wood and farm buildings at the side. But whilst we were wondering how to pass, a boy in a country blouse, but with a pair of military trousers, suddenly appeared, and lifted the cart aside. We thanked him and passed on, and that barricade was never used. But the adventures and misfortunes of the War Office Ambulance, on the same road, proved the truth of what we were led to suspect—that they were expected, and would not pass as scot-free as we did. The mark of suspicion was on them. They were going to Versailles to work in German lines, and the country people bore them no goodwill.

We reached St. Pierre-au-Louviers, and our old hostess received us with open arms; but the quiet village was changed now. A troop of mounted *gendarmes* were halting there. The roads were being barricaded, the bridge over the Seine mined, and the landlady's son had been called out in the last reserve. His state of utter despair was ludicrous. He put every dish he did not forget on the table with a deep sigh, and assured us he was quite 'discomposed.' His mother came in, and, pointing to him, begged us to observe what a hero he looked. 'Regard him, then, ladies; has he not the air of a grand captain?' We laughed and sympathised; it was all we could do.

At the station we found a guard of French soldiers of the line, armed, the first we had seen for many a long day. They all came forward to help us, and we were escorted into the train by a dear old sergeant, who seemed to think it his duty to take care of us. We reached Rouen that night, and found the Hôtel d'Angleterre in possession of the War Office Ambulance. The chiefs were dining in a private room, and the *infirmiers* and grooms in the *salle-à-manger*. They had just finished, and we were very glad, as they were a noisy lot. We sent off a telegram for one of the London papers, and, finding it was for one of French sympathies, it reached safely. We sent to tell Lord Bury we were there, just arrived from Versailles; and as I had known him when he was but a little boy, and we were from the same county, I thought he might be glad to see us, and we had several valuable hints we could have given him.

However, the *garçon* returned, and said, 'my lord was at dinner;' and though we did not leave till ten or eleven next day, he never asked to see us, so our information remained untold. We had no wish to intrude upon him, but it was a pity; for had they known, as we did, the feeling up the road, they would not have risked going on, as they did. Mr. Thomas, in a letter dated November 17, and published in the '*Times*,' gives an account of the loss of waggons, and stores, on that very route, three weeks later, intended for their use at Versailles; and all along, from the first report of their coming, the very fact of so large an ambulance going into German lines was a cause of suspicion and distrust among the country people. Even on this occasion we should not have been surprised to hear they had lost their horses.

The *francs-tireurs* were on the sharp look-out for these at least, and we had been asked at Mantes, Vernon, and St. Pierre-au-Louviers when they were coming. We did not know. We had not even heard if the ambulance had left England, only that it was expected at Versailles, so we were in ignorance; and, had we known, we assuredly should not have betrayed our countrymen. But we were only women, we were supposed to be friendly, and we picked up a good deal as we came along. Whatever we knew or did not know, we could not converse upon it with the class of men, however respectable, who sat round the long table of the Hôtel d'Angleterre, and our attempt to see the chief failed.

Failing Lord Bury, we tried to see Dr. Guy. He was at breakfast, and we were told could not be disturbed; so, we felt we had done our duty. We could not lose the train, and we hoped they could take care of themselves; but we did hear in London they had lost their horses on that very journey, and we simply remarked, 'We could have told them so.'

From Rouen to Amiens and Calais all was plain sailing, and we crossed by the night boat, had a very bad passage, and reached London, several hours late, on the 19th of October. All that day, after we recovered from the effects of our voyage, which was not till late, we passed in going to see Mrs. Pratt and Mr. Motley. This eminent statesman received us with his own peculiar courtesy, and promised to aid us by himself speaking to Count Bernstorff, begging us to call there the next morning. We saw the principal members of the Ladies' Committee for the Relief of French Distress.

All gave us hearty welcome and every help in their power. Till we had seen what chance there was of obtaining the desired leave, we had nothing to ask from any committee, for money and stores awaited us in Paris. However, next day we communicated with Messrs. Piesse and Lubin and Mr. Rimmel, the active members of two French committees, as to what aid they could give, if required. Were we to try and express our sense of all the kindness we received, we should fail. Only those working as hard as we were know what a blessing a little sympathy is.

We then called at the Prussian Embassy. Mr. Motley was there; but no words of ours are needed to prove how good and true and kind, to friend and foe alike, are Count and Countess Bernstorff. The count said Mr. Motley had well pleaded our cause, and he would do what he could. Quite delighted at this prospect of success, and the warm interest taken in the matter by Mr. Motley and Count Bernstorff, we drove off to a telegraph office, were assured we could telegraph to Orléans, through the British Embassy at Tours, and accordingly sent one off, pleasing ourselves with the idea what a relief it would be to Dr. Pratt. In this very telegram, too, we told him we had a hope of money and stores, if this failed.

Thus, no step of our progress was intentionally concealed from him, and we knew we had his sanction to use our own judgment in all we did. We wrote that night also to him and to the secretary of our British Committee, to say we had been detained too late that day to call, as we had hoped to do, in St. Martin's Place, but should be there next morning. I got a private note from one of the officials begging me to do so, as they were affronted, we had not been there before, and an anonymous scrap also from the office, begging me 'to go there directly, there was something up.' What, we could not imagine; and next day, accompanied by the Rev. Hubert MacLaughlin, Louise's father, we went down.

Captain Burgess received us with a warm welcome, and expressed no surprise we had not been there before. At this time Colonel Loyd-Lindsay had not returned. I told Captain Burgess what our business in London was, and what steps we had taken-this in public, before several of the clerks, and we both also said we would not take up their time, as we had nothing to ask till we received a reply as to Paris. He said, 'They won't let you go in.' We said, 'Then we will come and bother you for money and stores.' His answer was, 'I will do what I can for you,' and he himself was most friendly.

I also gave him Dr. Pratt's list of the ambulance, and begged him to submit that request to the committee. He said he would, but that he did not think they would take those gentlemen upon their staff. On this occasion, too, we saw several of the ladies, wearing gold lockets with a white enamel shield and a Red Cross upon them, and, to our surprise, were each presented with one. We have heard since that some of those who had picked *charpie* had silver medals with a Red Cross sent to them, a distinction in this case somewhat cheaply earned.

Next day I sent for some money (33*l.*) which the committee owed me, with a full account of how it had been expended. I was answered that the account should be submitted to the committee, and in the evening came a letter to say it was correct, and how did I wish the money to be paid? As we were going to see the committee again, I waited to receive it till I did so. The following evening came a letter from Countess Bernstorff, saying that the National Society did not express the wish we should enter Paris, and therefore, as it was an application that could only be made under special circumstances, in this instance it could not be done; but she told us further that the Bishop of Orléans had applied for assistance, and we should find 'full scope there for our devotion to the sick and wounded.'

Nothing could be more graceful and generous than this asking help for a French bishop. Now it became our duty to seek for money and stores, and Louise and myself went down to St. Martin's Lane. Captain Burgess was there, so were Lord Shaftesbury and Colonel Loyd-Lindsay; but though we particularly asked to see them, Captain Burgess did not attempt even to mention the fact of our presence there to them, and Colonel Loyd Lindsay brushed against us as he passed out of the room without taking the slightest notice of us. I asked first for my money; but the account had got into some pigeon-hole, and the affair could not be settled then. We asked for assistance for Dr. Pratt, and Captain Burgess replied, 'It is utterly useless; the Committee will not give it.'

I asked why? what had the ambulance done that the society would not support it? Captain Burgess replied, 'Simply, they have struck the American Ambulance off the list of those they intend to supplement.' Louise asked why they had done this? Captain Burgess answered, 'Oh! there is no reason, only they cannot support all. They have a right to choose which they will support, and as regards the request to put their men on our list, they will not do it.'

I said, 'Have you asked them?'

He replied, 'Yes, and they have refused.'

I said, 'At least, you will give them some stores. Here is the list of those which Dr. Pratt requested me to ask for,' showing him my pocket book.

He said, 'We are not aware you are authorised to act for Dr. Pratt.'

I was utterly astounded, and so was Louise, and we said, 'Do you think we should come here and say so, if we were not authorised?'

Captain Burgess said, 'But we don't officially know you are in London!'

This was startling. Can anybody write an essay on how to make your presence officially known, except by going down to an office in the very dress we had been ordered to wear, and announcing ourselves as come to see the committee on business, and having already had official communications addressed to my lodgings in London as regarded the debt they owed me. I laughed and said, 'Well, here we are, and here is the list;' and I explained how and when it had been given me. He looked at it and said, 'How do we know this is Dr. Pratt's handwriting?' I answered, 'Look at the page by the side of the list. There is his wife's address in London, written in the same hand.'

Captain Burgess said again, 'But we don't know that it is any of it in his handwriting.' Then indeed, I confess, my blood was up. I had worked with Captain Burgess and Captain Furley in getting up the Society before Colonel Loyd-Lindsay joined it. We had both served them faithfully, and this was a cruel insult. I said, 'Good heavens! Captain Burgess, do you mean to say we should come here asking for money under false pretences, with a forged list of stores?' He made no answer. I took my brassard out of my pocket and said, 'Take back this brassard, which has never been a protection or an honour, for we were obliged to leave it off at Versailles. If I could do this thing, I am not worthy to work under your Society. If you have accused me falsely, you are not worthy I should work under you.'

He refused to take it, saying, 'Oh, that is all nonsense.'

Angry as I was, I would not lose a chance of helping our ambulance, and I said, 'If you doubt me, will you give Dr. Pratt something if he comes himself to ask for it. Captain Burgess?'

'Not even if he comes himself,' he answered.

I remarked, 'Well, it is all very extraordinary. Will you submit it to the committee, at least?'

He said, 'Yes, I will; but it will be of no use.'

I said, 'I shall call tomorrow for an answer;' and we left, feeling we had been treated in a most unworthy way, grumbling about red tape and the state of things in general of the committee, as women will, especially when chafing under such absurd and uncalled-for injustice.

But kinder friends, more trusting hearts, awaited us. The good people of Putney gave us all the stores they had collected since they had sent out to Sedan, and all the balance of the money in hand, 40*l*.—this for the use of any ambulance we might work with, as they had heard of such quantities of stores getting ruined by damp in the vaults of St. Martin's Church, such waste of money in St. Martin's Place, that they preferred giving to those who would put to practical and instant use all that was sent.

From the committee in Red Lion Square, from Mr. Von Glehn in the City, from the Hon. Miss Rushout of Onslow Square, from Lady

Theodore Grosvenor, from the ample stores of Messrs. Piesse and Lubin, from Mr. Edward Walford, and the local committee at Hampstead, came help in new and valuable clothing, lint, wadding, and medicines; 30*l.* of the Putney money we spent in medical necessaries; and Louise's experience in hospital training, the judicious selection she made, and the trouble she took in going to purchase them from the Civil Service Stores in the City at less than half-price, placed us in possession of what would have cost the committee probably something like 100*l.* Messrs. Piesse and Lubin gave us a case of amputation instruments especially for the Anglo American Ambulance, the only thing so especially given for them, except the splendid donation of the French Committee in the City, the secretary of which is M. Pierrard, who gave 200*l.* for the Anglo-Americans, solely on condition that it should be used for French wounded alone, and through the kind interest and introduction of M. Eugene Rimmel.

We wrote an appeal to the public for assistance, as we had been requested, but deferred inserting it till we had received the National Society's decided reply. We worked hard all day, and next morning went for the committee's answer. Captain Burgess said, 'It has not come on for consideration yet.' I said we had already received promises of help, and we should start for Orléans as soon as possible. That we were also requested to form an ambulance near Angers, but of course should keep our promise, and take to Dr. Pratt whatever we could procure for him. We both added that we presumed that, as Captain Brackenbury had attached us for service to them, the committee would sanction our continuing to work with them. Captain Burgess said, 'Oh yes, of course; I don't see why not.'

I said, 'You will kindly, then, see for our free passes to Dover.'

He said, 'You shall have them. When do you think of going?'

Louise answered, 'As soon as we collect our bales and boxes and get off. There is no time to lose. There will be hot fighting round Orléans.'

I said, 'I'll send for my money.'

Captain Burgess replied, 'Oh, that account has passed the committee; you shall have it,' and we left.

That evening I received a letter saying the committee declined to support the ambulance. I wrote a remonstrance on the injustice of this, and begged them to reconsider their decision before I appealed to the public. The answer to this was a letter dismissing me from the society, signed by Captain Burgess, and saying, 'I am directed by the committee to request you will consider yourself as released from your allegiance to the society;' no reason being given. This I declined, as he had refused to accept my resignation. Louise then wrote and asked for her free pass to Dover, and she got an answer, saying it was not necessary for her to proceed in the society's service again abroad. Now, we had signed a formidable legal document by which our services were engaged for the whole of the war, our daily personal expenses being paid, so that we were advised that neither party could dissolve the engagement without mutual consent. I then received a letter more civilly worded, saying, 'they were not prepared to discuss the legal terms of their contract; they would pay the money I was owed when it was sent for;' and we hoped the matter was ended.

On the 2nd of November, Captain MacLaughlin, R.A., called to say we were about to start, and to try and make some terms with them. He took with him the copy of the appeal about to be inserted in the papers, and urged them to send a sum of money for the ambulance, and so end the discussion. By this time Mrs. Pratt had identified her husband's handwriting, and acknowledged it, by bringing us to take to him, one article he had asked for on the list, a large American flag. So, there could be no pretext for disavowing it. All was in vain, and Captain MacLaughlin returned, saying that they were obstinately determined to refuse.

We wrote to the President, the Prince of Wales, explaining the position of affairs—a letter which we heard long afterwards was forwarded at his desire to the committee—and having sent off the appeal to be inserted in the papers, we prepared for our start. We bought a large Union Jack—how useful it was afterwards the sequel will show. The committee would not even give us that, and on the 3rd of November all was ready; the heavy baggage, twenty-three bales and boxes, at Charing Cross, ready to go by the 6 p.m. train, and our farewells said to all who had so nobly aided our struggle for the ambulance.

At 1 p.m., having no time to go myself, I sent Mr. Francis Hartley for my money, with a properly-signed receipt for the committee. He was detained three hours, and at 4 p.m. returned with no money, but a note from Colonel Loyd-Lindsay himself, in part of which he said, 'If you will only give me your assurance that you are not going to Orléans to join the Anglo-American Ambulance, I will submit your letter to the committee'—what letter I know not, as every letter I had written had been addressed to the committee, and surely should have been submitted to them before any replies were sent. My account had passed and the order had been given to pay me, so it could not be that.

It must have been the final remonstrance I wrote against our being virtually accused of having asked for money under false pretences. This was addressed, as I have said, to the committee, and should have been laid before them, without trying to make me give any promise or enter into any arrangement with the chairman.

I sent Mr. Francis Hartley again to ask for my money. The Rev. Randolph MacLaughlin went with him, and we drove to the Charing Cross Station to register our baggage. The gentlemen came back; they could not get the money, and at 5.30 p.m. I went myself with Mr. MacLaughlin. I saw Captain Burgess. He said it was too late; Colonel Loyd-Lindsay was gone, and had left no cheque. At that instant I caught sight of the colonel going down a staircase. I ran after him; but he was too quick for me, and vanished. I told Captain Burgess I thought they had all behaved very badly, but I shook hands with him, and said I knew and felt we were going to do better work than ever we had done or could do under them; and so, we parted.

I saved the train by a few minutes, and left injunctions with Mr. Hartley to get the money and send it after me to Tours. What passed after we left seems to be that they gave endless trouble, and refused to pay the money unless my solicitor would give them an acquittance for anything else they might owe me. This he was not empowered to do, and represented that it had nothing to do with the debt I claimed. Captain Burgess spoke very hastily on several occasions to Mr. Francis Hartley, so much so that at last my solicitor went himself, and in Captain Burgess's presence told Colonel Loyd-Lindsay that Mr. Hartley was a young gentleman of as good birth and education as any of them then there, and that he had been treated with 'very scant courtesy.' Colonel Loyd-Lindsay was civil, and said he was sure Captain Burgess did not mean to be insulting, and he had a cheque ready for my solicitor. It is a pity it was not given without all this trouble.

Captain Burgess excused himself by saying he had only received 'a vague request for payment.' This, after his own statement that the accounts had passed the committee, and having had a stamped receipt sent by the hand of an articled clerk, with written authority to receive the sum for me, was but a poor excuse. However, there that matter ended, though the delay rendered the money useless to me till after the armistice was declared, and cost me a perilous journey to Bourges to try and cash the cheque which was sent about a fortnight after I reached Orléans.

CHAPTER 21

The Army of the Loire

The train rushed out of Charing Cross Station; the glaring lights faded into darkness. We were off to the help of those who so sorely needed it, alone and unaided, save by God and our own hearts. No doubt of success crossed our minds. We went in a cause too sacred for human prejudice and error to risk its failure, and, cost what it might, we resolved to reach Orléans with the money and stores. How thankful we dreamed they would be to see us-those who had sent us for the help we were bringing. They could leave the German lines; they could go where their own society sent them. The British National Society had cast them off. Well, we could do without that Society now; and so, in simple truth and honour, we went back to the friends we had left on that sad day at Versailles.

The tide was so low when we reached Calais that the heavy baggage could not be landed, and we had to wait till noon. We procured a sealed waggon, registered the baggage straight through to Rouen, and met with the greatest kindness and consideration from everyone. We arrived at Rouen at 6 p.m., and leaving our waggon at the station, drove to the Hôtel d'Angleterre, and were warmly welcomed. We stumbled over two, triangular tin boxes in the hall, and on them read the names of two English military officers. It turned out they were military commissioners sent out to join the Army of the Loire, and going on as we were next day, as far as they could—the termination of all journeys in those times.

We had just read a very amusing article in one of the daily papers, entitled 'In search of the Army of the Loire,' or something very like it; and we wondered if these gentlemen would be more fortunate than the unlucky special correspondent. All the way from Calais we had heard of the Army of the North, but where was the Army of the Loire? We had seen the railway stations fortified, the walls of the engine-houses crenelled for musketry, and the windows of the waiting-rooms tightly dosed up with planks; everywhere men drilling, and beginning to clothe themselves in military costume. Some had caps, some belts, some red stripes down their trousers; but everyone had something to show he was going to be a soldier. On every blank wall, in town and village, were placards calling the people to rise *en masse* and drive out 'the invading hordes of the Goths.' Rouen was no exception to this, but we noticed a vast improvement in the National Guards and Mobiles. One fortnight had given them much of the appearance of regular troops, and all were now armed.

Our heavy baggage, about four thousand pounds' weight, was brought across the city in a two-horse waggon, and safely got into the train. We procured another sealed waggon, and registered it through to Tours. As far as Rouen the baggage had come free, but here we found we must pay for it; but only quarter tariff, if we could procure an order from the office of the French International Society. It was too late to do that, and the station-master most kindly gave us a little note to pass the baggage on to Tours, and pay there when we had got an order.

We reached Le Mans very late at night, the detentions on the road being numerous. It was very quiet and silent; not a vestige of even a sentinel to be seen, but at daybreak drums and trumpets announced the presence of soldiers. We looked out; the scene was most picturesque. Men in every variety of uniform were crowding the streets, conspicuous among them the grey and red of the pontifical *Zouaves*. It was Sunday; but there was no regular church parade. The cathedral, however, was full of kneeling worshippers, soldiers greatly predominating; and there the pontifical *Zouave* and the Garibaldian volunteer, the Breton peasant and the long-descended *franc-tireur* captain of La Vendee, prayed side by side for their well-beloved and suffering France.

On the boulevard by the cathedral we met a body of small, active men, with bronzed complexions and brown cloth blouses, fastened in round the waist by a strong untanned leather belt. They wrapped their short-hooded capes about them, and shivered in the faint winter sunlight. I asked them where they came from, and they told me from Algiers, from the French colonies there, to fight for the dear mother country. 'We have crossed the sea, *Madame*,' said one of their sergeants, 'we have marched on foot from Marseilles, and we are going to Berlin.' He said it so gravely and simply that it was quite touching. The sons of these Algerian farmers may some day pass through Le Mans to

Berlin; but of these poor fellows too many fill soldiers' graves on the battlefields of the Loire.

But strange and most appropriate was the parade-ground of the *francs-tireurs* of Cathelineau. It was on the old Place Vianme. There, where Cathelineau fell in the moment of victory, fighting for the Bourbons; there, where his Vendeans, despairing and dismayed at their leader's fall, retreated from the position they had won, the grandson of the dead hero, the General Cathelineau of today, mustered around him the descendants of the men who had fought and fell, on that very spot, on that fatal day, to march again against a foe. The *fleur-de-lis*, and the white cockade, were replaced by the tricolour, but the enemy now was a foreign invader, and royalist and republican could fight side by side in this common cause.

Their dress was perfect for irregular troops. The men wore black cloth tunics and trousers bound with blue, blue scarfs around the waist, and black slouching hats, with a raven's plume fastened by a small tricolour cockade. The officers wore their scarfs over the shoulder, and had high boots and black gauntlet gloves. The rank was marked by a small gold star, embroidered on the sleeve, one, two, or three, as depended on the rank. Both officers and men were of a very superior class.

They were accompanied by a small, well organised regimental ambulance, under the management of Madame Cathelineau. She had a husband and two sons in the corps, and many, very many, friends and neighbours, and with two other Vendean ladies she followed the regiment in a carriage, accompanied by a couple of light store-waggons, to be at hand to nurse the wounded of the corps, in case of need. It was quite a model little ambulance, just what an ambulance should be—the nucleus of work able to be expanded to any extent that occasion may require.

One thing struck us as peculiar and beautiful—the deeply religious tone of the whole corps. English people, not considering the intense innate faith of the Breton nature in 'things unseen,' might have considered it superstitious to wear, as they all did, a crimson heart, embroidered on black cloth, and attached to the tunic, with the words written below it, '*Arrête! le coeur de Jésus est ici.*' Perhaps it was so; but the idea that the presence of the Saviour in the heart of the soldier would turn aside the balls and be his shield in the hour of danger is, after all, a very beautiful one, and that was but the outward expression of that ideal. Every good man has the same belief in Divine protection; and this was only their simple way of evidencing their trust in Him who 'could cover their head in the day of battle.'

Interesting as Le Mans was, we could not linger there, and that afternoon reached Tours. Here we had to halt, waiting for the letters of credit which were to meet us there. Besides, the railroad only 'circulated,' as the French call going on a straight road, as far as Blois, and how to proceed was a difficulty; for beyond were the Prussians, and the proprietors of horses and waggons did not care to take them into German lines, at the risk of having them 'required' for the service of the German Army.

We decided, however, that we would go to Blois, leave our baggage there, and get on into Orléans ourselves. As far as the German outposts at Beaugency we could get some sort of conveyance, and then there would be a walk of nine miles. This could be done in three or four hours. We should find the Anglo-American Ambulance there, and their waggons could come up to Blois for the stores. This plan was, however, disarranged by rumours of fighting round Orléans. If this were true, and the Germans pushed on to Blois, the baggage would not be safe there during the combat. We would wait a day and see. All that day came different rumours of victory and defeat, but night closed in without any decided intelligence.

Next morning, however, a general air of hilarity pervaded high and low. Bavarian and Prussian prisoners were brought in, and everyone started up from the *table d'hôte* breakfast to look at such an unaccustomed sight. At last came the despatch affixed to the walls and read by joyous crowds. Von der Tann had been defeated with loss and the French were in Orléans, the first to enter being part of the Cathelineau corps which had preceded the division we saw at Le Mans to the front. The Army of the Loire was found, and its first public appearance had been a glorious success.

Tours was a gay city that day. The Rue Royale was a mass of soldiers of the line. *Gardes Mobiles* and *francs-tireurs* all mixed together. Thousands passed up and down it with a light step and a cheerful air. Victory had dawned at last upon the arms of France. As I watched the thronging multitude, I regretted the strictly military costume of our volunteers. These men were so simply and cheaply dressed; their tunics sat so loosely and easily; all was for service, not show. Yet many preserved some trace of the peculiar costume of their various provinces. The *francs-tireurs* from the Pyrenees wore the flat woollen *berretta* and white tassel still used by the peasantry there; and the men from Brittany and La Vendée had the half-Tyrolese hat and cock's plume of their native woodland country. One corps was dressed in black velvet, with a violet scarf round the waist.

We derived much amusement from hearing that a friend had been offered some stray boxes belonging to the British National Society. This had been our lot. We might have accumulated a good deal of baggage at various stations all along the road from Calais to Le Mans, which was lying about at the various railroad stations. A good deal of it was addressed to a Colonel Cox. I wonder if he ever got it. One box at Le Mans looked most tempting. It seemed to be a case of instruments, and we had none for ourselves.

At Vernon some baggage, sent there *en route* to Versailles, had been burned when the Prussians made their first raid upon the town, and the station caught fire; and really it would hardly have been a sin, on the speculation that some such event might occur here before the colonel claimed his box—and it had been lying there a long time—to have *borrowed* it or 'required' it till the end of the war. But we left it there, and only hope all the stray packages got somewhere at last where their contents would be useful.

Next day we went on to Blois; our baggage was to follow by the first train that came through. M. de Villeneuve, of the French International, had been himself to Orléans, and ascertained that the traffic on the line would be resumed as soon as the bridge at Beaugency was repaired, and the workmen were there already, so that we should get it into Orléans as soon as if we took it on by road. Blois was quiet; neither French nor German armies had passed there.

It was very interesting to see the grand old castle prepared to receive the wounded. It could accommodate 600. In the great Council Hall there were 80 beds, but at present all were empty. At Tours we had also seen the old castle of Plessis-le-Tours making ready for an ambulance. It was not only that they had space in these places for wounded, but it was supposed to be a means of securing them from occupation by the Germans. In many instances it failed, but the Château de Blois does not appear to have been suffered, and Plessis-le-Tours was but an empty, half-ruined, half restored house.

It was only on the afternoon of the next day that trains began to run through to Orléans. The first was a special, containing M. Gambetta and two or three of his ministers; the second, a few hours later, a train of ammunition and forage; but there was no hope of passenger trains for several days. We had made acquaintance, fortunately, with a very civil *intendant militaire*, whose duty it was to arrange the military traffic, and he, when we had explained our great wish to get into Orléans, said at once that being on such an errand gave us the full right to go on, if possible, and he would apply to the station master to put on one passenger-carriage. The station-master refused; nothing would induce him to help anybody in any way. The *intendant* had no power to force him to give us the accommodation of a carriage, but took down his name, to make a formal complaint of his conduct to the directors, and himself helped to get us into a baggage-waggon, which was the best thing he could do for us.

A wounded officer going to an ambulance at Orléans, a surgeon on the way to join his regiment, and two or three workmen, who got out at various places on the line, composed the party. When we came near Beaugency the guard showed us a ruined windmill. The story of it was that it had been used as a signal-post by the Prussians; the turning of the mill-sails one way warned their outposts of the presence of the French in force, whilst when they turned the other it was safe for the *Uhlans* to advance.

A party of ingenious *francs-tireurs*, perceiving some connection between the action of the mill-sails and that of the Prussian cavalry, took possession of the mill, found that the millers were Prussian soldiers, and having dispossessed them of their situations (how, the relater knew not, whether as prisoners or dead), they resolved to try the effect of working the mill-sails their own way. They turned them in the direction that betokened safety, and a cavalry picquet of some forty or fifty White Cuirassiers came riding up the road. A volley was fired from behind the hedges which bordered the way, with such fatal precision that they left twenty-one dead on the spot.

The bridge over which we passed, by a temporary and apparently not very safe wooden flooring, had been completely destroyed; the centre arch had been blown up and left a yawning chasm, rather terrible to look at from the frail platform over which we were passing. The peasants pointed out as we went on to Meung, or more properly Mehun-sur-Loire, the distant country where far away on our left the battle had been fought at 'a village called Coulmiers.' We did not think then how that name would represent the solitary great victory of France. All was hope and exultation. The Army of the Loire was in Orléans. Had we not seen its divisions at Le Mans and Tours, all well-armed, all ready to fight to the death for France? A few days more, and they would advance on Paris. There would be a grand sortie, and Paris would be relieved before that *coquin* 'Frederick Charles' could arrive;

and if he did, so much the better—he would be caught between two armies and ground to powder. So, they talked on, full of hope and confidence in the victorious army of the Loire.

Orléans was reached at last. Our guard refused to accept even a couple of *francs* for all his civility, and ordered one of the luggage-van attendants to take ourselves and our bags to the best hotel. We had to walk through the station, which, during the German occupation, had been used as a guard-house and ambulance. Very dirty and miserable it must have been. It had been occupied for German wounded from the first battles of October 11th and 12th, when Orléans was taken by the Germans, and now the French authorities had ordered their evacuation to some place in the town, as they intended to restore the station to its original purpose.

As we came out on the boulevard beyond, we met Dr. Tilghman, one of our surgeons. He gave us a warm welcome, said he had got the telegram we had sent from Blois, but had no idea we could get through that day; that they had had the station as an ambulance, and very rough work it had been, but that they had got a house for sixty wounded, all that were left to them then, and that Dr. Pratt had gone to England for money and stores, everything being exhausted. In the Rue Bannière, the High Street of Orléans, we met two more of our friends, and they accompanied us in search of rooms, which we at last found in the Hôtel d'Orléans.

CHAPTER 22

The Only Victory

The morning of the 12th November was a bright sunny day. The Orléans world was abroad in gay costume. The bells of the cathedral, silenced since the Germans entered the city, rang out a gay carillon, and scarlet *kepis* and trousers, gold epaulettes and bright blue overcoats, with a little dandy hood, were flashing about in all directions. At last we had found the headquarters of the Army of the Loire. The statue of Jeanne d'Arc, in the Place Martroi, was hung with wreaths of flowers and *immortelles*, and a crown of crystal beads was placed on her head; but, having been somewhat swept aside, probably by the wind, it hung slanting over one eye, and gave the 'Immortal Maid' a decidedly dissipated appearance.

It was our first day amongst the French Army, and the cheerfulness of all around us, the quick, active step of the soldiery, and courteous manners, were quite refreshing. Good M. and Madame Pillion, the landlord and landlady; made us as comfortable as the crowded state of the hotel would permit, and from one or two of our ambulance we heard how sudden and unexpected had been the entry of the French. The gentlemen were not over charmed; they had been most kindly received by the German officials, had been hand in glove with the Bavarian officers, and gave us glowing accounts of the splendid house on the Quai du Chatelet, which had been allotted to them, and the magnificent requisitions of food and wine and all luxuries which had been granted them.

We rather wondered, now the French had come back, if the owners of the house would not return too; and then what would become of the splendid quarters? Also, we thought they had got Germanised, for they had adopted white *kepis* bound with black—the Prussian colours, which I cannot say I liked so well as the blue cap and Red

Cross of yore. They had been requested to wear no brassards, as the Prussians did not like them. They had not seen the battle, but how the retaking of Orléans was effected was, as they said, a very easily understood thing.

On the 8th of November the Germans discovered the main body of the Army of the Loire in the neighbourhood of Vendôme. Their own force at Orléans was weakened by the detaching of General von Wittich and 15,000 men to occupy Châteaudun and Chartres, and General Von der Tann found himself in a dangerous position. He sent the baggage to the rear on the Paris road, and marched out to meet the advancing enemy. Next day, the 9th, the battle began near Coulmiers. It was a place of good omen for the French, for there 'the Maid' defeated our English troops, commanded by Sir John Falstaff. The battle lasted all day, the French marine infantry and artillery particularly distinguishing themselves. At dusk the Germans retreated towards Artenay, on the Paris road, which they reached next morning, and were there joined by General von Wittich and a body of Bavarian cavalry who had been left in Orléans.

The French rested for the night on the field they had won, not knowing that Orléans was evacuated. On the morning of the 12th Cathelineau and his corps of *francs-tireurs* pushed on up to the gates, or rather entrance, of Orléans. To their surprise, no opposition met them. The German sentinels had been posted as usual the evening before, and were quite as much astonished to see the French as the French were not to see the Germans. Of course, they were all taken prisoners, and Cathelineau took possession of the city. During the morning the rest of the French Army marched in. Then, during that day, was the opportunity to have pushed forward and cut a road through Von der Tann's broken and dispirited army to Paris.

One hundred and forty-two German officers fell at Coulmiers, dead or wounded. From this their loss may be judged. They assert it to have been only 700 killed and wounded, but more, far more, than that number were buried, and still more brought into the ambulances of Orléans. The burying parties affirm that they interred four Germans for every Frenchman, and the French losses were severe—2,000 hors de combat by their own account.

On the 11th the Germans further retreated to Toury and the French advanced to Artenay, too late, for reinforcements were rapidly coming up, and the German Army withdrew to Epernon, about thirty miles from Versailles, leaving the French in quiet possession of Orléans and its immediate neighbourhood. Before quitting this subject we may remark that in a letter in the '*Times*,' dated from Tours, November 18, and called Central France, the writer says of the Germans, as regards their losses in this battle, that there is evidently concealment on their side, and that not more than 100 dead bodies were found on the field.

He did not know, as we knew and proved afterwards, that large numbers of dead were burned in the lonely farms around, and not only then, but in the later battles of the first week in December. In Orléans, over 1,000 German wounded were left in their military ambulances, so utterly deserted that for twenty-four hours no one went near them, not being aware that surgeons, *infirmiers*, and all, had gone. It was the compassionate French people who, discovering this, gave notice of it to their parish priests, and it being brought to the bishop, he ordered the Mother of the Novices in the Convent of St. Aignan, Mère Thérèse de la Croix, to go round herself, and make arrangements for the nursing of every one of these deserted ambulances.

In one the meat for the soup was found ready chopped, but the fire was unlighted, the attendants all gone, and the hundred poor fellows left to the chance of discovery by some good Samaritan. Long before night French Sisters and French civil surgeons were giving the kindest care to their helpless enemies—enemies no longer now wounded, and left to their mercy.

But one pretty little romantic incident may please some of our readers. A young Bavarian officer had been quartered in a distinguished French family, and there, in spite of their different nationalities, 'love was still the lord of all.' He left with his regiment to fight at Coulmiers. When all was lost, and it seemed too probable that, in the chance of war, he might never see Orléans again till peace was declared, if his life were spared so long, he obtained a few hours' leave, and rushed back to bid his lady-love farewell. He lingered, as lovers will, and was made prisoner by the French. He was sent to Pau, and we give the sequel here. When peace was declared, and he was free, the faithful soldier came back to Orléans, and his fidelity met its reward. The marriage has by this time been celebrated, and even the Orleanais, bitterly as they object to intermarriages with the enemy, can but smile and say, after all, 'He is only a Bavarian, and he loved her so well.'

So quiet and noiseless was the entry of the French, that the inhabitants, looking from, their windows, could hardly believe their eyes; but when they discovered the truth, they gave themselves up to the wildest expressions of joy. But to their honour be it said that every wounded man and prisoner met with the kindest treatment. Fifty Germans were nursed in the bishop's own palace, and the fact of the universal charity of the inhabitants of Orléans to their helpless enemies has been testified to by the German generals and principal medical officers. There is no single instance of cruelty or neglect established against anyone in Orléans during the space of the French occupation. We found our quarters at the Hôtel d'Orléans rather noisy, and resolved to seek for private lodgings.

Dr. Pratt was in England, and till his return Dr. Tilghman said he could not employ us, as he had opened a letter from Colonel Loyd-Lindsay to Dr. Pratt (which letter he did not show us), and he dare not, in the face of that, ask us to work under them, till Dr. Pratt returned. We replied we had done the work in England Dr. Pratt had sent us to do, we had brought out the money for him, and stores we could give him if we worked with him; but we begged Dr. Tilghman distinctly to understand that our services were required in three other quarters. We should wait Dr. Pratt's return, and if he did not require us accept one of these offers; but we felt in honour bound to keep our promises first. I asked if Dr. Tilghman had not expected us. He said, 'Yes; it was Colonel Loyd-Lindsay's letter that prevented his putting us at once on work.'

Now, we were beginning to think that we could do better service attached to one of the bishop's ambulances, and rather hoped we should be released. Next day we presented ourselves to a gentleman high in the French International, who had called upon us directly we arrived, and on our saying we had brought money for the Anglo-American Ambulance, he said they had left the city. They had been ordered to do so by French authority. We had some trouble to convince him they were still there. Not to enter into details, we left with the honest conviction that for us it would be better to take some other service. We went to the palace.

The celebrated Monseigneur Dupanloup received us most kindly, and next day we went, at his desire and request, to the Convent of St.-Marc, where he had an ambulance, and where he begged for our assistance, at least till we were obliged, if we were really compelled by honour to do so, to return to our old ambulance, the Anglo-American. A charming sister, the Mother of the novices, came to fetch us, in a light covered car, drawn by a white pony named Cocotte. We drove down a street, past the palace, or *évêché*, as it was called, across the boulevard, over a bridge that crossed the railway, down a road with houses and gardens each side, the Faubourg St.-Marc till we came to a high blank wall, as it seemed, with a large door in the centre.

The coachman, or rather driver, Pierre, rang the bell; the door opened as of itself by a cord pulled in the lodge at the side, and we found ourselves in a covered entrance, a square court-yard before us, with trees and shrubs and a statue of the Virgin in the centre, and beyond a very large white house, four storeys high, with many windows. On our right a wing only two storeys high, on our left a low covered passage leading from the main buildings to those through which we had entered, and which we now saw were also a two-storied range, the lower windows opening on a passage below the level of the courtyard. We entered the central building by a glass door, and we were in a corridor with a pavement of black and white marble; opposite to us another glass door, opening into the interior of the house, the little hall going through to a large garden; on our right, two small rooms, on our left, a wide staircase of polished oak descending to the basement and ascending to the top of the house, and beyond it another small room.

The lower floor, except this centre part, consisted of two large halls and a room at the further end on the left. These two large halls were already arranged for wounded, also the room beyond, and were called afterwards, when all was organised, the Salle St.-George (for French), the Salle St.-Aignan (for Germans), whilst the room beyond was for very bad cases. The two small rooms inside the hall-door were first a room for preparing linen, and used also for operations; and the second, looking into the garden, *la petite ambulance anglaise* for *sous-officiers* (French), the one other opposite being for *sous-officiers* (German); and this, when we first arrived, was all that was used—19 beds in Salle St.-George, 21 in Salle St.-Aignan, and 8 in the two small rooms, 48 in all.

We ascended the stairs to the third floor, and were shown three nice rooms, one for each of us and one for the stores, when they arrived, and were then taken down to a snug and comfortable parlour, where an elegant little lunch was prepared. We were delighted with the house and its capabilities, and resolved, if possible, to establish an ambulance on a larger scale, or rather assist the good Sisters to develop the one they had. We told them we must await Dr. Pratt's return before we could decide, and meantime we held consultation as to the capabilities of the house.

Two more rooms upstairs on the first floor could be prepared for wounded, two others in the infirmary, in the entrance block of buildings, and eight beds in a large wooden building that had been used as a chapel, thence called La Chapelle-de-Bois; and there was a possibility, if required, of more rooms in the gardener's house opening into the stable-yard, and in a schoolhouse now occupied as a military post by the French. These two were afterwards called the "*Basse-Cour*" and "*La Poste*," and the day came too soon when all were crowded with wounded. Thus, we have an idea of the Maison Mère, as our house was called, to distinguish it from the Maison Marie across the garden, which opened on to the other faubourg, the Faubourg Bourgogne, and this house, too, which belonged to our convent, was also prepared for wounded.

Both convents were educational establishments—the Maison Mère at St.-Marc for a first-class education, and the Maison Marie, Faubourg Bourgogne, for poor scholars and orphans. Some thirty or forty Sisters lived in the two houses, and a more cheerful, friendly, kind-hearted set we never could wish to live amongst—no gloom, no bigotry, no distrust. They received the strangers with open arms, and in twenty-four hours we were part and parcel of the establishment, and a friendship and affection sprang up betwixt many of the Sisters and ourselves that will last while life endures. There was a large building used as a washhouse or 'lingerie,' and a kitchen that could cook for a hundred, so we started with unusual advantages. Linen, medicines, and money were all that was needed to enlarge the ambulance and make it most efficient, and then we could proceed; and we anxiously waited our chief's return to know what we were to do.

The city meantime was rapidly filling with troops. General d'Aurelle de Paladines had his headquarters there, and daily received reinforcements. Everything was gay and cheerful, and no one doubted of ultimate victory. Arms and ammunition arrived by every train, and long convoys of heavy artillery blocked the roads. The French gun factories turned out 200 rifles and six cannon every day, and by November 11th, 215,000 Remington rifles and 26,000,000 cartridges had been landed at Havre from America. Everything foreboded the great struggle so soon to come off. The Lycée, the Grand Seminary, the Little Seminary, the Casernes St.-Jean, St.-Charles, and d'Étapes, were all fitted up as ambulances; also, the Convents of St. Mart, Ste. Marie, the Visitation, the Recouvrance, the Sacré Coeur, the Little Sisters of the Poor, and many others.

With the troops came many ambulance corps. The splendid arrangements of the Ambulance de Lyon may be especially noticed. Every man was unpaid; they took the simplest requisitions, and lived in the humblest lodgings, though all were men well known in the hospitals of Lyons. The Ambulances du Puy-de-Dôme, du Midi, and several others, took up their headquarters in Orléans, and sent detachments with the army for field service. The bishop addressed an eloquent appeal to the ladies of Orléans to aid in the good work, and they at first proposed to occupy and fit up the unused Church of St. Euverte; but a committee of medical men of Orléans decided that it was unhealthy, that it could not be sufficiently warmed or ventilated, and was unfit for hospital use. In the face of this it was taken up by the Anglo-American Ambulance, a very large sum expended in arranging it; but, as we shall see, the opinion of the medical men of the place was, after all, correct.

A great number of other ambulances were formed, and began to fill fast with cases of dysentery, fever, rheumatism, and smallpox, and aid to support present and coming efforts was earnestly sought for on all sides. Then was the time to have sent into Orléans some of the vast store of supplies the British Society possessed; but none arrived. There was a rumour of a depot to be formed at this centre of action; but it never was done. Colonel Reilly met us in the courtyard of the Hôtel d'Orléans, and told us he had received a telegram from Colonel Loyd-Lindsay, authorising him to give away 1,000*l.*; and we consulted together who was to have it. It ended in 200*l.* being given to the bishop, 300*l.* to the Anglo-American, and the rest to some of the French Ambulances in the field—the 5th International, a very celebrated one, being included.

Every day some band or other played in the Place Martroi, and every day, and twice a day, official announcements, written in the crookedest of hands, were stuck up on the gate of the *mairie*, to be devoured by the admiring crowd. The result was universal confusion as to what was going on. All that we could find out was that Prince Frederick Charles was at Montargis (which, by the way, he left 8,000 *francs* in debt for extras over and above requisitions), and that daily skirmishes occurred all over the department with varying success.

The Prussians advanced on Artenay and were repulsed, shelled Neuville and were driven back, leaving eighty prisoners in the hands of the 29th of the line, whom we met being marched into Orléans, looking rather cheerful than otherwise, and evidently glad to be out of it. We began to wonder how long all this would go on. Every day was a repetition of the day before.

We had some trouble to get our baggage, but M. de la Thouanne, of the French International, went off to Tours and sent it down to Orléans. It had been piled in the Tours station for several days, and one gentleman wrote to Messrs. Piesse and Lubin, whose names were marked on the bales, to know if he could not take possession of it. This was declined with thanks, and it arrived safely at the convent in time to be of the greatest service. Meantime we heard, to our sorrow and annoyance, that Dr. Pratt in London had disowned us as his authorised agents, and, hearing he had arrived, we sent for him. He delayed calling for several days, and then came alone. We declined to see him except in the presence of his staff, and he returned next day with Drs. May, Tilghman, and M'Kellar.

He expressed his sincere regret for what he had done; told us that his wife and family wept bitterly when his letter appeared in the *Times*, and reproached him for his conduct; that he had fully authorised us to do all we had done but ask aid from the British Society, except as regarded the putting his men on their staff, and was quite conscious that in his flurry, excitement, and distress at Versailles he had not explained this to us, nor made any exception, and he promised to write a letter to the *Times*, stating this. So, we shook hands, trusting to his honour. They had only sixty German wounded then, but were about to open the Church of St. Euverte for French wounded; we therefore gave them over the money sent by the French Committee, and settled that, for the next few days at all events, until the church was opened and the wounded really came in, we should remain where we were, to assist in the bishop's ambulance, and decide afterwards, when we saw what work there was.

The following morning, he called again, accompanied by Mr. Olliffe, and brought the copy of the letter. We mutually agreed to the alteration of a sentence, and it was to be sent to Mrs. Pratt, to forward through a friend to the *Times*. The baggage was, by agreement, to remain till we had decided where to work. Thus, ended the last week of November. The storm was gathering, and we watched the course of events with intense interest. On Monday, November 28, the main body of the army was to advance by Patay and Artenay, and on the day before a grand military mass was to be celebrated in the Cathedral of Ste. Croix, to pray for and bless the arms of France. This was the opening scene of that week so truly called the Week of Battle.

CHAPTER 23

The Week of Battle

The sun shone very brightly on that Sunday morning, November 27th. The streets were crowded with men, women, and children, in holiday costume. Peasants from surrounding villages had come in to meet some brother or son in *la jeune armée*; the women in clean white caps, and the men in gay waistcoats and head-dresses of various colour and form. *Zouaves* lounged along with their red *fez* on the back of their heads, and artillery officers dashed about in all directions, bound on imperative and imaginary errands. It was towards the cathedral that the stream of people set in. There every chair was occupied and the aisles filled with soldiery; the nave was lined with sailors from the frigate *Jeanne d'Arc*, their drawn cutlasses on their shoulders; the choir was reserved for officers and the National Guard; and when at nine o'clock the clanging of the bells ceased, there was not a vacant space in the church.

The general and his staff had entered by a side door, and Mass commenced, the bishop officiating. The service was very short, and the music, which was executed by the band of the National Guards, very fine; but the crowning effect was when, after the consecration, the bishop turned to the kneeling crowd and raised the Host, in blessing, high above his head. The sailors dropped on one knee, lowering their cutlasses on the pavement with a clash, and a breathless silence ensued, whilst every eye was fixed on that central figure standing on the steps of the high altar, the sunlight striking on his silver hair and rich robes—a silence broken by soft, exquisite, plaintive music, so touching that it was a relief when the bishop turned away, the sailors and soldiers sprang up and lowered their arms, and we breathed again.

It was soon over after this. The band broke into a splendid triumphal march, and General d'Aurelle de Paladines, followed by his staff, came down the nave, looking hopeful and cheerful. Did he believe in victory then, or did he know how the lines were closing round him, and the road to Paris was blocked by the Red Prince and his veteran army? We saw amidst the officers who followed the general the familiar dress of our own Royal Artillery, and we hoped that no stray shot would hit the gallant military *attaché*, whose kindly ways and frank face had already won the goodwill of the French soldiery.

On Monday the city was half emptied of troops. We received a few slightly wounded men from some outpost skirmishes, and made all preparations for the coming week. Rations were allowed by the town for each wounded or sick man. They had been very liberal during the German rule. There was plenty then, and the conquerors did not care what the town might have to pay afterwards. It was managed on a very regular system; orders were issued for the things required, signed by the surgeon of the ambulance, and countersigned at the *mairie*. This order, being presented to the tradesman, was cashed by him in the article he dealt in; and when presented at the *mairie* after the war was over, was to be paid from the funds of the town.

When the expenditure exceeds the income, these funds have to be raised by extra local taxes. Therefore, as the tradespeople have to pay these extra taxes, it was literally giving their things away, for they had to supply the funds by which they themselves were to be paid. It is not surprising, therefore, that the *maire* struck off many items which the German *commandant de place* had sanctioned. Good wine, choice vegetables, poultry, and fruit, for the tables of the surgeons of some of the ambulances, were no longer given, and I met an *infirmier* of one of them who, showing me his dishonoured cheque for sundry dainties, said he thought the *maire* was right.

Gentlemen should not come to help and cost the poor French such a sum to keep; but what his masters would say he did not know, and just as they were going to have a dinner-party, too! We had had wine, meat, bread, butter, milk, coffee, sugar, and vegetables granted, so many ounces for each man; now all was cut off, except bread and meat, the wood for firing and kitchen use being reduced by half, and the vegetables also to one *sou* per man.

It was a hard struggle to get on. The good Sisters used their own vegetables. We bought two casks of wine and some firewood, but how we lamented over the stores so wasted in other places, and the money thrown away in telegrams and odds and ends! Fifty pounds would have enabled us then to lay in a stock that would have been invaluable of sugar, candles, wood, wine, soap, coffee, and extract of meat. With that sum we could have kept the whole ambulance in plenty for the winter. We had money of our own; but the cheque, sent at last by the National Society, instead of the gold which I ought to have had in London, was useless, and we were obliged to husband our resources.

That day, too, came a piteous request from the French ladies at Caserne d'Étapes for help. Seven hundred wounded and sick were there, and very little *charpie*, very few bandages, no carbolic acid, no shirts, no drawers, no linen pieces for dressings. The Germans had taken everything during their occupation. Not even a lancet could be bought in the city, and medicines were most rare, and frightfully dear. They had applied, through the bishop, to the British Committee. The bishop had received a few bales of linen from them, brought out by a special messenger; and there was little or nothing at Tours. Could we, would we help them? The French Society was utterly overwhelmed, and they were in despair. We could not refuse. Cocotte was harnessed to the convent cart, and we took them what we felt we could spare. (We had already sent a provision to the bishop.) Their delight and gratitude were unbounded.

All this time Orléans was being put in a state of defence. The bridges over the Loire were mined, trenches were dug, and batteries planted, though everyone said the Germans would never come back there. On the Tuesday I went out to see. Close by our house was the Church of St. Marc, a quiet little village church. In the yard was a bivouac of troopers who rode up and down the fields, superintending the workmen. Women were pulling up the vine-stakes and placing them crossways, to hinder the advance of cavalry, they said.

My idea was that it was not probable cavalry would charge up a slope against a mud wall, for such was the face of the entrenchment, and that the stakes would be just as useful against infantry. They must have been pulled up before any body of men, unless mounted on stilts, could have marched over the ground. There had been rain every night, and the ground was a perfect bog. The soft mud clung to my boots, till I slipped and slided about, and my companion, a good-natured, chatty, peasant woman, decided that those 'dogs of Prussians would be well tired out before they came near the rifles of the boys hidden in the trenches.'

We walked as far as the great battery which the sailors were constructing, and we admired the huge 'marine pieces,' as the ship guns were called, which they were placing in position. The battery was on a slight rise, and overlooked the ground beyond the trenches. They told us the forest of Orléans was so fortified that it was impassable: the roads were cut, and ambuscades made in every direction. But as there were ways and means of getting at Orléans round about the forest without coming through it, I never had the profound faith in that forest as an impassable obstacle to Prince Frederick Charles that the natives had.

We met a surgeon of the Anglo-American Ambulance, and he told us how he and a friend, on hearing of the fighting at Neuville the preceding Thursday, had gone out to look for wounded, had found quarters in the village inn, and there, in the stable, was the body of a Prussian officer evidently of high position. He had been brought in terribly wounded, and survived but a few minutes. A herald with a white flag arrived and claimed the body, and it was identified as that of Count Plater. Reports were current of a victory of the French at Beaune-le-Rolande, a town beyond the forest in the direction of Montargis; but it was said that Prince Frederick Charles was at Pithiviers in great force. All the afternoon crowds besieged the *mairie* in search of news, and muddy dragoons rode in from the front with various orders.

There were in the Maison Marie, our other house in the Faubourg Bourgogne, many Bavarian wounded. On going over there we found that they were ordered to leave Orléans by the evening train. They were all in a state of great distress and alarm; and the Mother Superior begged me to explain to them where they were going. She had provided a loaf of bread and a flask of wine for each man, and their fear and regret were that they were leaving their quiet resting-place, and were to be sent to rejoin their regiments. I endeavoured as gently as possible to explain that being prisoners they would be sent to the south of France, to Pau, there to remain during the war, or till exchanged.

To my astonishment, one stalwart sergeant seized my hand and nearly embraced me, and the rest uttered violent exclamations of joy. 'To Pau! to Pau! hurrah! Not to the front; not to fight again. *Bismarck caput! Bismarck caput!*' This mysterious phrase, I afterwards discovered, is supposed to be derived from '*coupe tête*' (cut his head off). It was always used about Bismarck by the German soldiers, as he was a special object of detestation, and also with regard to everyone else they disliked, or to express death; for instance: 'Where is Franz? Has he rejoined his regiment?'

'*Nein, meine Schwester; er ist caput*' (No, my sister; he is dead).

I said to my Bavarian friends, 'So, then, you would rather be prisoners than fight?'

'Surely,' said my friend; 'poor Bavarians always first in fight, last at supper. When we gain, brave Germans always conquerors; when we were beaten at Orléans, stupid Bavarians, all their fault. Only let us get home to the wives and children in Bavaria; see if we fight any more for Bismarck *caput*.'

And this sentiment, in various forms, we heard over and over again. The poor fellows bade us a most grateful and friendly farewell, the good Mother rushing from one to the other, to see that Carl had his bread, and Adolph was well wrapped up round the throat, and Johann had his stick (he was a little lame still), and lamenting over her patients as if they had been countrymen and sons.

We heard that the armies were facing each other in a long line extending over many miles of country. Now I wish specially to notice the utter ignorance in which we of Orléans lived as to all that passed outside. We read on the *affiches* on the *mairie* wall of a succession of small victories, of convoys cut off, and prisoners taken. We knew Prince Frederick Charles was at Montargis or Pithiviers, or thereabouts; but of all the military movements that took place around Orléans we were and are profoundly ignorant. We can but give our own impressions of what we saw. Certainly, everyone was full of hope and confidence, and never for a moment believed the Army of the Loire could be defeated. On the 30th (Wednesday) the telegrams spoke of a repulse of the Germans at Beaune-le-Rolande.

After our morning's work we went out into the town, and found troops and artillery passing through it to the front. We saw a lady who arrived from Tours to go to Montargis, and found it impossible to get a carriage. Whilst she was still lamenting her hard fate, a gentleman entered the hotel where we had called in search of letters, and their meeting was most enthusiastic. It was her husband. He had come in from Montargis, intending to go to Tours, for the purpose of telling her that all the roads were cut, and she could not reach her home. It must be left to the mercy of the invaders.

We heard that the French had withdrawn from Beaune, even after their victory, and it seemed to us the Germans were approaching; but this was indignantly denied. We heard, too, that wounded were hourly expected, and waited till 11 p.m.; then, thinking it too late, went to bed and to sleep. But at 1 a.m. a Sister rushed into the room. There were three or four carts of wounded come; would we come down?

We dressed in haste. How cold it was! how bitterly the December wind blew in as we opened the court-yard door! There, indeed, were four large waggons full of wounded men. The drivers were holding lanterns by the horses' heads, and the *infirmiers*, of whom, at that time, we had but three, were handing out knapsacks and muskets.

The poor creatures were half frozen with an eleven hours' journey in a biting frost. It was with difficulty we could get them into the house. They were, of course, not the worst wounded—those could not be removed for a day or two—but some who that night seemed but little hurt were with us for three months afterwards, still almost helpless invalids. What a ragged, muddy, dirty, miserable lot they looked, as they leant against the walls, or lay down on the floor, in the dim gas-light. Fires were soon blazing in the kitchen and infirmary, and we took them one by one and pointed out their beds. Hot soup was brought, and we would have taken off their coats and boots and re-dressed their wounds, but fatigue overpowered them, and the head nursing Sister and ourselves decided to let them lie as they were and sleep till morning.

This was now the 1st of December. Having settled our patients for the night, or rather morning, we went back to our room, very cold and very tired. The usual routine of inspecting the wounds took place about 10 a.m., and we prepared clean shirts for all the men as soon as they were washed and dressed; but about 11 a.m. more wounded were sent in, and it was only possible to dress the wounds, with the prospect of making them comfortable before evening. Just after dinner came a sudden order for every man who could travel to be evacuated. Many wounded were expected, and the Orléans Ambulances must be cleared at once. Now that they were rested and refreshed, most of them found themselves able to go to the train. Two or three remained, and were transferred to one of the large halls, and the infirmary was again empty.

Later in the day we went into the city. A huge crowd surrounded the *mairie*, and the good news flew from lip to lip. Ducrot had made a successful sortie from Paris; Prince Frederick Charles was retreating before the Army of the Loire; the French outposts were at Tivernon, a station on the Orléans Railway beyond Tours; the two generals, D'Aurelle de Paladines and Ducrot, would crush the Prince's army between them. The greatest enthusiasm prevailed, and the most confident opinions were given on every side that in three weeks the Germans would be driven across the Rhine. Some even went so far as to say that the King of Prussia had evacuated Versailles, which was occupied by General Trochu, and had withdrawn to Rheims.

The streets presented a singular appearance workmen in muddy trousers and jackets going to and from the trenches, half-equipped *Gardes Mobiles* coming in by every road and every train, all anxious to go to the front, and D'Aurelle de Paladines! his name on every lip, the hero, the saviour! We took home a great many daily journals—the '*Loiret*,' the '*Impartial du Loiret*,' and the '*Gazette nationale*'—and our entrance into the long halls of the ambulance was the signal for a scene of joy that was overpowering. Whilst I read the despatch aloud, and Louise handed round the papers to those too ill to move, all who could rise from their bed crowded round me and greeted every paragraph of Gambetta's florid despatch with almost tearful delight.

It was impossible, being English, not to feel French just then. It might have been an English hospital; it might have been the third edition of some evening paper; it might have told how Kent and Sussex were evacuated by an invader, how London was freed, and some great English general had cut his way through the lines, and some other great general leading our Volunteers, our *francs-tireurs*, our citizen soldiers, side by side with regiments just come from India, and corps of colonists from Australia and New Zealand and Canada, were beating back the foreign foe, and soon we should see them recrossing the Channel, and we should be left in peace. And so, we cried '*Vive la France!*' and shook hands all round *à l'anglaise*, and were very happy. To their honour be it spoken, the Bavarians and Prussians entered into the Frenchmen's joy. The war would be over, they should go home; and home to a German is more than glory.

It was a very happy evening in the ambulance and in the city too. But next day told a different tale. It was a bright sunny morning, and about nine o'clock the Mother Superior came to tell us the bishop had ordered a three days' exposition of the Sacrament, that prayers might be continually offered for the triumph of the French arms; also, that the flags were to be immediately put up on the cathedral towers, in honour of the victory already announced. But even as she spoke a sullen sound came on the sunny air, the low, deep, distant booming of cannon. How could the Germans be so near if indeed it were true that they were in full retreat?

There was no time to speculate on this, for the arrival of wounded was announced, and going down we found every hall and corridor crowded—poor fellows! some lying on the ground, their heads on their knapsacks, some with folded arms, half sleeping on the long table in the centre, all weary, dirty, and hungry. They had heard of no victory by Paris; they only knew of their own retreat from Beaune-le-Rolande before Prince Frederick Charles, ordered to fight in retreat before they were defeated, when they had beaten back the attacking enemy from the positions they held, and they muttered dark threats against the authors of such treason.

One by one we examined their wounds and dressed them; the worst cases were put to bed, the others prepared as far as we could to be sent on that afternoon to the rear. Amongst them was a captain of National Guards. He had been wounded at Beaune-le-Rolande, and placed in a house close by, which had been made an ambulance. The Prussians had fired on this house, it was burned, and the poor wounded crawled out to another place of shelter. That, too, was fired on and burned, in spite of the Red-Cross flag. Again, they escaped to a third place of refuge, and from thence, were brought in country waggons to us.

For the truth of this several men of his corps who were with him answered also. About two o'clock, just as we were thinking of littering down the long corridors with straw for the wounded, every bed being full, the *intendant militaire*, M. de la Cape, came down to say every man who could safely leave must go by the train at three o'clock. This was utterly unexpected, and a scene of confusion ensued. The coats and boots of all had been sent to be cleaned and their shirts to be washed, to be ready for next day; but some idea got abroad, and it was a true one, as it turned out, that the Germans were advancing very fast.

The low booming of the cannon was distinctly heard, and, as we found afterwards, there was hard fighting at Bazoches des-Hautes, so every man was anxious to get away beyond the possible reach of the Germans, and even those whose wounds were serious, if they were in the shoulder or arm, insisted on their perfect ability to travel any would; nothing should stop him. It was evident to us that to do so would be fatal to him, and Louise, with the greatest promptitude and decision, caught hold of his trousers, just as he was about to rise from his bed, and with her huge scissors slit them up at the side, rendering it impossible for him to put them on.

It was an effectual preventive, and often afterwards he said he owed her his life, and used to tell the tale of her cutting up his trousers with the greatest enjoyment. That he never resented his captivity is proved by a very grateful letter we received from him, signed 'For life, your devoted and grateful friend.' One poor boy, too, we grieved for. He had been in the ambulance since October, he was very delicate and little used to rough it, and 'Emile' was the spoiled child of the whole convent. He was nobly born and highly educated, but had run away from home, and was only a corporal in the Chasseurs de Vincennes, and it may be imagined how little he relished leaving his comfortable quarters for an uncertain railway journey and a possible night at the station.

We wrapped him up in a knitted vest and a flannel shirt, a huge comforter, and everything we could get on under his uniform, and he started with the rest. After they were all off we discovered that two men who certainly had smallpox, and had been ordered by the surgeon to the Hôtel-Dieu, had succeeded in escaping. They would not remain in Orléans, to run the risk of being made prisoners, and they had avoided the little cart prepared to take them to hospital, and where they had gone to no one knew.

Louise and myself, later in the day, went into the city. It was crowded with peasantry from the neighbourhood, who had fled from the advancing Prussians, for that advancing they were there was no doubt; but still we tried to believe it could not be, and to think that what we were told was true. D'Aurelle de Paladines was retreating, certainly; but it was only a feint to draw the enemy within reach of the heavy siege-guns planted around Orléans. The Place d'Étapes was full of waggons bringing in fresh wounded, and everything looked disturbed and disquieted. We went into the cathedral; a few solitary worshippers were there—women mostly, dressed in mourning.

The Sacrament was exposed on the high altar, and on the second step was a *prie-dieu* covered with purple velvet, and a little behind it, on either side, two others. At the centre one knelt the good bishop, so motionless that it was impossible to believe it was a living man, his white head bent down in his hands; he was absorbed in most intense prayer, his two grand vicars kneeling at the other *prie-dieus*. We watched him for some time; there was not the faintest motion, not even a rustle of his purple robe.

The old familiar scene came back forcibly as we looked at his earnest, rapt figure. The soldiers of Israel were fighting in the plain, and their prophet and leader was pleading on the mountain top that the God of Israel would arise and save his people in their hour of need. He had blessed them before they left for the battle; he was praying for them now—if not to return victorious, to die as Christians and soldiers should.

We left the church feeling that, even if all were lost, France had something left still in that grand old man, with his fervent faith and his gallant disposition, his brilliant intellect and his loving, gentle heart. We went home sadly, for the foreshadowing of sorrow was upon us. The noise of the distant cannon had ceased; but what might tomorrow bring forth? To our surprise, we found Emile. That *enfant gâté*, having discovered that there was no chance of his starting before noon next day, had quietly come back, to have, as he expressed it, a good supper and a good night's rest.

There were so many German prisoners going, and so many other wounded and sick, that the trains for that day were all filled. I must say that it confirmed our impression that things were going badly in front, or the 'powers that be' would not have been so anxious to send everybody to the rear. We resolved to hoist our Union Jack next morning, and so be prepared for any event under its friendly shelter, and having ordered a pole on which to fix it, retired for the night with the comfortable conviction that, come what might, we should be able to hold our own against all comers.

CHAPTER 24

Le Dimanche Noir

It was quite dark on Friday evening before the noise of the cannonade ceased. The poor people in the cottages around us were all in a terrible state of alarm. Many left and went beyond the Loire. One poor old man arrived at the convent door late in the evening; he led by the bridle a rough pony, harnessed to a rougher cart, containing the household goods, amongst them a mattress of blue and white check, on which sat an old woman with a copper saucepan in her hand. They begged for shelter in the convent, but it was impossible, crowded as it was with wounded; for they had been coming in all the evening.

There was no room for anyone else, and had the report spread abroad that safety was to be found in the convent of St. Marc, we should have been overcrowded with refugees. So, we had to request the poor old couple to go on into Orléans, escorted by a stalwart *infirmier*. We, as I have said, retired to rest, and slept so soundly we did not even hear the arrival of more carts of wounded, as when they came at 6 a.m. all the world was up and stirring, ourselves excepted; we were not actually wanted, and the good Sisters would not wake us.

At eight o'clock next morning, when our coffee was brought, the thunder of the cannon began again louder than ever. We almost thought it must be our batteries close by opening fire, but the postman informed us it was beyond Chevilly, eight miles off on the Paris road, and that we should hear it nearer, for General d'Aurelle de Paladines was drawing the Germans under the fire of the 'marine pieces,' and that we should see them crushed. After the morning's work we went into the city. It was very empty.

Orderlies rode at a rapid rate up and down the streets, and the Lyonnaise Ambulance passed us going to the front in splendid order, the waggons for the wounded being properly covered in, as was necessary in so sharp a frost, and the surgeons and dressers marching by the side, with all surgical and medical requirements in a large case or bag suspended from a leather belt, which crossed another supporting a *havre-sac* with the day's provisions. They were followed by a light cart covered with oilcloth, in which were their stores. About ten minutes afterwards the Ambulance du Puy-de-Dôme went down the street and out by the Faubourg Bannière in similar order. Every man wore the Red-Cross on his cap and the brassard on his arm, and both ambulances were accompanied by their chaplains, priests in broad beaver hats and *soutanes* well tucked up through the belt and *havre-sac* over the shoulder.

We saw many carts coming in from the country with peasants flying from their homes before the Prussian advance, and trains were being rapidly despatched to Tours one after the other, regardless of timetables, crowded with fugitives wounded. The boom of the cannon went on, sometimes seeming more distant, sometimes nearer, and all sorts of rumours were in circulation as to the result of the battle evidently going on all around us. Our convent was full with wounded, so was the second house in the Faubourg Bourgogne, 'Maison Marie.' The continual noise of the cannonade had rendered everybody excited and nervous, and we were not sorry when, after the early dinner, came a fresh order to send off every man we could.

As we crossed the courtyard to the infirmary to see to this, the sound of the firing was nearer than ever, the ground actually vibrated under our feet. The sun had gone in, the sky was overcast, and a chill wind whistled through the leafless branches. Nothing more dreary and desolate could be imagined than the ceaseless thunder of the cannon, the poor sick and wounded huddling on their clothes to escape the advancing enemy, the cold, biting wind, and the gloomy sky. The spoiled child Emile still refused to go. Louise and I told him we fully believed the Prussians were rapidly gaining ground, and the city might be taken that night. It was perhaps his last chance of freedom, and we urged him to go.

At last he consented, strapped on his knapsack, and went up the road after his comrades. The wind whirled up the dust in clouds, and just as they were hidden from sight a report so loud that it shook the very window-frames startled the Mother Superior and the good Sisters. Only two men were left in the infirmary, which looked upon the road, and it was thought best to remove them into the main building, for fear of shells. Under the convent were great vaults on which part of it was built; they were in the garden and covered deep by earth, certainly bomb-proof, and here we could resort in case the shells came too near.

There were very few patients now in the wards, and those who were left begged us to go out and get some information for them. We did not think the firing sufficiently close to render the streets dangerous, and we went to the Hôtel d'Orléans, to know if the English *attaché* were there, and what he could tell us. He had breakfasted there, and ridden out to the general's headquarters. These said headquarters, we found, were considerably nearer Orléans than they had been. All to us looked like a retreat, but we were assured it was not so.

How very empty the streets looked! Most of the shops were shut; not a soldier to be seen; all were at the front. There was a general air of doubt and depression abroad which contradicted the *affiche* at the *mairie*, that by news received from the general in command all went well, and the final result of the struggle could not be doubtful. It was well known too, by this time, that the victorious sortie from Paris was but an invention of some imaginative brain, and one poor, shivering citizen, looking at the placard still affixed to the wall, and signed by 'Pèreira, *Préfet du Loiret*,' said, with a bitter smile, 'See how they deceive us! Not M. Pereira, he is too good a man, but *ce Monsieur Gambetta—là!*'

It was getting dark as we entered the Cathedral. The seven lamps were burning before the Chapel of the Sacrament in the right transept, and many lighted tapers before the Shrine of the Virgin on the left, placed there by sad and loving hearts, whose dear ones were where those terrible guns were firing. Suddenly, yet sharply, their echo rang through the vaulted cathedral, and poor, frightened women and children, cowering by some great pillar, would start and look around them, as if expecting to see some shell fall crashing through the roof. But the bishop still knelt there before the High Altar, as if he had never stirred from his position since the day before, still bowed and motionless, with the faint light shining on his grey head, and his vicars kneeling behind him.

Only the Sunday before, amidst sunlight and music and crowds of worshippers, he had blessed the Army of the Loire in his Saviour's name; and now, in the closing twilight, in the lonely, deserted cathedral, with that ominous sound echoing through it, instead of the rich tones of the organ, he knelt in a wordless agony of prayer for the salvation of the land he loved, the fair city he ruled over, as God's minister, and the souls of the dying, even now gasping out their life on the dark, frozen battle-ground beyond the city walls. We lingered for some time, watching the scene, so touching in its sadness.

There was a small group of persons collected round a tall priest who was standing by a side chapel, talking vehemently, half aloud, and we crossed the nave to hear what it was. It seemed he was the *curé* of Chevilly. He had come to Orléans with the sacramental plate and other church valuables, and he told us how his little house was turned into a fortified place, the walls pierced for musketry, and a battery of nineteen siege-pieces planted in his garden. 'You will observe, *Mesdames*,' he continued, 'these very circumstances expose my poor house and garden to a return fire.'

I asked where the Germans were. 'Not in Chevilly when I left it,' he replied; 'but I suspect they are in it now.'

'The sound of the firing is nearer,' I said; 'but can they ever take Orléans, with all those heavy guns and trenches lined with riflemen around it?'

'*Ma chère Dame*,' answered the good *curé*, 'the cannon in my garden are the largest imagination can conceive; if they pass those, they'll pass anything, and listen; even as I speak, you hear how near the firing comes. I have no doubt they have taken Chevilly, and you will have them here very soon.'

Two or three women wept and wrung their hands at hearing this, and we thought it best to go home directly. If the Germans were coming on so fast the streets might be dangerous soon. As we crossed the bridge, we stopped to speak to some men who were gathered there, watching and listening. They pointed out the smoke rising up in the distance, and told us the firing was coming very close.

Some hundred yards down the line, on our left hand, another bridge traversed the railroad by the Faubourg Bourgogne, and over this, to our astonishment, we saw strong batteries of artillery passing into the town, coming back from the front, for the battle was on the three sides of Orléans (the Paris side of the Loire), and enclosed the city like a semicircle. We all walked by the bank to the other bridge, and one of the men, an *employé* of the *Octroi*, or local custom duties office, asked an officer who was riding by the side of a gun how all went on. I thought his answer very unsatisfactory, though they did not. He simply said, 'Very well on our side, but we must hope still better on the other. We go to strengthen the front by Cercottes and Chevilly.'

It was certain by this that the result of the day's fighting was that the Germans had come considerably nearer the city; and as for the wonderful crushing of them which was to take place when D'Aurelle de Paladines had drawn them under the fire of the 'marine pieces,' I did not believe in it. I quite agreed with the *curé*, if they could pass them at Chevilly they could pass them at Orléans; and besides, if they were allowed to come so near as under the fire of these batteries, and were pleased to try and silence them by returning it, our position would be by no means a comfortable one. They would not be two miles from the city, and their shot, and shell, would easily reach, at all events, the outskirts in which we were situated.

We hoped and believed that the Red-Cross flag floating from the topmost roof might prevent their firing on the house, and we were glad to see that our Union-Jack was floating gaily and conspicuously from it, with the tricolour on one side and the ambulance flag on the other. Experience had taught us to have more faith in its rainbow crosses than in all the Geneva flags that were waving in the city, for there was a perfect outbreak of them. We were thus guarded as far as possible from long shots, and to provide against any sudden invasion of the convents during a storming of the town in the night, when the English flag might not be so visible, was our next care.

Now, we had a Bavarian *infirmier* named Matthias, the best-natured, best-tempered fellow in the world. He had been gardener in a Bavarian convent, and considered that he had been especially blessed and protected by Providence in having been slightly wounded and sent to a convent, where he had been made *infirmier* to the German wounded, and where '*Bismarck caput*' could not send him to rejoin his regiment and tramp through mud and snow, 'with no supper,' as he used emphatically to add, to carry a heavy rifle and fire it off at nobody in particular, with the certainty of being shot by his general's orders if he did not fight, and the chance of being shot by the French if he did. Matthias was of a pacific disposition, with a perpetual grin on his broad, flat face.

He detested his uniform, and would wear any disgraceful old jacket rather than put it on. I now explained to him he must dress in full uniform, helmet and all, and sit in the porter's lodge, in case the city was taken, to explain to any German marauders it was a hospital, and that there were German wounded there; but Matthias refused, weeping bitterly. He should be taken by the Germans; he should be sent back to his regiment. No, never; he would not put on his uniform clothes, he would hide in the '*lingerie*.' 'The *fraulein* (myself) could sit in the lodge, with the big English flag; that would be *gut*' (good).

And so Master Matthias walked off, installed himself in the French Hall, and announced his intention of forgetting how to speak German if his countrymen came; and there he remained, helping the wounded most actively, and administering consolation and soup together, by shaking his head and saying in compassionate tones, '*Ah, Bismarck caput!*' as much as to say, 'My poor friend, it is all his fault!'

At nightfall the cannonade ceased. Many wounded came in; but they had little to tell, except that they had been fighting in retreat, and they believed the Prussians were in Chevilly. From the upper windows we saw, in the far distance, the red glare in the sky, that told its sad tale of burning homesteads and ruined farms; but all was silence now, except the roll of the carts on the frozen road bringing in their sad load of pain and suffering. Lights were still gleaming from the windows of the convent chapel, where the evening prayer was going on, and the wounded listened to the soft sounds of the singing with a quiet air of repose. It seemed to soothe their over-excited nerves and lull their pains.

It was such a contrast, those warm, well lighted halls, those white-sheeted comfortable beds, the good warm soup, the glass of cooling wine and water, the kind attendants round them, forestalling every wish and changing the position of the pillows under their weary heads, to the scene of a few hours before, the confusion of the battle, the smoke, the noise, then the sudden, sharp pang, the half-muddy half-frozen earth for a bed, and the fear of being trampled down in some sudden charge of friend or foe, or being left there through the long winter night, to be frozen to death, as so many were whose wounds were comparatively trifling. Nothing disturbed the quiet of the night, and Sunday morning came in again bright and sunny, and seeming to inspire hope even in the half-despairing hearts of the Orléanais.

From early morning wounded had been brought in, and our house was again quite full. They all told us that the Army of the Loire was concentrated round Orléans, and the battle this day would be fought in the last trenches. Pleasant news this for us, considering that the last trenches were about 400 yards from us, and the great marine battery about 900. At ten we went to the cathedral. High Mass was being celebrated, but the congregation was a very scanty one.

Up to this time there had been no firing, but just as the Consecration was taking place came a report like a sharp clap of thunder. Everyone started and looked around. Louise said it was the banging of the great west door, so distinct and close by was the sound. It came again and again, and I could not understand why the sacristan should be perpetually opening and shutting the door;—but in one of the pauses came a long, low rattle—the firing of a *mitrailleuse*.

The door fiction was instantly dispelled; we knew the enemy were close by, and the great siege-pieces had opened fire. Many rose and left the cathedral. We stayed to the end of the service, and all through prayer and psalm came that terrible accompaniment, that voice of war and terror. How strangely it mingled with the chanting of the 'Gloria in Excelsis!' Peace on earth! goodwill to men! What a mockery Christian practice is sometimes of Christian doctrine.

As we came out of the cathedral and descended the broad steps leading to the Place Ste. Croix, we saw that the city was in confusion and dismay. We passed the *mairie*. There was no fresh *affiche* with its deceitful tale of victory; a picquet of dragoons were lounging in the courtyard, but what news they had brought from the front was not made public. We went across the broad boulevard, and found a battalion of *Zouaves* encamped upon it. They had lighted fires, and were boiling soup. They had come in from Beaune-le-Rolande, and were, after breakfast, to go on to St.-Jean-le-Braye, a *faubourg* close by Orléans.

Having heard that the station was still full of sick and wounded, evacuated from the hospitals and ambulances, and for whom there had not been room enough in the train, we went there to see if any of our men were left, and if they had had anything for breakfast. We found at least a couple of thousand men, in the waiting-rooms, on the platform, everywhere where they could find standing room. One train had just gone off. Another was being formed, and into this the men rushed, leaving the badly wounded to be assisted into first-class carriages. An officer of high rank was carried past us by two soldiers, and placed in a compartment.

I said to Louise as I saw it, 'This is a retreat; if there were an hour to spare, the colonel would not be hurried off in that condition.' Besides, we saw fresh wounded, who under other circumstances would at least have been sent into ambulance for twenty-four hours, to have their wounds looked to. They had been hastily attended to on the field, but needed much more careful bandaging to enable them to travel in comfort. Our men were all gone; went at four in the morning, an officer of the staff told us; and all, as we saw, had a good basin of soup and a large slice of bread.

Amongst those still remaining were two decidedly full of smallpox.

It is too probable that by such means the disease was spread, as was the case in Orléans and around it. A little common precaution would have obviated this. The men should have been sent back to the Hôtel-Dieu, the civil hospital, which was prepared for such cases. When we left the station, we went to the Hôtel d'Orléans. Madame Pillion, the kind landlady, told us Colonel Reilly had come in from the front, had his breakfast, ordered his carriage to be ready at a moment's notice, and had ridden out again to St.-Jean-le-Braye. We all agreed that General d'Aurelle de Paladines having fixed his headquarters so close to Orléans looked very much as if he had been forced back upon his inner line of defence.

Of course we were all ignorant of what was passing outside, of the general's telegram to Gambetta at Tours to say he must evacuate Orléans, and his later decision to defend it; but what we did see from the hotel windows was that the street was a block of artillery and provision waggons, carts with stores of all kinds, baggage, ammunition and guns, retreating down the street, to cross the bridge at the end which spanned the Loire. Several bystanders remarked on this as looking as if the army was in retreat, and sending on its heavy baggage to save it from falling into the hands of the enemy; but an officer standing there denied it.

He said all was going on well, but that the general considered, as the battle was to be fought so close to the town, and as the heavy baggage is always in the rear, it would be better not to encumber the streets with it, but to send it across the river. We quite agreed in the indignant question of one lady, why the general could not have fought the Prussians a few miles off, instead of exposing the town to a chance of bombardment? It did seem very bad management, certainly.

The crowd in the streets increased every minute, the noise of the cannonade was louder and louder, and we could hear the rattle of musketry. We went home; fresh wounded men were being brought in, dressed, and sent off every minute. At last the halls were again cleared of all but the very seriously wounded, and we sat down to lunch with what appetite we could, resolved that, at all events, God helping us, we would try in this hour of danger to be a help and support to those around us, and to prove that English courage was not a mere fable of romance.

CHAPTER 25

Under the Shadow of the Union Jack

It was a very long Sunday afternoon, that 4th of December; the rainy Sundays of our childhood were not so long, nor yet broken by incidents so sad. The sound of firing was all around us now, and three or four times the great doors of the convent were opened to admit wounded men shot down close by the house. To go out in the garden would not have been wise, for the rifle-balls were whizzing all round. So, we waited, the bright sunshine streaming into our room, and, except for the noise, everything seeming still and quiet. Louise wrote letters in spite of my assurances that the post did not go; and I arranged my few clothes in the drawers. Why I do not know, except that it was difficult to fix the mind on any one given subject.

About 3 p.m. there was a violent ringing at the door-bell, and one of the chaplains rushed in. Orders had been received to take the Host from all the altars and conceal it; and this we thought looked very bad. As we were talking to the Sister at the gate, a battalion of *Gardes Mobiles* came by at the double. A sergeant lingered, and asked for a glass of water. He told us they were going into the trenches; the Prussians were close by; the town would be defended to the last. Probably it would be bombarded. This intelligence spread some dismay. There were thirty children in the house—the remnant of the Sisters' school. It would be well to put them in safety; and the good Mother Superior ordered that all the Sisters and children should assemble in the underground refectory, except those in attendance on the wounded.

Louise and myself mounted up to a dormitory on the fourth floor, and from thence watched the battle. On our right and also facing us were the trenches lined with men, firing over the low earth-bank. We could not distinguish the Prussians, there was too much smoke, and they were apparently in the low wood which bounded our view to the NE. On the SE., houses and shrubberies concealed both defence and attack. On the N. and NW. we could perceive the marine batteries firing rapidly, their fire being replied to by the Prussian guns, which we could not, of course, see. The hottest of the battle was close to us, though, in the Faubourg Bannière. Had it not been for the stern reality of the whole scene, and the inevitable death and suffering that was being worked out, it would have been a beautiful sight to watch the flight of the shells as they soared in a graceful curve through the clear blue sky above, leaving rings of white smoke in the air.

These rings, when darkness came on, were more beautiful still, for they then showed themselves in rings of fire. Sometimes the shell burst in the air, scattering its pieces about, sometimes plunged into the soft ground, throwing up a shower of brown earth and green turf, and sometimes crashed down amidst buildings; and then, when the smoke and dust cleared off, great gaps were to be seen, where it had torn its passage through roof and rafter.

A house just opposite us, about 500 yards away in the fields, was almost entirely destroyed. One shot fell in our garden, close to the '*lingerie*,' but did no damage. Smoke soon veiled the whole scene below, but it hung low, and up above it was the deep blue sky. We had got used to the roar of cannon and rattle of musketry, and could calmly watch the battle. No wounded were removed from the field till towards dusk, and then they principally came in by the Faubourg Bourgogne, and into the other house.

The possibility of our being wounded, or the house itself struck, did not enter our minds. It was more than possible, it was probable; for, as an officer of the English Army, who came after the peace to see the defences, remarked to us, we were in a most exposed position. The supper in the halls and our dinner were served, as usual, about half-past six. As few as possible of the Sisters remained above ground—it was unnecessary, and they had the children to care for. But all who had duties to perform went about them quietly and regularly.

At about seven the cannonade ceased; several wounded were brought in, and spoke positively of the bombardment of the city, which would commence in a few hours. The third trenches were not taken, nor the batteries, and would be defended to the last. They were utterly ignorant that the defence was prolonged into the night only to cover the retreat of the main body of the army across the Loire. Darkness had now closed in, and for a little while there was quiet. About 9 p.m. we were startled by renewed firing quite close to us. It was very violent, but ceased in an hour; and we heard next day that it was caused by the storming of the railroad-Station, which, across the fields, was very near to us, though we had to drive to it through the city, and also that then the marine battery we had seen firing had been captured.

The surrender of Orléans by General Martin de Pallières is well known. He capitulated after D'Aurelle de Paladines and the greater part of the Army of the Loire, with all their baggage, ammunition, and stores, had safely crossed the Loire. They did not blow up the bridges behind them, which were ready mined. Had they done so, the pursuit would have been checked for many days, as a hard frost had set in, and ice was coming down the Loire in huge blocks. To cross by pontoon bridges would have been difficult and dangerous, and much reproach was afterwards bestowed by the French on such bungling management. It strengthened, too, the idea of treachery, for, to this day, there is no soldier of that defeated army, no citizen of Orléans, who would not tell you the town might have been defended much better, held much longer, and even, that had it been honestly done by, it was nearly impregnable, owing to the forest, and the river, and the trenches.

When the noise of the firing had died away, we went to sleep; we were very tired, and the ambulance was about half empty. By military order we had sent out every man who could crawl, and though the last train had left Orléans at 3 p.m., several walked across the railway bridge and gained the other shore of the river.

It was broad daylight before we woke. A good Sister brought us, in our coffee, and I asked, 'What news?'

'The very worst,' she answered; 'the Germans are in the city!'

'Impossible!' we said. 'When did they come in? Was there no more fighting after ten o'clock last night?'

'No,' she said; 'the general surrendered, and the Prussians came in at midnight, the postman told us. He begs to inform you there is no more post.'

'Well,' I said, 'on the whole, I think I'll get up. We may have them here, and Matthias is probably hidden among the piles of linen.'

Dressing at such a time is not a prolonged operation, and we soon descended to the hall below.

Some freshly wounded men had just come in, one so shot in the hand that amputation of the finger was necessary, and the surgeon was not there. Hearing there was one at Ste. Marie, the other house, I said I would go and fetch him, whilst Louise occupied herself in dressing the wounded; but one of the Sisters begged me not, saying that the firing was still going on and balls whizzing about the garden. This I could not believe, and started off. I passed through our garden and came out on the paddock, at the end of which was the vineyard, and just beyond it the trenches. Surely enough, balls were whizzing about and shots being fired in all directions. However, I could not turn back.

I had just reached the low door opening in the wall which divided the garden of Ste. Marie from the paddock, when something whistled close by my head and struck the wall in front. I knew it was a bullet, and that it had probably fallen at the foot of the wall; but under the circumstances I thought it best not to stop and look for it, so I went on my way, and met the Mother Superior and the chaplain coming over to St. Marc's to see how we all got on, and to tell us they were so overcrowded with wounded they wished to transfer some into the Maison Mere. I told them to go back; it was useless exposing themselves to these stray shots. We had thirty vacant beds, and I would go and find the surgeon, send him over, and follow myself with the wounded. If the Prussians met a posse of French soldiery crossing the gardens (and they might at any moment enter by the vineyard), there would be trouble unless someone attached to the ambulance were with them.

I found the surgeon very busy in his sad work. His comrades were out in the trenches; but he himself, being attached to a *franc-tireur* corps, feared even his profession might not be respected, and had taken shelter there. He asked me to escort him across the garden, and I proposed that, as we had so many wounded, he should be attached to us as resident surgeon. The President of the French International could appoint him. M. Emanuel Dupoux and myself walked back to St. Marc's, and from that day till he left, just before Christmas, he stayed with us, and proved himself one of the most talented and skilful of surgeons, and a splendid operator. Then I went back again and brought over the wounded, and then went off into the city, to arrange about going out to the field to bring in any who might be lying there.

The firing had ceased; it was the Prussians firing at French soldiers attempting to escape by the *faubourgs*. All was safe now, but how miserable! As I stepped out of the wicket door, I saw the helmets of the Prussian sentinels on the bridge; the road was strewed with knapsacks, arms, and accoutrements. I reached the Hôtel d'Orléans. All was confusion; the Grand Duke of Mecklenburg was there, and *aides-de-camp* and orderlies rushing about. I took away several letters which were waiting for me, and went down the street to the Place Martroi. Everywhere arms, belts, and knapsacks were strewed about. The retreat must have been very sudden at the last; indeed, Madame Pillion, at the Hotel, told me they had all gone to bed and to sleep when the Germans thundered at the windows and doors and took entire possession of the house. Every shop was shut, very few civilians in the streets. They were full of soldiery, infantry and cavalry, the horsemen, as usual, riding on the side pavements, and store-waggons and guns were clattering down towards the Loire.

The cathedral was the saddest sight. Within it were congregated the prisoners, 4,000 of them; the porches were full of them, pressing against the iron gates and begging for bread and tobacco. I did not go in, but hastened on to St. Euverte to find Père Guerin, one of our chaplains, and ask him where we had better go. He told me the fields immediately around the town had been well searched, but we should do good service by going out to Cercottes, and he would go with us. I found all at home quiet; the wounded had been attended to.

So, we summoned the long waggon from the other house, harnessed a horse to a large covered carriage we had, and Père Guerin, la Mère Marie-Therese de la Croix, Louise, myself, and the surgeon started off for Cercottes. It was bitterly cold, and the road blocked with Prussian columns. At last we got free of them and came out on the battle ground. A light snow had come on, everything looked dreary; here and there were dark heaps, from which we turned away our looks. It was too late to help them, and we must first attend to the living.

We reached Cercottes at last, a small village of one street. There were wounded in every house, and in the little sacristy of the church. The *curé* came up to us as we halted in the street, and begged us to take away three very badly wounded who were lying on straw in the sacristy. We entered the church. It was entirely desecrated, full of filth, and the High Altar had black bottles and unexploded cartridges lying on and about it. The poor *curé* had nothing to give the wounded; the Germans had taken away all his bread and two casks of red wine. He had found three sacks of rice in the railway station, and these he had very wisely taken, and the grains of rice, softened in a little tepid water, were all they had had for twenty-four hours.

We went into his little presbytery, and there, in an upper room, were all his helpless parishioners, who had not fled into the woods. An old man of eighty lay gasping in the *curé's* bed, little children were cowering around the spark of fire, and weeping women huddled in every corner, and here they were all sheltered by their priest. We left bread and wine, as much as we could spare, and a little money, to buy anything that could be bought; we took away his wounded, and a German officer who came up to see what the strangers were about ordered his men to assist us. We showed him that we had two poor German wounded already in the carriage; he seemed very pleased, and politely said he was sure they would be well nursed.

We then searched some stables and out houses, selected all we could take, and dressed the wounds of the others, giving them bread and wine and promising to return next day. One poor lad, a Swiss, of the Foreign Legion, was mounted on the box of our carriage, the surgeon going in the waggon with the wounded, and this boy was severely frost bitten in the foot. Louise, seeing he had not been properly bandaged, stopped the carriage, pulled out her materials, and dressed the foot then and there, wrapping it well up. He did not forget it, for three months afterwards I met on the stairs a bright, rosy lad, who smiled and greeted me. 'Who are you, *mon garçon?*' I asked.

'*S'il vous plait, madame, je suis le garçon de Mademoiselle Louise!*' was the answer.

'*Mon enfant,*' I said, utterly astounded, 'what do you mean?'

He then told me he was the boy whose foot she had dressed at Cercottes. He had been put in the little house, 'La Poste,' where it was very dark, and I did not recognise him in his new clothes, for he had been made *infirmier* and invested in a certain grey jacket, one of a lot sent out from Putney, which was the pride of all their hearts.

We had a long, slow drive back, not improved by the fact that Pierre, who was ahead with the waggon, chose to turn down a side way, and bumped us over the roughest road I ever drove upon. Père Guerin, putting his head out of the window, called to him and informed him he was a man utterly devoid of common sense; he would ruin the carriage, jolt us, and, what was far worse, the wounded. It was too late to turn back, but we were very thankful to see the convent lights before us.

Just before we left Cercottes we met two of the surgeons of the Anglo-American Ambulance. Dr Tilghman came up to me and implored me for God's sake to go on to Chevilly. There were eighty wounded in the *mairie* there, and they had had no bread since Saturday, no wine, and no soup, only grains of rice. I told him we were already laden with wounded, and had given away all our bread and wine, and asked him why he was on foot, and why he had not brought out their waggons. He told me they were afraid the Prussians would seize their horses. I replied I doubted that; they had not in any way interfered with us. It would be too late to return from Orléans to Chevilly that night, the gates would be shut; but we would come out with a store next day. But next day we found how very scarce bread was. We sent down to Pomme-du-Pin another of our ambulances, and found they by chance had had a double supply, and could give us five or six huge loaves.

I went off to the Hôtel d'Orléans, and Madame Pillion most kindly seized upon my idea, and sent a waiter to find all the broken bread. The Germans were very wasteful, and the breakfast table just deserted was strewed with whole and half-loaves. All was collected and put into great bags. I transferred it to the little cart, hid it up carefully under a railroad rug, and went back delighted. Louise volunteered to remain with the wounded, but the surgeon begged me to go, as I spoke German, and we started at noon. We drove through Cercottes, and stopped at the stable where we had left our wounded. One was dead, the others removed by the Ambulance Lyonnaise, and we pressed on to Chevilly. Sad traces of the fight were left on every side; the dead were yet unburied, but the snow had covered them with a pure white shroud. Chevilly looked as sad as Cercottes. All the inhabitants had fled. Every house was occupied by wounded or soldiery.

We reached the *mairie*; but I will not shock those who may read this in quiet English homes by a description of what the state of that house was! Even the kitchen was full of wounded. The mayor's wife was actively employed, aided by two Sisters of St.-Paul-de-Chartres, in nursing them, and the village doctor was there. They had nothing to eat, no medicines, no mattresses, no blankets; all fared alike, and I felt the tears rushing to my eyes as I thought of the stores in St. Martin's Place, and those dying here for want of them.

And with these terrible conflicts foreseen during the past three weeks, no agent had been sent out, no depot established! When will Englishmen on a committee learn to think and act for themselves and those who have entrusted their gifts to them, and not indolently confide all to the care of two or three men, however active and energetic? When will they insist on a voice in the disposal of their own money? And when will they claim a full and true account, with vouchers and receipts for the expenditure of every shilling of it?

We did all we could, and fainting men raised themselves in their bloodstained straw, and seemed to gain new life from a draught of wine.

We had medicines and materials with us, and thus could make the sufferers comfortable for the day. We prayed them to try and clean up the place a little. We would relieve the overcrowded rooms by taking away some wounded and send out more stores next day. As I was trying to dress a wounded man in his great-coat, to come away, an English voice struck my ear. It was a Sister of St. Paul; she came from my own county, she had known my people, and we met as if we had been old friends. She and two other Sisters had had the charge of the village school, but a bomb had fallen in their house. The Prussians had taken possession of it, and they had sought refuge at the *mairie*. We heard the full details of their misery later.

We reached home with our cargo of suffering, and found that, sundry Prussians had presented themselves at our doors, claiming food, forage, and quarters; but seeing the Union Jack, to which Matthias called their attention, they had retreated. I was conscious that the Union-Jack bought in Orléans which floated over the other house was a very dubious sort of one, so I went over there, and found, to my horror, sixty soldiers occupying the kitchen, and even turning the French wounded out of their beds. To cook for the ambulance was impossible, and, summoning Mère Therese, I started for the *prefecture*, to find Prince Frederick Charles. A most gentlemanly *aide-de-camp* received us, and took my letter in to the prince, who was, fortunately, at home. I had asked for a safe conduct—that is, an order that no men should be quartered, no horses stabled, in either of the houses, but that they should be kept as an ambulance.

My friend returned in a few minutes with a mystic scrawl on a piece of paper—the prince could not give the order himself, but this paper would procure it from the Prussian *commandant de place*. It was kindly and courteously done, and in doing it the prince rendered us a service for which we never ceased to feel and express our gratitude. Armed with this, we went off to the *commandant's* bureau, and were lost in a struggling crowd. Men and women with complaints of having too many men quartered upon them, of ill-treatment by the soldiery, dragoons with despatches, pushing everybody aside, swearing, shrieking, struggling all around, made it anything but pleasant.

Seeing an officer of rank pressing through, I caught hold of his arm and showed him my paper. He immediately caught hold of me, I caught hold of the Sister, and shouting to the sentinel to open the door, he fairly fought us through, and we emerged, breathless and disarranged, before the Prussian colonel.

A very few words explained. A copy of the note we had was taken. I was asked for how many houses I claimed protection. I replied two—the Convent Faubourg St. Marc, the Convent Faubourg Bourgogne, and their stables and outhouses. A paper was written out and given to me, and as I was thanking the colonel and leaving, he called me back, and said, 'Has *Madame*, by chance, any vacant beds; if so, will she receive our wounded?'

'Surely,' I replied, 'we have got vacant beds. May I place twenty at the permanent disposal of Your Excellency?'

He shook hands warmly, and the best possible understanding was arrived at. I told him of the sixty men who had quartered themselves upon us, and he shouted to a fierce-looking, though small, lieutenant to take a guard, go down directly, and turn them out. Not to be outdone in courtesy, we begged they might remain till seven o'clock, so as to have their supper before leaving; but he would not hear of it, and once more thanking him I left.

As we crossed the Place Ste.-Croix we saw a stir amongst the poor prisoners in the front of the cathedral, and went in to see if there was any help we could render to anyone. What a scene it was! The whole church was full of a thick smoke, caused by the fires the soldiers, both guards and prisoners, had lighted to keep themselves warm. The pavement was inches deep in dirt; the smell was frightful. The chairs had been burned up for firewood; many had been covered with red velvet. The choir, being surrounded by stalls, and having high iron gates in front, had fared a little better. Still every altar was desecrated. The sacristan wept as he pointed out the ruin wrought in the side chapels, and one or two priests lingered about the desolate shrines in tears.

Cartridges were occasionally thrown into the fires, and exploded with a loud noise. We felt some uncertainty as to where the bullets might go. We stood in sadness and horror, listening to the fearful noises around. Amidst them came the tones of the organ, which a German *Landwehr* man was playing, harsh and discordant. The keys were touched by no experienced or gentle hand; and it seemed to shriek out a wild lament over the desecration of the holy place. The lamps were extinguished. The House of God was deserted by its Lord, and given up, as He was, to the hands of wicked men. It was indeed the 'abomination of desolation in high places.'

Presently came a loud, guttural shout. It summoned the prisoners to muster and march. Many did not understand it, and the Prussians soldiers struck them with their muskets, pulled them about roughly, kicked them into the ranks, and yelled fearfully at them. I remonstrated with one of the guard, told him the day might come when, in the fortune of war, he himself might be a prisoner, and begged him to be patient. He instantly desisted, said it was only they were so stupid, and if I could tell them what to do it would be good. I did explain to the poor fellows that they must fall in and march out of the cathedral, on their way to Germany; and seeing I was translating for the guard, an officer came up and, touching his helmet, asked me to come with him and explain that all really too ill to march, lame, wounded, or footsore, were to come with me to the gate of the choir, and sit by the fires there till the rest were gone, when they would be taken to Caserne St.-Charles.

This I did, and seeing several poor fellows wearily limping away, I ran after them and sent them off to the haven of refuge by the choir. The good Sister kept watch there over our flock of some fifty or sixty men. One lad of fifteen who was not very footsore, but looked very ill, we told to take off his shoe and tie up his foot; he might pass muster, and be spared a five miles' march in a bitter wind. We stood till all were gone, explaining to the guards, who as they passed ordered them, not too gently, to rise and go on, that the captain's orders were, these men were for ambulances.

A little decision always settled the question, and seeing the Sister's black robes and my grey dress with the silver shield and Red Cross on the collar, they imagined we were going to take them with us, desisted from attempting to take them away, and ended by going after the others. The poor wretches actually clung to us, imploring us to save them, to have them left here for a while. The cold night march, the uncertain end of the journey, any misery in Orléans, was preferable to that. We stayed till they were taken away to the Caserne St.-Charles in carts, and walked home sad and depressed.

We found Mère St.-Joseph at Faubourg Bourgogne in a state of tearful delight and gratitude; all the Prussian soldiers in the house had been ordered away by a guard. But since they had left twenty fresh ones had taken possession of a large schoolroom, next door, belonging to the convent, and were clamouring for supper. So, there we went, and I found my gentlemen breaking up the benches for firewood and very insolent. I addressed a *sous-officier*, showed him the safe-conduct, and begged them all to get out. They refused, saying they were sick men for the ambulance.

'In that case,' I said, 'pray stay; but you are aware that, being in ambulance, you must comply with ambulance rules, or I must report you for punishment.'

'True, *meine Schwester*, we are ready,' said they; 'only we shall eat, shall we not?'

'Certainly,' I answered; 'but when we have sick men here, we close the shutters, as the windows look into the street.' ('Close them, *ma soeur*,' addressing one who was with me.) 'Also, we take their boots and coats, and they must directly go to bed.' ('*Infirmier*, take these good gentlemen's boots.') 'You shall have some soup at eight o'clock; but I see you are all fatigued and feverish, and I shall administer a strong dose of cooling medicine all round. I shall go and seek it and return in ten minutes,' and out I walked.

As I expected, I heard a burst of German oaths—for they swear fearfully—an immense shuffling succeeded, and in five minutes out trooped my twenty patients, and walked off to seek better quarters than in *l'Ambulance Anglaise*. A roar of laughter from all followed their exit, in which two or three newly arrived and really sick Germans joined heartily; and so closed the day in peace and security which had opened so anxiously and stormily, and by ten o'clock friend and foe, wounded and sick, aged men, paralysed women, poor orphans, and wearied sisters, 600 souls in all, were resting safely under the shadow of the Union Jack.

CHAPTER 26

A Lost Battlefield

Before driving to Chevilly, as we had promised, on the morrow, it was necessary to go into the city to buy more bread. The town looked very sad. The shops were still closed; a Prussian order had been issued commanding them to be opened, on pain of fine and imprisonment, and this had been complied with by keeping up the shutters of the windows and just taking down those of the doors. Many had been much pillaged, and naturally were afraid to display their goods.

On every door in the place were white chalk-marks, to efface which was a heavy crime, and these showed how many men, and of what regiment, were to be quartered there; but in too many instances the houses had been entered by bands of soldiers forty or fifty in number, whom nothing could dispossess, and as these unwelcome visitors claimed not only lodging and fire, but the best of food and wine, in unlimited quantity, it may be imagined what utter ruin it was to the poor citizens. A refusal was met by the blow of a musket, or the miserable proprietor being turned into the streets.

One old man of eighty was taken out of his bed, to make room for a German corporal, and placed on some straw in the open courtyard, the snow falling fast. He was dead before morning broke—gone to bear witness against his cruel foes before the Judgment Throne. A poor artisan pleaded that he had been two months out of work, and had no means of procuring bread even for his own children. 'We must have meat and wine,' was the answer.

'If you have no money, you must go in debt for them.'

'No one will give me credit,' said the workman; 'I could never pay.'

'Show us the shop,' answered the sergeant, 'we'll settle that;' and the unfortunate shopkeeper named had to supply the workman on credit with articles he never would have bought for himself.

But what could be done with a dozen Prussians in the shop, filling their pockets with everything that struck their fancy—a bottle of wine in one hand and a revolver in the other!

Lord Palmerston, in his *Journal of a Tour to France in 1815*, remarks on the Prussian system of plunder as then in force as contrasted with the English rules for requisitions. The Prussians then, as now, made requisitions by order of their officers for the support of their troops whilst the English stated their wants to a commissary, Lord Palmerston says:

> Who applied to the agents of the French Government for the articles required, and the supply being made through channels known to the people, and by authorities recognised by them, the burden was not felt to be so oppressive as if the exaction had been made by the immediate order of an enemy, and at the caprice of individual officers. The consequence was, that, though both Prussians and ourselves lived equally at the expense of the country, the first are detested and the latter liked. On the march to Paris Blücher's army crossed the line Wellington meant to take, they having got before him while he halted at Cambray. He advanced through a line of country which the Prussians had been actually starved out of, and yet found no difficulty in obtaining supplies. The inhabitants who had deserted their villages at the approach of the Prussians returned the moment our troops came up, and confidence being restored, provisions followed, of course.

He says also:

> Wherever we passed we heard complaints of the Prussians, who seem to have behaved roughly; at the same time, when asked for details, with the exception of some particular cases of individual excess, they appeared to have chiefly confined themselves to heavy contributions.

They did not do this at Orléans, and they also added heavy money contributions. Seeing in what a state of terror and danger all the people were, we went to the *évêche*, intending to ask the bishop to entrust any valuables to us. We entered the wide-open gates. The old porter and his wife were weeping. In spite of there being 100 wounded in the house—50 French and 50 German—the general of a division had taken possession of it, it was turned into quarters, and resembled a barrack. There was no one to announce us. We crossed the courtyard, and entered the hall. It was full of soldiers. Turning off, we went through the little private chapel, where all was dark and quiet, one solitary lamp still burning before the altar, up a back staircase, and so through to the first floor, where were the bishop's rooms. Chaplains, servants, all were gone; we came into the ante-room of the bishop's library, where he usually received visitors, and here we met a grand vicar in tears, a little carpet bag in his hand. His bedroom had been taken possession of by a German lieutenant, his two watches and some linen shirts stolen, and his purse with some money in it. He was going to seek a roof to cover him in the town.

Shocked and disgusted, we stood still, consulting what to do—how to announce ourselves to the bishop, indeed where to find him—when we heard a voice speaking loudly and harshly in the next room. We listened; it was certainly a Prussian, but the tones were not those to use in the presence of a man so high in rank, of such world-wide reputation, as Monseigneur Dupanloup. The door suddenly opened, and a tall, beardless boy in uniform came out, followed by the bishop, in his violet *soutane*, the very picture of an aged and dignified priest. He was remonstrating with the officer that this room was his own library. He could not have officers sleeping there. He had been kept awake till three in the morning by the shouting and singing going on in the room down below him, and to have it here was impossible.

But the boy answered sharply, in very bad French, 'But you must; no nonsense with us; do you hear that? Three beds to be made up in this room by five o'clock this evening, or you will be the worse for it.'

'*Mais Monsieur*,' said the poor bishop, mildly—'

Do you hear me?' broke in the officer, raising *his clenched fist* as he spoke. 'Three beds here tonight; you know what you have to do; mind that it is done. Do you hear?'

The poor bishop leaned against the door, saying in a faint voice, '*Monsieur, je ne peux plus*' (Sir, I can bear no more), and, catching hold of the arm of a chaplain, tottered back into his room.

If ever I longed to be a man and a soldier, just for five minutes, it was then; but I was only a woman, and I looked the Prussian full in the face as he passed me, saying in German, 'You brute, they shall know of this in England.'

He looked very foolish and said, 'I was ordered by the general.'

'You have done well,' I answered. 'I am happy to see how you Germans honour an old man and a priest.'

He walked out cursing and muttering, and, not liking to intrude on such sorrow as the bishop's, we left.

After about an hour's rest we started with the good Père Guerin for Cercottes and Chevilly. Just before reaching Cercottes we overtook the Mayor of Chevilly, and gave over to him the stores we had brought, which saved us a four miles further journey on a bitter day. A light snow was falling and the frost was intense. As we came to the entrance of the village, we saw in the corner of a field that bordered the road a deep trench, and round it forty or fifty dead bodies, all French. We did not halt, but drove on to the presbytery, and the *curé* came out to greet us. He begged us to go to a farmhouse about a mile off across the fields; where three officers were lying seriously wounded, who had begged to be transported into Orléans.

Père Guerin suggested that the *curé* should show us the way, and I requested him to get into the carriage. Poor fellow, he looked at his torn *soutane* and his muddy sabots and apologised; he would go on the box, he was not in a state to drive with a lady. I only felt he was worth a dozen dandy grey-gloved curates, and I got out, saying, 'If he would not get in, I would not.' So, with many words of gratitude for a simple courtesy he mounted, and we started. He told us he had been helping to dig the trench we had seen. He had buried forty Germans that morning at the other end of the village. All the dead he could find left unburied had been collected, and this afternoon he hoped to inter the French.

At this juncture the road got so bad that I preferred to walk, and a very short cut across the fields brought us to the courtyard gate of the old farm. Here we met a surgeon who introduced himself as one of the Fifth Ambulance. We explained our errand, and he regretted we had not arrived the day before. They had been obliged to amputate in all the cases; and, therefore, removal for fourteen or fifteen days would be impossible; but he thanked us most sincerely for the offer to receive the patients at the end of that time, and asked us for some wine for them.

We entered the farm; it was very sad and dreary. In one room lay a young officer fresh from the amputation-table. He smiled and seemed glad to see us. Just then his comrade was brought in, hardly recovered from the effect of the chloroform, and placed on a rude mattress beside him, and the third was still under the surgeon's knife. And here the sufferers must remain for a fortnight with the scantiest of comfort; yet the farmer's family and a bright, intelligent *infirmier* left by the ambulance were there, and would doubtless, under the surgeon's direction, prove valuable nurses.

We left what wine we could spare, then visited another farm, where also were amputated men, and finally returned to the presbytery. Here the *curé* got out, and seeing a woman leaning against the wall asked if she had cleaned out the church. In a shrill scream she instantly demanded, 'Did M. le Curé wish to sacrifice her to those fiendish Prussians? They had dirtied the church; doubtless it pleased them best dirty. Should she interfere? Names of all the saints, no; she was going back to the forest till the dogs of Germans were gone.' And off she walked. The *curé* called after her in vain, and addressed an indignant protest to two old women and a child, declaring Mass should be celebrated next morning, *coûte que coûte,* and when he came back from burying the French, he would clean the church himself. Probably he did; he had energy enough for anything.

I drove on alone to where the path rejoined the high road, my two companions crossing a field to see if a white heap under a tree was a dead man or not. Down by the trench round which lay the bodies I was struck by the appearance of one, he looked so calm and quiet, so little hurt; his arm was in splints of English make. He had died from cold and exposure, not the effect of his wound. Another mobile by his side had his trousers cut up and his leg bandaged; he, too, was slightly wounded. On the bandage was a mark I recognised; it was one of the splendid supply sent from Putney, some of which we had given for the use of surgeons and wounded in Caserne d'Étapes. One man had his head clean shot off, and close by lay a captain of the Foreign Legion, fearfully wounded.

But I will not shock our readers by details. They had been dead several days, but owing to the severe frost showed no signs of decomposition; and there they lay, ranged round the open grave, victims of a cruel war prolonged by a king's ambition, when he might have had a peace more honourable to him in the eyes of Europe than all the victories won after Sedan; and looking on these pale, bloodstained corpses I thought of a day when they will stand before the Great White Throne, and their death on this needless battlefield will call for vengeance on the heads of emperors and statesmen, who looked on them, breathing, living men, as mere machines to minister to their glory or their ambition. What will be the answer to the question asked then, 'Where is thy brother?'

Could that scene have been transferred to canvas, what a lesson it would have taught! The long grey road, the poplar stumps, the fields powdered with a light snow, the black forest in the background, the branches tossing in the bleak north wind, the leaden sky above, the corpses ranged around the grave, with the fresh upturned mound of earth beside it, and the three solitary figures standing by it, wondering where were the homes awaiting those pale forms and where were the women who loved them. Would they ever know of this grave?

The *curé* stood bare-headed and silent by the trench while Père Guerin, stooping over the officer's body tried if by chance he recognised the face. In vain. Every care had been taken to collect the papers found upon the bodies; but his had been too well plundered. Probably his pocket-book had contained notes, and all had been taken together. He was to be buried on the top of the others, so that if by chance at any time search were made by his friends the body might be easily identified. There they lay in the closing twilight, and no one to bury them. The men the *curé* expected failed him, and there was no one to lower the bodies into the tomb.

In despair he appealed to the Prussian guard, and two or three stolid, good-natured soldiers offered to assist; and so, we left them to their sad task, and drove on to another lonely house where we were told a solitary wounded man awaited help. We found him, a young *Zouave*, most kindly tended by the farmer and his wife. He, was severely wounded in the leg by a ball which had struck him on the Saturday morning. He had crawled into the forest, remained there till dusk, and then made his way to this farm, which was just on the outskirts. He was very lonely, and gladly accepted the offer of going into our ambulance, and with this patient we started for Orléans, and in due time reached the convent.

During all these days we had heard heavy firing on the other side of the Loire, and were aware that fighting was going on round Beaugency, where General Chanzy was said to be defending the way to Tours and Le Mans. The history of those battles is told in the newspapers of the 16th and 17th December.

We heard the booming of the guns, but saw nothing of the battles beyond the usual sad result—hundreds of waggons full of wounded and a few squads of prisoners. Every bed we had was occupied. M. Emanuel Dupoux, our surgeon, had his hands full, the surgeons of the Puy-de-Dôme Ambulance were in Ste. Marie, and those of the Lyonnaise at Pomme du-Pin. A Spanish noble volunteered to be our secretary, and a Savoyard gentleman our chief *infirmier*. We had no paid service, yet all went on splendidly.

Now and then Prussian soldiers presented themselves and claimed quarters, but soon withdrew. On one occasion Louise and myself were summoned into the stable-yard by the cry, 'Here are the Prussians!' and arriving there found half-a-dozen dragoons trying to turn out our two poor old white ponies and insinuate their big horses into the little stable. I sent a Sister flying for the safe-conduct, which was kept at Ste. Marie, as most exposed to danger, being on the high road from Gien, and told my friends they could not come in there. The sergeant, a boy of eighteen or twenty, persisted that he would. The weather was bitter, his horses must have shelter.

I went into the stable, seized the bridles of our two ponies, who had only just been taken out of harness, and said they were for the service of the ambulance, and should not be turned into the cold. The sergeant grew furious, and insisted on going into the gardener's house, a small one-storey cottage, to see if he could not screw his own special great beast in there. I told him that that was the house for smallpox cases; he was welcome to sleep there himself, if he liked. He replied, 'He would not do that, he would not be murdered; but his horse should sleep there.'

I grew tired of all this nonsense and said, 'To finish this affair, get out, horse and all.'

On this he drew a remarkably long sword and brandished it ferociously about me. Louise stood by, watching the scene with much amusement, and sundry Sisters clung round her, declaring I should be killed; but she knew better, and coolly said, 'Oh dear no; *Mademoiselle* is quite competent to take care of herself.' I felt very indignant, and seizing the boy's wrist I twisted his sword out of his hand with a jerk. It was quite new and very bright, and I gave it back, congratulating him on the opportunity he had of trying it for the first time on a woman. His companions began to laugh at him, and just then the Sister arrived breathless with the safe conduct.

'Now,' I said to the sergeant, 'you see I might punish you very severely for this. You saw the Red Cross marked on the doors, and the words "*Ambulance Anglaise*"; but if you will go away directly, I shall not complain to Prince Frederick Charles.' He hesitated, and I seized his horse's bridle and led him to the gate. 'Get out,' I said, 'and never let us see you here again, you stupid boy!' He did get out, and his companions followed him, and never from that day had we any annoyance. The poor Sisters gave a sigh of relief, Louise and I retired upon our laurels to the calm of our own room, and so ended the defeat of the *Uhlans* in the Convent of St. Marc.

We were now getting uneasy; our gold was running short. The 33*l*. due to me by the National Society, instead of being paid me in London in time to get it in *napoleons*, had been sent after me in a cheque, that no one would look at. I consulted everybody, and was told I could get it at Tours or Bourges. Now, this was a three days' journey, and I hesitated; but we saw the men needing wine, tobacco, and vegetables, that only ready money could procure; we wanted instruments, too, and other business had to be transacted; so we resolved that Louise should remain to guard the two houses against all comers, and I should go to Bourges. Lord Lyons had left Tours, but was reported to be there. I went to the Prussian *commandant de place* and asked for a safe-conduct to Tours.

He said certainly, but I must go round by Versailles and Rouen. To this I replied, 'Nonsense! Do look at your map. Really, I cannot afford to go that roundabout way.'

He turned round, studied a map, and said, '*Madame*, you are right; Versailles is out of the way; Will you go to Nantes?'

'Now, why should I go to Nantes?' I remonstrated. 'I have no business there.'

'Well, *Madame*, you see you might give intelligence of what is going on in our lines if you went straight to Tours. If ten days have passed before you reach it anything you say will be of no use.'

'Colonel,' I said, 'if I am a spy, I could go straight to Rouen, and be in French lines in thirty-six hours. Spies have plenty of money; I have none. I wish to go to the nearest point in French lines, and I intend to go. Please to give me a safe-conduct.'

The colonel burst out laughing, and said, 'Well, I must write that you go to Nantes; but you may go which way you please.'

'Thank you,' I said; and not pledging myself to visit the ancient Breton city, I took my precious bit of paper, written in blue ink and dried with gold dust, and walked off. We have that piece of hieroglyphics still. It was never looked at, and shall be framed and glazed as a trophy.

So far so good; but how to get out of Orléans. The railroad did not run, there were no diligences. The Prussians had seized all the horses and carriages, and though I saw our friends of the Anglo-American always driving about in a basket *phaeton*, it was not the sort of vehicle for a three days' journey, even if they could have spared it. I went to the President of the French International, on the speculation of borrowing an ambulance waggon, to which our two white ponies might have been harnessed, and there met a very gentlemanly Frenchman, a civilian, who was imploring M. Dubois d'Angers to ask for a safe-conduct for him out of Prussian lines.

This M. Dubois d'Angers said he could not do, and the young man was evidently '*au désespoir.*' I stated my wish, and he sprang forward and said, 'I have a carriage and horses. If *Madame* will permit me to accompany her, I will not only take her to Tours or Bourges, but she shall have my carriage and horses to return to Orléans.' Here was an offer. I asked simply, 'But what has *Monsieur* done to be so anxious to get away?' He turned to M. Dubois d'Angers, and most gracefully begged the honour of a presentation.

It was done, and M. Maxime G—then explained that he had expressed himself too freely in the presence of a Bavarian officer. He had justified Gambetta, whose personal friend he was, in his policy of *guerre à outrance*, he had had a hint that his arrest, though he had never fought against the Prussians, was more than probable, and he only prayed to be able to rejoin his wife and child at Pau. I told him that though I would not be responsible for his safety, I should be very thankful for his carriage and escort, and could conceive no reason why I should not accept it. And so, it was arranged; at eight next morning I was to be ready for our somewhat perilous journey.

When I got back, I found our surgeon in a woeful way. He had been told that, having served with *francs-tireurs*, even his profession would not be respected. He was resolved to leave Orléans, and begged us to accept his substitute. Dr. Bertier, of the *Garde Mobile* of Savoie, who would remain as our surgeon. Next morning, I presented myself, and found at the door M. Emanuel Dupoux and M. S—, a merchant of Chambery, all resolved to accompany me. At eight M. Maxime G— arrived with a nice closed carriage, drawn by only one horse. Alas! the Prussians had stolen the other the night before. It was no time for lengthened *adieux*; difficulty and danger had to be faced, Prussian guards, French outposts, and camp-followers, so with a gay wave of the hand we started.

The 14th of December was a bright morning, all looked cheerful; it was a good omen for our expedition. As we drove along the quay by the Loire, M. Emanuel Dupoux and M. S— gave me their loaded revolvers, which I put one in each pocket of my dress. It was necessary to have them, yet to have been found with arms might have drawn suspicion on the gentlemen. The little Union-Jack on the carriage blew out in the fresh morning air as we drove over the bridge and past the guard. Not a question was asked, the sentinels there paced up and down, and only gave a glance at the carriage, then down the other bank, and past the sentinels at the outpost. They did not even look at us; we breathed again, and drove merrily on through the lonely, desolate Sologne. We had fairly left Orléans behind us, and were on our way to Vierzon, from whence a line of railroad branches either to Bourges or Tours.

Chapter 27

The Army of the Vosges

The Sologne is a dreary waste of country, scattered stunted shrubs breaking the monotony of a barren, sandy heath. There is marsh land, too, upon it, where lonely pools look like oases in the desert. A few villages and farms are scattered about it; and the railway from Orléans to Vierzon runs through it, while that from Orléans to Gien runs on the other side of the Loire, which bounds this melancholy region to the east. At La Mothe Beauvron is a farm that did belong to the emperor; he bought land about that place to try if it could not be reclaimed, and the experiment answered; but all the rest is left in its primitive state of desolation.

We avoided both the high road by the river and the Imperial Route by the side of the railway, and struck our course right through the heart of the Sologne, midway between the two. I do not suppose English travellers ever went that way; I know no reason why they should. There is nothing to see, and no possible object to be gained by so doing; but, in our case, according to good information sent to us from Vierzon, we should keep clear of Prussian outposts. We might meet a few *Uhlans*, but they would be simply on a foraging excursion, and have no authority to stop travellers with an English flag.

We went quietly along, every now and then meeting a peasant, who invariably informed our coachman that a camp of at least ten thousand Prussians lay only five miles off, and my friends were slightly nervous. I had no fear for myself, and all went well till we arrived near Vannes. As we were drawing near, Henri, our coachman, turned round, and made most frightful and unintelligible faces, which M. Maxime G—translated into '*Uhlans*,' and looking out, sure enough there they were, at least eight or nine, clustered round a forge, where the smith was shoeing one of their horses. Henri said, 'We are lost.'

The gentlemen were fidgety, to say the least of it; but it was arranged that I should answer all questions, and, pulling out my safe-conduct, I prepared for the encounter. 'Drive on slowly and steadily, Henri,' I said, 'and take no notice of the Prussians.' Henri did so; my heart beat a little fast; we neared them, were up to there, passed them, and drove up the street. We were about to rejoice, when I saw two in full array, lance in rest, and little flags fluttering in the wind, one on each side of the road, keeping watch on the entrance from the Vierzon side. Henri grew pale. 'Drive on,' I said, 'don't stop,' and on we went. The *Uhlans* smiled and saluted us, but asked no questions; and we were a couple of miles away before we could realise we had passed the last outpost and were free. It was evident, by the watch they kept on the road before them, that they expected the enemy from that side.

In a couple of hours, we reached a small village called 'Isdes,' and halted to rest our poor old horse. We drove into the yard of a small village inn—how clearly even now the scene rises before me. I can see the low shed opposite the house, with a couple of carts standing in it, the straw heaped about the place, and the group of peasants who came around to ask news of Orléans. One amongst them, an intelligent-looking man of thirty, in a blue blouse, was presented as the mayor.

M. Maxime G— was well known in the district, having a nice estate near Orléans, and he invited the mayor to take a glass of wine with us in the long, dark kitchen of the *auberge*. The mayor told us that *Uhlans* had paid a visit to the village about a week before. Their coming had been preceded by the arrival of a man, calling himself 'George,' driving a fine pair of horses in a light country waggon, and proclaiming himself to be in search of two carriage horses, stolen from his master's property, near Gien, by the Prussians.

This strange tale seems to have excited no suspicion, and the simple peasants asked what news he brought from his part of the country. He said he had met *Uhlans* everywhere; they would shortly come there. How much hay and corn was there stored in the village? It had better be hidden. Some, still unsuspecting, answered him; several, however, kept silence, and the result proved their wisdom.

Next day came a troop of *Uhlans*, and 'required' the hay and corn that had been pointed out exactly from those people who had spoken of their stores. The same had happened in a neighbouring village. M. Maxime G— instantly exclaimed, 'That man is a spy; we shall have him on our track; he will be here today. Be sure he is just ahead of those *Uhlans* we saw at Vannes, and if he find the coast clear here he'll bring them on.'

The words were hardly spoken before the mayor sprang up. '*Le voila!*' and, sure enough, a man drove into the yard with the fine horses and light waggon they had been describing to us, and, flinging the rope reins to a stable-boy, jumped down and began to bluster about, asking if there were Prussians there. M. Maxime G—, M. Emanuel Dupoux, and M. S—withdrew with the mayor, and a consultation was held. It ended in M. Emanuel going to order out our weary horse, and requesting me to be ready for a start. Then they went into the yard and confronted the newcomer.

I saw him through the window, a fine man, about forty years of age, six feet high, with dark, curly hair and a rosy complexion. He wore a dark blue woollen guernsey and fustian trousers, and a crimson handkerchief twisted round his throat. He seemed very excited, and was pulling out more papers and passports and certificates than ever any honest man travelled with. His last passport was only a conditional one. A request from the mayor of some commune in Alsace addressed to the mayor of the first town still in French possession to furnish George (I forget his other name) with a passport, if he thought proper so to do. The rest were certificates of character from various masters he had served. He spoke German very well. This he accounted for by being a native of Alsace, but his story about his master's horses was very vague, and whilst fumbling with his papers one fell out. M. Emanuel seized it. It was a German cheque on a banker at Hamburg.

That settled the matter. The mayor took M. Maxime G— aside, and I caught the words, 'Keep him safe, or he'll bring the *Uhlans* upon you and us.' Two strong peasants placed themselves on either side of George, and the gentlemen and the mayor withdrew with some dozen peasants, and held conference in the long shed. George saw that his fate hung in the balance, and, catching sight of me, suddenly dashed up the steps down which I was coming to get into the carriage, and began with trembling hands to show me his papers. M. Emanuel ran forward, and called me to get in quick. I did so; the coachman mounted, and the carriage was driven out of the yard. I looked back as we halted in the lane. I saw the crowd close round George; I heard loud voices. I saw our friends disengage themselves, followed by the mayor, who shook hands with M. Maxime G— saying, 'Yes, it must be, for the safety of all.'

The gentlemen got in, and we drove up a cross lane leading to Cerdon, thus leaving the road we had been traversing before, so that, supposing the villagers were true and silent, all trace of our way would be lost. The road was a short, steep ascent to a sandy down. As we reached the top, I heard the ring of half-a-dozen rifles, and I saw the gentlemen look at each other, but no remark was made. But I knew what it was, and that George would give no more information to the *Uhlans* waiting at Vannes.

It was a dreary drive to Cerdon. The road in one place had been cut, but a lad who accompanied us from Isdes showed us a path cunningly hidden by bending down brushwood where, if we got out and walked, our carriage could pass. It rained hard, but there was no help for it, and as we were getting out, we saw a strange sight in such a journey. There came along the road a neatly-dressed woman with a Red-Cross brassard on her arm, driving a very good horse in a light covered cart. She was evidently much frightened at us, and M. Maxime G——, going up, politely saluted her, and asked her what she was doing there all alone, and what assistance we could be.

She, too, pulled out a paper; but this time it was correct. She was servant in a very large farm about ten miles off. The Prussians were hourly expected, and her master had told her to take his best horse and his cart to Bourges, to save them from the *Uhlans*. She wanted to pass on, and was most grateful for being shown the side-path round the obstruction. Her horse was young and fresh, ours old, lame, and tired, so that when we rejoined the high road we soon lost sight of her.

We had intended to sleep at Aubigny, but at Cerdon our horse was so done up we could get no farther. Cerdon was another miserable village. The mayor; an old friend of M. Maxime G——'s father, arrived to call upon us, with two or three of his acquaintances. They heard the tale of George's arrival at Vannes, and expressed themselves delighted that he was not likely to pay them another visit. So wild and lonely was this Sologne village, that I was not sorry to find two of our party were to sleep in the room adjoining mine, and M. Maxime G—— and his coachman in a little room at the foot of the staircase. The loaded revolvers were placed under my pillow, ready to be handed out if required, and, forgetting danger and hardship, I slept soundly.

We found next morning we were only an hour from Aubigny, a pretty little town, entered by a bridge over a narrow, clear stream. Here Henri, the coachman, insisted upon stopping for half an hour, in spite of our remonstrances. We strolled through the town, and saw several mediaeval houses and an interesting old castle, now an ambulance, with a picturesque entrance gateway. I know nothing of its history.

Murray does not even name the town; yet it is well worth a visit. The only direction I can give is that it is in the midst of the Sologne. We halted again at a village on the high road, where M. Emanuel and myself agreed it would be better that the party should sleep. We were not far from Bourges, and by an early start should be there in good time next day. But Henri was obstinate; it would be impossible; the inn at Henrichemont was the best about there; it was a little farther on, and would shorten the stage next day.

We were over-persuaded, and went on. We found we were taken a good way to the left, and, therefore, a little further from Bourges, which was straight before us; and, as we guessed, the circumstance of our quitting the direct road and coming round by Henrichemont, for no apparent purpose, brought suspicion upon us.

Henrichemont is a pretty town, with a handsome central market-place. But we were no sooner in the hotel than I found we were taken for Prussian spies. Henri, too, was stupidly mysterious. He had been told, on the best authority, that Prussians were between us and Bourges; and he made matters worse by refusing to tell his master's name. Whilst we were at dinner the mayor was announced. His manner was very peculiar; he said he came to inform us that a sortie had been made from Paris; that Versailles was occupied by the French, and King William flying for his life to Rheims. How did we like that? My companions said truthfully, very much indeed if it were true; but it seemed too good news to be credible. The mayor looked sulky, and walked out, saying the *sous-préfet* would be there in the morning.

Very early next day M. Emanuel went to see the *sous-préfet*, and came back indignant at his insulting manner. However, the authorities could find no pretext for detaining us, myself especially, in consequence of my English passport, and we started. I begged Henri to go straight to Bourges, and he promised he would. We had not left Henrichemont an hour before we saw, in the dip of the road, a large body of cavalry. My friends grew very nervous. It would be too hard to be so near freedom and fail at the eleventh hour. I looked out. I caught a gleam of scarlet.

'French *Cuirassiers!*' I cried.

M. S— looked out, and gave a shout of ecstasy. '*Nous sommes libres!*' was all he could say.

We drove on; we passed the troops, and it was a comfortable feeling that five hundred good sabres were between us and the Prussian lines. Henri, imagining all safe, insisted on halting for luncheon at a small town crowded with troops; and here again the gentlemen were taken for Prussian spies, and were in a very bad temper at their reception by their countrymen. But the truth was, the whole affair was considered so extraordinary—how we could possibly get out of Prussian lines unquestioned and unchallenged, and come in safety through the lonely district of the Sologne; that it was difficult for them to believe in our tale of having quietly driven out of Orléans to go to Bourges as if it were a summer day's excursion.

We reached Bourges at last. The high road was blocked by artillery going to join General Bourbaki's headquarters at La Charité, near Nevers. Infantry, cavalry, artillery, waggons of ammunition and provision, Mobiles, *francs-tireurs*, all were there. We asked what *corps d'armée* it was. 'The 18th,' was the answer; 'part of the Army of the Vosges.' Bourges was crowded with troops; but, fortunately, owing to the lucky chance of my being recognised by the mistress of the hotel, I obtained a small room. Having taken possession of it, I went out to try and cash my unlucky cheque. In vain. I was assured by two bankers that under present circumstances it was impossible; I might get it done at Poitiers. Lord Lyons was at Bordeaux, there I should be sure to succeed; but to go to Bordeaux to find thirty-three pounds was absurd. I bestowed a hearty grumble on the British Committee and their utter want of forethought, and gave it up.

Had this been my only business my expedition would have been a failure; but it was not. Just the day before Orléans was closed in, I had received a letter informing me of 500*l.* worth of stores sent out by an agent to be confided to us, to form an ambulance for the Army of the Vosges. They were to come to Tours. Since then we had heard nothing of them, and it was clearly our duty to see they were not lost. At Bourges I heard English stores had passed through and gone to 'headquarters' at Autun. General Garibaldi was still there, and there I could hear where the stores were, and if we were wanted. I found I could get by Nevers to Autun, and resolved to go on next day. My three friends begged me to dine with them at the *table d'hôte*, a farewell dinner, and I did so. Their joy and gratitude were most touching, and when next morning early I started for Autun they all escorted me to the railway station.

We got to Nevers at noon, and here we had to make a long stop. I engaged a *commissionnaire* to show me the town, which he did by going full speed up and down the streets, saying as he went, 'That's a church, that's the Hôtel de Ville, that's an hotel,' and not proposing going inside any of them. The cathedral was remarkably dirty and not very beautiful, and the town not much worth a visit. There were very few soldiers in it, only National Guards being drilled. All the troops were being sent to La Charité.

When I returned to the hotel, I found a young Englishman there who had come out with a few bales from the British National Society, which, as there were no wounded at Nevers, was a superfluous proceeding. He could not give me change for my cheque, to my great disappointment. He talked of going back to England *via* Poitiers. It is rather a round-about way, but doubtless he arrived safe at last. In the evening I started for Autun. The scenery was lovely, and the mountains of the Vosges showed themselves in the distance. It was quite dark, however, before we reached our destination. I could find neither *fiacre* nor porter, so, asking my way to the best hotel, I set off to find it.

But under General Garibaldi's rule early hours prevailed. It was barely ten o'clock, yet not a soul was in the streets, not a sound to be heard. The hotel was closed, but when I knocked the door was opened. To my dismay, they had not a vacant room. I tried two others with the same ill success, and, tired and weary, I sat down on a bench in the kitchen of the last one, and begged them to let me stay there till morning.

The good woman was about to consent, when an Italian *franc-tireur*, who, seeing the light, came in, insisted that I was a spy: and must go to the guardhouse till the *préfet* could be found. There was only one resource. I said, 'Very well, take me to the general.' At first, he refused, but I persisted, and we set off. How weary and dispirited I felt! and how utterly disgusted when, entering a small cabaret, my captor told me to come in and wait while he and a companion who had joined him drank absinthe. This I positively declined, and a boy *Garde Mobile* who was passing stopped and asked me what it was all about. I explained; he was most indignant, and told the *francs-tireurs*, if I was a spy, I ought to be taken directly to the *préfecture*, and he should go with me himself as far.

Poor lad! he had to march to La Charité at three in the morning, but he came with us to the gate of the *préfecture*, where, to my relief, I saw a sentinel. My captor began to look very foolish, and the sentinel told us to go into the hall. We entered a brightly-lighted vestibule. An officer dozing on a bench sprang up, I instantly addressed him, and begging me to sit down, he ran upstairs and brought back a most elegant, courteous old man in a fine crimson flannel shirt and gold sword-belt around his waist. I never heard his name, but his fatherly kindness I cannot easily forget. I told him my errand, showed him my letters of introduction, and he turned quickly round to the *franc-tireur*, demanding by what right he had dared to arrest a lady with a letter to the general and an English passport. The man shuffled and tried to explain, but the officer ordered him out, assuring him that in the morning he should be taught a lesson in the difference between an English lady and a Prussian spy, and so dismissed him.

What I was to do was now the question. It appears that after the retreat was sounded at nine p.m. all pleasure and business ceased, and the inhabitants of the *préfecture* were in their first sleep, though it was not eleven o'clock. The general allowed neither drinking nor gambling, his own habits, so singularly quiet and even Spartan in their simplicity, were copied by his officers, and the discipline of his *corps d'armée* was far superior to that of the new French levies.

A few words of consultation between the two officers resulted in the elder one offering me his bedroom, a dark closet opening off the first-floor corridor. The bed was a heap of straw; no light was possible, it would have been dangerous in so small a space, but weary as I was it was most inviting. I laid down on the straw, the kind old officer covered me up with a huge military cloak, and saying, 'Rest quietly, *Madame*; under the general's roof you are perfectly safe,' bade me a kind goodnight, and withdrew.

Dawn was just breaking when the opening of the door aroused me. It was my old friend. He took me into a room opposite, where was the officer on guard, reading by a table, with his revolver in front of him; and my kind friend, who, I found, had passed the night on a chair in the corridor, retired for an hour's sleep on the straw in the closet. The officer begged me to sit awhile by the blazing fire and tell him all the news. There was not much that he did not know, except the difficulty of getting provisions and wood in Orléans. About seven he summoned a young officer and told him to take me to the best hotel, 'La Poste.' I should there find an English lady who could give me all the information I sought about the stores and the ambulance work, and with my young escort I again sallied forth.

Madame M. W— was not up. I arranged to return to the *préfecture* and see the general, and then the kind landlady found me a recently vacated room, where I made myself look as respectable as possible under the circumstances, and enjoyed some hot coffee. I then went back to the *préfecture*, and on my way bought a pair of gloves, for the purpose of a chat with some inhabitants. I spoke with several tradespeople and heard but one account, how very orderly the general's troops were. It was utterly untrue that the *évêche* at Autun had been invaded by the soldiers. No annoyance of any sort had been suffered by the bishop, or priests. The churches had not been desecrated, the daily services continued as usual, and the *préfecture* had been offered to the general by the *sous-préfet*.

All this I saw and ascertained for myself, and I cannot too much reprehend the practice of those who, from personal prejudice against General Garibaldi, accuse him of acts which never took place, and which accusations they know themselves to be wholly and wilfully false. His own personal character needs no defence from me. His purity of life, his kindness of heart, his generous, unselfish disposition, are acknowledged even by his bitterest enemies, and that they believe him to be mistaken in his course of action is no excuse for cruel and wilful slander. No town that I saw in military occupation was one half so well organised as Autun, and there were no complaints of depredations committed in the villages around.

It is not my place to enter into any disquisition as to the rights or wrongs of his fighting for France; but it is well to remember, he alone of all the generals during the war never lost a French gun, and that he alone took a Prussian standard and saved his whole *corps d'armée*. He carried out his charge of blocking the road to Lyons, and whether the Germans meant to go or not, we all know that they never did get there. I was not surprised at what I heard. In 1867, at Rome, I had been told of the ravages and sacrilege committed by the Garibaldini. I visited every place. I found it utterly untrue, except at Monte Rotundo, which had been taken by storm.

Nor can I conceive how those who, on the scantiest evidence, call out against the Garibaldini as mere brigands, can reconcile their virtuous horror at such things with the quiet way in which they find excuses for the massacre at Bazeilles and the cruelties of the German troops in the occupied provinces. War is very terrible, but General Garibaldi never made it unnecessarily so, and the next generation, coolly looking back on the events of this, will do full justice to '*Il Generale.*'

I found at the *préfecture* that he was ill in bed, but I saw General Canzio. I was received in a salon, in which the furniture remained in its proper place, a noteworthy fact, as contrasted with a Prussian occupation! Several *aides-de-camp* were sitting reading round a central table.

Their dress was soldier-like and simple: a fine scarlet shirt fastened with gold buttons, open at the throat, to show a white shirt and cravat, grey trousers with a crimson stripe, and half-boots, a patent leather sword-belt and slings; gauntlet gloves, a large grey cloak, and a fur cap completed the costume. They were quiet, gentlemanly men, and General Canzio looked so very English that his face seemed familiar to me. He said the stores had arrived safe, and in our absence had been transferred to Madame M. W— for the use of the ambulances. Our help would be most welcome, if we could give it. Would I go and consult with her? This was very satisfactory. The loss of so many valuable stores would have been very provoking, and would have entailed a long hunt for them. So that they were safe and in use, it mattered little who gave them away or what *corps d'armée* had them.

Another *aide-de-camp* escorted me to Madame M. W—. Her reception was most warm and cordial; she only regretted I had not knocked her up the night before, and insisted on giving me some luncheon. She most kindly asked me to stay with her till the next day, but, having discovered the stores, I was anxious to return. I found that she was managing the ambulance work, and perfectly competent to do so. They had very few wounded at present, and it must depend on circumstances whether our assistance would be needed. We arranged that at all events, till further events occurred, there was more work to be done at Orléans. Her kindness and my luncheon quite refreshed me.

We laughed over my miseries of the night before, and at noon she drove me down to the station, and I started for Nevers. I slept there that night. It was most lovely weather—quite warm and spring-like. I sat with the windows open, enjoying it, and hoped to find it the same at Orléans; but I was cruelly undeceived.

I reached Bourges next day. At Sanscaize, the junction from La Charité, some French officers got into the train, and one greeted me as a friend. He had been in our ambulance at Sedan, and preserved a most grateful recollection of the skill and kindness of Dr. Tilghman, and the good nursing he had had there. He had been sent to Mézières and the north of France as a hopeless invalid, but he had wonderfully recovered, and though the wound in his thigh was yet unhealed, he was able to rejoin, not his regiment—they were all dead or in Prussia—but the depot, as the nucleus of a new one. He had some fifty men with him, and was especially annoyed at their want of order. They would get out of the train at every stop, and he had to descend and order them in.

Close by Bourges we had a two hours' delay. The railroad runs on an embankment above the level of the road, which was on the right hand. Beyond that road, on the crest of a rising slope, was another road, and on our left hand another, all leading towards Nevers. These three roads were a mass of troops going to La Charité, of every kind and sort. Even the *spahis* of Africa were there, with their broad stirrups, their red morocco boots, their curved sabres and white *burnous*. It was reported that they carried a terrible weapon—a lasso with a steel hook at the end, with which to catch unwary Prussians, and drag them from their horses through the dirt. I never heard of its being used.

Thousands and thousands of men passed us, some already foot-sore from being badly shod, and lagging behind. Those bad boots and shoes were the ruin of France. One lot was found with brown paper soles. Soldiers could not march and fight lame and crippled from want of proper boots. If ever England goes to war, which God forbid, let there be special care taken that the boots and shoes of our brave fellows are well-made, strong-soled, and easy fitting, and we shall avoid one cause of French defeats.

We got weary of waiting. The gate across the railway was kept closed, but we saw a break in one of the long columns, and, escorted by my military friends, I availed myself of that, and walked into Bourges. The first man I met in the streets was M. S——, gorgeously costumed as *commandant* of *Gardes Mobiles*. How changed he was from the shabby, depressed man who had travelled with us from Orléans. His good-natured countenance was beaming with smiles as he presented me to his general, who said in his graceful French way, 'I thank you, *Madame*, for having given back a sword to France.' He looked so happy that it was quite a pleasure to see him. M. Emanuel, too, was there; he was going back to his home; and M. Maxime G——had already left, to rejoin his wife.

I found, however, he had left his carriage and Henri, and next morning I started on my return to Orléans. A poor coachman begged for a lift. His well-authenticated story was a strange one. A countess from Alsace had borrowed the carriage and horses of this poor man's master to take her to Bourges. The Prussian *commandant* had sent them all round by Nevers; however, they got there at last, and here my lady presented the carriage and horses to a French general on receiving a consideration of two-thirds of their value, and gave the coachman a *napoleon* to get back with. He would have had to walk, but I gladly consented to his occupying the other seat on the box. He was obliged to get back to Orléans to explain what had happened as soon as possible, and brought with him all the necessary papers to enable his master to prosecute the said countess.

Before leaving Bourges, I went to the *préfecture* to ask for a safe-conduct, and was referred to the *commandant de place*. Finding that I should have been detained too late, I resolved to start without it. Henri's parents lived at Romorantin, half-way to Orléans. He was well known on the road, and my German safe-conduct secured us from all danger from Prussian picquets. It was, however, nearly noon before we drove out of Bourges, and still on every street, on every road around the town, we saw the apparently countless thousands of the Army of the Vosges.

CHAPTER 28

Convent Life at Orleans

We passed out of Bourges unchallenged, and drove away by the road to Vierzon. We reached that place before sunset, and found it had been occupied by the Prussians, but evacuated, and the belief was, there was none of the enemy nearer than the outposts round Orléans. There was a very small garrison of French troops in the town, but a great many *trainards* or lingerers from the battalions which had passed through on their way to Bourges and Nevers. We made no halt here, but pushed on to a village some miles beyond, called Mennetou, where we stayed while the horse was shod. The *auberge*, though humble, was very respectable, and I advised sleeping there, thinking it better to remain where evidently no suspicion was entertained of our being Prussian spies, rather than go farther, to encounter, perhaps, all the trouble and delay of such an accusation; but Henri was sure that he could reach his father's house at Romorantin that night, and there we should be quite safe from annoyance.

So, on we went; it was dark when we entered another small village, full of lingerers from the main body of the army. I told Henri to drive straight through, but he would stop to find intelligence, as he said, and to take a glass of cognac, as I saw; and while the carriage was standing in the street, a man, looking like a miller or baker, came up to the window, and began to cross-question me. I answered him frankly, and thought I had got rid of him. I saw him go into the *auberge*, and a few minutes after Henri came out and said they would not allow our carriage to go on; we must go to the *maire*.

I was very much disgusted, and told Henri it was all his fault; had we driven quietly through we should have attracted no attention, and this would not have occurred. I found our accuser did not accompany us, only an energetic patriot, who, on being asked what authority he had to interfere, vanished in the darkness.

We found the mayor at supper with his wife. He was very nervous, especially when I showed my English passport, with the royal arms flourishing upon it. He caught sight, however, of the Prussian *visé*, and remarked it was German; what was it about, and I had to explain that the passport was visaed for all countries, including Russia, Turkey, Italy, and Spain, as he might see, English being free to travel anywhere, and, taking the offensive upon myself, I demanded by what right any Frenchman, seeing, as the miller had done, my passport, and knowing the coachman who was driving me to be an inhabitant of a town five miles off, dare stop me on my way. The mayor made many humble apologies, and ordered a servant to go back with us to the carriage and see us off, and to seek for the miller, to punish his unauthorised interference. The miller, however, was nowhere visible. The indignant eloquence of the other coachman who had remained with the carriage had convinced the crowd of our not being Prussian spies, and we drove on again without further hindrance. All this made it very late before we entered Romorantin.

Henri's father was knocked up, and, astonished as he was, gave us a most cordial reception. He was delighted to see his son, and thanked me much for coming round by Romorantin, to give the family that pleasure. Under their hospitable roof I slept honoured and secure, and before awoke next morning they had seen the *sous-préfet*, and obtained a safe-conduct from him to go, if possible, to Orléans. I did hope our troubles were ended; but not so.

We left Romorantin at eleven a.m. It was a quiet-looking town. About three hundred Prussian dragoons had passed through, and demanded food for themselves and forage for their horses, which was given, and they departed, and no others had, up to that time, arrived. We were going steadily along the road, hoping to reach Caumont-sur-Tharonne by dinner-time, for there the other coachman was well known, and we should probably be free from annoyance; but as we came near Châteauvieux we met an old farmer and his wife jogging along in a cart, and they told us that a bridge just ahead had been blown up, and we must turn off the high road into the marshes below, cross the stream, which was very shallow, and so arrive on the other side of the bridge to rejoin the road.

Our poor old horse was so lame and tired, and his shoulder so sore, that I felt convinced he never could drag the carriage through the boggy ground, and so the farmer thought, and then he most kindly offered, if we would wait till he had deposited his wife, to send his man back with his horse, to help ours through. So steep was the bank, I preferred to get out and walk—the carriage coming after, drawn by the two horses, tandem fashion, and plunging about in a most uncomfortable way. I should have continued my march on foot, but the water grew too deep, and, with many misgivings, I got into the carriage. Every moment I thought we should be over, but the drivers urged on the horses, and we got safely over the stream and marsh. I offered a trifling recompense, but it was refused. The farmer would take nothing for helping an English lady who was nursing his countrymen.

When we reached Châteauvieux, our poor horse was half dead. We must sleep there, and we pulled up at the inn. But hardly had I sat down by the kitchen fire to wait till a room was ready for me, when Henri entered to say the landlord would not allow us to remain as being suspicious, characters. I spoke to him, and trying to convince him I was not a Prussian spy, I pulled out the English brassard, which, though I did not wear, I had in my pocket.

He flew into a fury. He had had gentlemen there with that band—they were ambulance men, they had come with the Prussians. They had dined, had forage for their horses and beds for themselves, and next day, when he presented his bill, refused to pay, saying they had a right to requisitions. By the description of the waggons, I knew they could not be Anglo-Americans, nor do I know to what ambulance they belonged. However, their conduct was our misfortune. All remonstrance was vain; out we must go. The horse must be led at footpace to Caumont, and we must walk; it was only four miles, but the sleet was falling fast.

At this juncture I remembered that in the *château* from which the village took its name, and which was just opposite the inn, lived two French nobles—the Laselles—brothers in-law of Marshal MacMahon, and sons of an English mother, and I resolved to ask them if they could not send me on to Caumont. I went accordingly to the *château*. Madame de Laselles was absent, but the *vicomte* and his brother were only in the grounds, and would be back directly. The servants—pretty-looking, active girls—were most sympathising, and placed me close to the wood fire blazing in the huge kitchen fireplace. Presently a tall, gentlemanly man entered, bringing some fish he had caught.

I rose and explained my tale: he said his brother, M. Arthur de Laselles, was mayor of the commune and the man in authority, but he himself would go with me to the *auberge*, to try to bring the man to reason. We found the poor horse harnessed, and Henri and the coachman ready for our walk. The *vicomte* spoke very severely to the landlord, who persisted in his refusal to take us in. 'If your brother makes a requisition to me to lodge these people here, good; I must. If not, I refuse altogether.'

The *vicomte* turned to me, saying, 'it is certain, Madame, that you cannot remain here to be subject to this insolence. I request you will accept a dinner and bed at my *château*.' I thanked him most sincerely, apologised for the trouble I was giving, and accepted his hospitality as frankly as it was offered. He ordered the coachman to bring the carriage and horse to the stables of the *château*, and there we all proceeded. The *vicomte* and myself re-entered by the great kitchen, for the upper part of the house was kept closely barred.

There we found his brother, the mayor of the commune. I showed him my papers. He said they were as correct as possible. The innkeeper was a surly, drunken fellow, and must be punished. In opening my bag to get the papers out I pulled out a parcel of French newspapers only two days old.

'Can it be possible,' said the *vicomte*; 'are these new newspapers?'

I was very glad to hand them all over to my kind hosts, only asking to have them back in the morning, as I had promised the Bishop of Orléans to bring him some. The gentlemen took them, saying they had seen none for three weeks, nor heard one word of news outside their village, and became instantly immersed in their contents, whilst I was taken upstairs to a splendid room, where a bright wood fire was blazing. Dinner was soon announced, and my hosts' kindness made me feel quite at home.

I left the *château* at eight the next morning, the *vicomte* coming down to the carriage with me, and his brother giving me a fresh safe-conduct. I never had an opportunity to thank the Vicomte de Laselles for his courtesy and kindness, but I have not, nor ever shall forget it. All this trouble, however, depressed me much. It is so miserable to be an object of distrust, especially to those whose interests lie close at heart.

It froze hard, it snowed. I felt thoroughly cold, but I wrapped myself up as well as I could, and was half dozing, when a call from my coachman startled me. The carriage stopped, and looking up I saw an *Uhlan*, lance in hand, close to the window. I instantly began to get out the Prussian safe-conduct, but the trooper shook his head, and two or three others coming up behind him jabbered away at a furious rate.

'What do you want,' said I, 'if you will not look at Colonel Leuthold's safe-conduct?'

'Ah, *Madame* speaks German,' said the first *Uhlan*—a fair, mild-looking young man. Then came a short consultation between them all, and the first, riding up still closer, said mysteriously, pointing to the little Union-Jack I had flying from the carriage, '*Madame* is English?'

'Certainly,' I replied.

'That is good,' he went on; 'the English speak the truth. You will tell us the truth, will you not?'

'Yes,' I answered, very much puzzled, 'I will tell you the truth, or not answer at all. What is it you wish to know?'

'Ah! most worthy and gracious lady!' continued my friend, 'you see I am young; I want to go back to Stettin to my mother; we none of us wish to be killed. Will you tell us truly, are there any *francs-tireurs* on the road to Vierzon?'

'I will tell you truly, my friend,' I replied, infinitely amused. 'There are none as far as Romorantin. Beyond, I think there are, and you will not be safe.'

'We all thank you,' they shouted in chorus. 'A good voyage to you; we shall not leave La Ferté St.-Aubin.'

'Will you be so kind as to see,' I called out, 'that we are not taken for Prussian spies? We have been much troubled by that.'

'Leave it to us,' said my first friend. 'You will have no more trouble now we are here;' and sure enough we had no more.

At La Ferté St.-Aubin we halted for breakfast, and heard a ludicrous story of a Prussian general who arrived, ordered a superb dinner, good wine, and beds for himself and his staff, and when the bill was presented next day gave the poor woman an order on a banker in Berlin! Her husband, however, vowed that when peace came, he would go to Berlin and cash the cheque. I do hope it will not be returned marked 'no effects.' I should think it very likely.

At last Orléans came in sight. How I longed for the quiet convent and the warm welcome. It was really like going home. We drove over the bridge, which we heard had been blown up, and speculated how to cross the Loire if it were, down the Quai du Chatelet, across the railway bridge, and there was the English flag, floating bravely out over the convent gate, the tricolour on one side, the Red Cross on the other, and in a few moments more I was enthusiastically welcomed by Sisters, patients, *infirmiers*, and last, not least, Louise.

She told me all that occurred since I left. Our Spanish noble had left, and was to be replaced as secretary by an invalid *sous-lieutenant* of *Zouaves*, who was to have his permission from the Prussians. Dr. Bertier was still there, assisted by a Dr. Bock, a Prussian, from the Hospital La Charité at Berlin, who was so kind, so clever, and so pleasant, that he was as popular with the French as the Germans. Some few men had got much better and been sent away prisoners, they had been replaced by others, and a great evacuation of some twenty from St. Marc and twenty from Ste. Marie was to take place the Monday or Tuesday after Christmas Day. Beyond this there was no news.

One of the grand vicars, who had seen the carriage, came to call, and brought a message from the bishop to go and see him next day, if I could, and to him I lent two newspapers, which I heard of three weeks afterwards as having made the circuit of the town, and having been looked upon as great curiosities. Can we fancy such a state of things in a town of 50,000 inhabitants, and only seventy-five miles from Paris?—such an utter being cut off from the world outside, confined within the narrow circuit of the city, no letters, no newspapers, no railways, no diligences, no means of communication with the rest of France. We could come and go, we could send and get letters by the Feld-post (not that we got more than one or two at that time, and most of ours to home missed). We were English, but for the poor French there were no means of receiving intelligence or of leaving or entering the town.

It was well for us that hard work and much kindness from all around made us as happy as it was possible to be amidst sad scenes and some hardship, felt all the more keenly, perhaps, just at this Christmas time. It was so bitterly cold, and the house was warmed by hot-air pipes, and the furnaces would not burn wood. There was no coal or coke to be had. It required two Sisters to feed the kitchen stove with fuel, small pieces of brushwood, cut short, being the only ones that could be got into it, and they burnt up quickly. For us there were no Christmas chimes, the Germans did not allow any church bells to be rung; all were silenced, and the effect was very strange, especially on a Sunday.

On Christmas Eve we expended some of our remaining gold in the purchase of tobacco for the French wounded. The Germans had it from the stores of the Johanniter Ritter. Great preparations were made for the midnight Mass. We helped to decorate the chapel, and with difficulty found in the city two large pots of white heaths, and a huge bouquet of camellias, azaleas, and ferns. The chaplains went round the wards to see and converse with every man, and the Protestant Germans expressing a great wish to be present, special seats were reserved for them.

When at 11 p.m. the service commenced, the chapel was crowded. The music was conducted by the Sisters, and the '*Adeste Fideles*' was beautifully sung, all joining in it. The lights, the flowers, the incense, the dark robes of the Sisters, the uniforms of the soldiers, all made up a scene never to be forgotten. Several of the wounded were carried in on chairs, and when the administration of the Holy Communion commenced, it was a most touching sight. There French and Germans, everything of struggle and contest forgotten, enmity and hatred put away for the time, victor and vanquished, knelt side by side before their Lord. A wounded *Uhlan* was assisted up to the altar by a *Turco* and a *Chasseur d'Afrique*, and a *Garde Mobile* leant on the strong arm of a German dragoon. Such a realisation of 'Peace on earth, good will to men,' we shall never see again in this stormy, weary world.

The service over, mutual greetings in the corridor followed. The good Mother Superior had ordered a basin of warm strong soup to be served to every man. It was quickly carried into the wards by the *infirmiers*, and at 1 a.m. the whole house was quiet. It was the only place in Orléans where the midnight Mass was celebrated, and here it was done by special permission of the authorities and the bishop. The Germans kept Christmas Day gaily.

There were banquets at the *préfecture*, where were the headquarters of Prince Frederick Charles, and at the houses of various other Prussian officials, causing an enormous consumption of firewood and champagne, and a cutting down of all the tops of the fir-trees in the neighbourhood for Christmas trees. The Anglo-Americans had a dinner party, and the few English in Orléans tried to make believe it was Christmas Day in an attempt at English festivity and roast turkey and plum pudding. We passed it quietly enough. It is not a French *fête*, except in a religious point of view. They keep New Year's Day instead as a day of rejoicing.

On the 26th the proposed evacuation took place. About forty men went from our two houses, and ten from the Pomme-du-Pin. The journey was a most disastrous one; the poor men were placed in open waggons without seats. The snow fell fast, till it was up to their waists. Many died, and dead and living were wedged in side by side. It was sixteen days before they arrived at Stettin. It was found impossible to take them on farther, as originally designed, and they were taken out of the train and placed in hospitals and private houses there. There were about one thousand seven hundred in all. One poor fellow from Ste. Marie, a *Turco*, who could only speak Arabic, and who had been the amusement of all the patients, slipped in getting out, and, half-frozen as he was, was unable to help himself, fell under the wheels of the carriages, and was crushed to death.

After this orders were given for no more transport of prisoners in such severe weather. This week was cruelly cold. No coal was to be had; it was all kept for gas, as the Germans feared disturbances if the streets were left in the dark at night; but the worst of it was the scarcity of wood. The townspeople could not go out to get it, nor the country people bring it in. The first had no horses, they had all been taken, and the latter dare not run the risk of losing theirs. I paid eighty *francs* for wood enough for our one small bedroom, to last ten days. Provisions, too, were very scarce. The butcher often declared he had no meat; the tradesmen would always, if possible, avoid giving it on requisition. They had to pay ready money for the meat, and wait an uncertain time for repayment.

The Germans have enormous appetites, and, of course, helped themselves first, and there was little left for the rest. If I had had money instead of a useless cheque, I could have bought many things to eke out the scanty rations; but we had very little gold, and though at this time, through the kindness of Count Bernstorff, I received 30*l*. in Bank of England notes instead of the committee's cheque, they were just as useless; I could not get them changed.

Every day things got scarcer and scarcer. Tobacco could not be had for love or money, and the cold grew worse and worse. We tried our best to keep up the spirits of the men. Dominoes, draughts, cards, and games of different sorts were produced to pass away the weary day, and the chapel services, with their sweet music, were an unfailing source of interest. We heard no news, received no letters. Books and newspapers were strangers to us. Occasionally a visit from some of the English in Orléans enlivened us.

To tell the truth, we were all very badly off; yet our little money really seemed to last like the widow's cruise of oil. The men in our own two wards and all the *infirmiers* were always well dressed—the '*beaux messieurs*,' as they called themselves, of the establishment, and it was a great object to get transferred from the other halls to the *Salle Anglaise*—the '*Salle St.-George*,' as the Sisters had named it. Our lives were certainly very quiet, but not dull. Every day had its new object of interest and anxiety in the matter of clothes and food for our patients. We had such a splendid store that we pretty well supplied all the wards.

The Sisters were indefatigable; one in especial we must not forget, good Sister St.-Antoine, the head nurse. Every man in the ambulance loved her rosy, kindly face, and welcomed her with smiles as she trotted into the wards with her basket of materials on her arm, her robe tucked up, and her merry greeting: 'Now then, *mes enfants*, I am ready for you.' She always had two or three pets, usually boys, who became of course the *enfants gâtés* of the place, and when remonstrated with on spoiling them as she did with bread and jam, and begging little extras of shirts and tobacco for their special benefit, her reply was, looking sunnier than ever, 'But they are such babies, *chère demoiselle*, such little babies, and they like it so!' Her German pets were a difficulty; they used to impose upon her in every way, and one young rascal of a trooper declared that he would not go back to Berlin without her, which being translated, she only laughed, and begged me to assure him she meant to come to Berlin someday with the French Army, and would be sure to look out for him.

The most perfect harmony subsisted. We had put the Germans in one of the long halls all together, thinking they would prefer it; but the Hessians and Bavarians refused to sleep in the same room with the Prussians, so French wounded were mixed with them, and no single quarrel or dispute ever occurred. As for ourselves, the most perfect understanding existed between us and the Sisters. We all worked together, shared hardship and danger alike, and an affection and esteem sprang up which we trust will be life-long. They were so unaffectedly good, so truly religious, and full of faith, and trust, and resignation, in the darkest days, always cheerful and hopeful amidst all the terrible anxiety as to the fate of their Sisters, scattered over the Department of the Loiret in thirty dependent houses, that we could not help learning to sympathise in their joys and sorrows as if they had been our own and we had really belonged to the Sisterhood of St. Aignan.

And one remark more I must make: they were aware we were not members of their Church, but no attempt was ever made to 'convert' us. They saw that we showed every possible respect to their religious observances, that we urged upon the Catholic soldiers the performance of their duties, and they were content to accept us as we were, without enquiring narrowly into the differences in our creed. War does away with bigotry. It tries the stuff of which men's religion is made—whether it will bear the test of calmness in danger, cheerfulness in hardship, and self-sacrifice in a great and holy cause. Those qualities once proved, members of all faiths think of each other in a wide and noble spirit of gentle judgment. 'They are not far from the Kingdom of Heaven.'

The week passed away quietly and sadly. We heard rumours of a large army under General Chanzy coming down on Orléans by the way of Vendôme; again, that Bourbaki was moving rapidly across the Sologne by Tigy and Ferté St.-Aubin, and every hour we expected to hear 'the opening cannons roar.' We suffered much from cold, not personally, but the wards could not be made warm. An English officer then in Orléans, who had friends at headquarters, made every effort to get us an order for coals.

Prince Frederick Charles gave one, but in vain. The *commandant* refused; he dare not do it; he had superior orders from headquarters at Versailles. We, however, got an additional grant of wood, which, when there was any in Orléans, was of great use. Money got scarcer and scarcer with all of us. The poor Sisters had literally none. One day we saw the Sister who acted as porteress making shoes with serge soles. We remonstrated that on a damp day these soles would be like a sponge. 'Very true,' she said; 'but there is no money to buy leather with. The Sisters who wear these must stay within doors.'

We had a great loss, too. Cocotte, the white pony, died of cold and starvation, and we should not have been able to send into the town for the bread and meat, but that, luckily, Pierre, the convent coachman and gardener, had met a man a few days before with a wounded artillery horse. Pierre directly asked the man if he would part with his horse. He answered, 'Yes, for five *francs*.' The horse was brought home, cured, and took poor Cocotte's place. He was a singular creature; he objected to leave the city, except by the road he had entered, and if once he had stopped at a house or shop always insisted on stopping there again. Cocotte was buried in the paddock, and on my announcing the fact to some of the wounded men they exclaimed, 'What a pity it was! He would have stewed down so well with onions!'

Matthias, our Bavarian *infirmier*, and Paul, a French one, who drove 'M. Cinq-Francs,' as the new black horse was called, were two characters, especially Paul, who by sheer impudence established such friendly relations with the Prussian *commandant de place*, that he got extra rations of everything for the ambulance. Matthias aided him by praising the kindness shown to the German wounded, and his round, rosy, happy face bore evidence that he at least had no cause of complaint. He was a sharp boy, too. On one occasion an order was given for a sack of rice. On presenting it, this precious pair were informed there was no rice, on which Matthias, who could make Paul understand, requested his colleague to inform the grocer that he should take a sack of vermicelli instead, which he did, regardless of the difference in price, and for some days after the whole ambulance feasted on soup well thickened with vermicelli.

On the Wednesday in the Christmas week we were called downstairs to receive a Hessian general, who announced himself as come to see the English ladies and the ambulance on the part of Prince Louis. He went over every part of it, even the kitchen and laundry, spoke to all the patients, and on leaving turned to the three officers who accompanied him and said how delighted he was with everything. He then thanked the Mother Superior and ourselves for the great kindness shown to the German wounded, and said they seemed so very happy and contented, and in bidding us goodbye most courteously added, 'I shall tell the prince, ladies, and he will be pleased to write to his wife that her countrywomen have the best ambulance in Orléans.' I mention this here simply to show the kind friends who assisted us that their gifts were not wasted nor their trust misplaced.

We had a cheerful New Year's Day. I had actually bought a turkey and some good wine, hidden from German eyes in the deep recesses of a wine-merchant's cellar. It was a farewell banquet (?), too, to our kind friend Dr. Bertier, who was summoned to rejoin his regiment, and from whom we parted with sincere regret, and with this week we bade farewell, too, to quiet days in our convent life at Orléans.

Chapter 29

A Sad New Year

On the Tuesday after New Year's Day Dr. Bertier left us. We found it impossible to replace him by any French surgeon; all those attached to ambulances had vanished one by one into French lines; the last of all being Dr. Francois, a surgeon of the Ambulance Lyonnaise, who had been left with the wounded at Pomme-du-Pin. The ambulance had requested permission to return to Lyons. Most of its surgeons belonged to the great Hospital there—La Charité; and their time of leave was up. The German officials, regardless of the fact that Lyons, by way of Bourges, was but a three days' journey, even now, from Orléans, sent them round by Saarbruck and Basle; an eighteen days' journey, and even poor Dr. François had to make the same tour to get home. We could find no civilian doctor. All were too fully occupied, and we were, besides, quite satisfied with Dr. Bock.

On Wednesday, Prince Frederick Charles left with his headquarters to meet and, if possible, defeat the army of General Chanzy, which was advancing on Paris by Vendôme. The weather was terrible that week and the next, the snow fell heavily, and the sufferings of the soldiers on both sides must have been dreadful. Camping out under such circumstances must have been the death of many a brave man whom shot and shell had spared, and as for the wounded, unless found and taken off the field at once, there was not a hope for them. They would be hidden in the snow long before they were frozen to death.

On the Friday, to our deep regret, Dr. Bock received orders to take charge of the Caserne Place d'Étapes, and was superseded by Dr. Kröner, a gentlemanly little German, with whom we all got on perfectly. He did his best for everyone, and was very kind and considerate. So far so good. But the next week we were hastily summoned downstairs one morning and informed that a civil inspector and a physician inspector had been appointed, and that the ambulance was to be attached to the 9th *corps d'armée*; in short, we were to be turned into Germans altogether, and it was darkly hinted that one or both of us would be attached to this new-formed ambulance for service at the front with the Prussians.

Louise, the good Mother Superior, Mother St.-Joseph at Ste.-Marie, and myself were all equally determined that we would not be 'required' in this way; and whilst I went to get a copy of the safe-conduct which granted the two convents to *myself* alone, to be used as ambulances, Louise faced the new '*Ober Arzt*,' or head physician. That he had very properly been ordered to do service in the ambulance was probable—one surgeon was not enough for so many wounded—but that he had any right to take possession of our ambulance and ourselves was not so clear. Louise found him, as she said, 'bullying everybody! No other words could express it.' He was a Jew of most pronounced type, spoke very bad English and worse French, but fancied himself a splendid scholar in both, and Louise instantly attacked him.

By the time I arrived as a reinforcement the battle was won. Dr. Kröner was in roars of laughter, the Mother Superior mildly triumphant, and Dr. C— retreating, quoting as he went, in the worst of pronunciations, 'Rule, Britannia! Britannia rules the waves,' to which Louise emphatically rejoined, 'Yes; and "Britons never shall be slaves!"'

It was settled that we should remain as the *Ambulance Anglaise*, that our two halls should be always reserved for French wounded, and that both parties should render to each other all the assistance in their power. One thing he said to Louise she very soon put down, 'You two women cannot come here and make an ambulance;' to which she replied, 'That I don't care the least about; we *have* formed one, and we *shall* keep it.'

But from that day, though Dr. C— was a horrible fidget, he never attempted to interfere. If he only would have spoken German he would have been intelligible; but, no! he would show off his learning, and under the delusion that the louder he spoke the better he should be understood, he roared out the worst compound of European languages I ever heard, and thereby gained a character for ferocity of which, I do believe, he was utterly undeserving. Our first trouble with the little man was about *counterpanes*. There were about four green ones in the Salle St.-George to seventeen beds, and nothing would satisfy him but that all the coverlets should be green. Five or six more were found in other halls, and the inspector discovered some '*couver-*

tures vertes,' or, as he called them, '*goufertures fertes,*' at the Convent of the *Bon Pasteur* opposite, after having spent two hours searching for them in town.

He had formed this convent into an ambulance of his own, for only Germans, and thereby much annoyed the Mother Superior, who could not see why her poor French wounded were sent off to dreary barracks to be replaced by Prussian sick; and when Dr. C— blundered in, and demanded her green coverlets, which had been piled in the entrance-hall, ready for transportation to our establishment, she ordered them to be taken back into the wards, and defied him to remove them without her sanction.

Dr. C— came back considerably crestfallen. '*Mein Himmel!*' he groaned to me, 'what for are you Englander so intractable?' for the Mother of the *Bon Pasteur* was English, too. I advised him to take a civil message from us requesting the loan of the green counterpanes in exchange for some of our brown ones. It had its due effect, and this mighty affair was arranged after two days' constant worry, during which Dr. C— came and went so often that he gained for himself the name of 'the Wandering Jew,' which he retained to the last. He was at once the plague and the amusement of his subordinates, and Dr. Kröner's assistant, an intelligent German student, was especially delighted with the counterpane affair, and proposed suggesting to '*Le Juif errant*' to turf the halls, that the green grass might match the counterpanes.

We, however, finding Dr. C—'s weak side was to have everything, as he called it, 'aspect,' placed a bed at one end of the ward, the Salle St.-George, in which was a Frenchman seriously wounded in the arm, the worst arm case, and faced him at the other end with the worst wound in the leg. We dressed all the men who could not leave their beds in scarlet flannel jackets, and all who could hobble about in brown cloth ones, and when next Dr. C— arrived he went into a state of ecstasy, exclaiming, 'See now how beautiful! we are aspect now,' and from that day became quite good-tempered and very proud of the ambulance, which he praised in private and public with an absurd idea—it was all his formation and his management that had attained such brilliant results—an idea at which Dr. Bock and all the medical men who had been in it and seen it, long before Dr. C— left Saarbruck, laughed heartily.

Three German *infirmiers* came to reside in the house; they were very good-natured and very idle. They went round the wards with the doctor in the morning to take down names for evacuation; the Germans to rejoin their regiments—a process they particularly objected to (and no wonder in such weather)—and the French ready for the next transport of prisoners to Germany. They ate and drank and smoked, required the best of food and wine, and were particular as to having coffee, good bread, and honey at three p.m., to sustain fainting nature between dinner at twelve and supper at six. They lived a great deal better than any of us, and had far less to do; and they had each a soldier servant to wait upon them and clean their boots.

They were not above begging, though, and whenever they saw me bringing down socks and shirts for the wounded asked for some for themselves, and I sometimes complied with the request, as I found that, whenever I did so, the result was a distribution of cigars, good wine, fresh eggs, and stewed prunes to the French wounded. These stores were sent in by the German *intendance* for the use of the Germans; but we kept the *infirmiers* in good temper by giving them all we could and asking them to do noticing, and by this means procured a few extra luxuries for our poor Frenchmen. On the whole, we had no complaint whatever to make of them. They were quiet, respectful, and never interfered with us; very stern with their own men, but did not order the French about; and when they left, after the peace, spoke most highly of the way in which they had been treated at St. Marc.

Dr. C—insisted on having twenty more beds, and the good Mother Superior gave up the pretty private chapel of the community, which was on the floor above the public chapel, and it was devoted entirely to German wounded. It was a sad pity to dismantle it altogether, and the cost of restoring it to its original condition will be considerable. The altar was left. The German *infirmiers* enforced upon all comers the necessity of not in any way profaning it, and, moreover. Dr. C— ordered that no man should arise and walk about the room till after the seven o'clock Mass below was over, and during Vespers that they should sit quiet and make no noise by singing or talking, and so great is German discipline that the orders once given were never infringed. There were not beds, mattresses, and sheets enough for so many extra men, and Dr. C— sent in an application to the Knights of St. John, who had immense stores in the railway station.

It has been said that the English money, so much of which was given to the Knights of St. John, was equally distributed by them between Germans and French. It was not so; nor could it be expected. The 'Johanitter Ritter' are the great Hospitaller Order of Prussia. They are attached in that capacity to the German Army. They do not profess to be neutral or international. Nothing could be had from their stores in Orléans unless upon the order of a German physician, countersigned by Count Stolberg, one of their chiefs, and this was not given, naturally, to any ambulances that had not a German head, and was given for the use of the German wounded.

We were English; we had brought our own stores; we always gave to the Germans if, as it very rarely happened, they were not supplied from their own ample resources; and Dr. C— told us to take all he got and use it indifferently. But that was his personal kindness, not official orders. Our Civil Inspector was a very good-natured man, whom we called Bon-bon; first, because we never got comfortably at his unpronounceable German name, and secondly, because he was quartered at a celebrated *bon-bon* shop, where he distinguished himself by his quiet, regular habits and his kind, cheerful manner. His entertainers were violently French, and never attempted to conceal their feelings; but Herr Bon-bon took it all in good part, lived on terms of the greatest friendship with the whole family, breakfasting and dining with them every day, and when he departed was universally respected and lamented.

Whether it was that we were peculiarly fortunate in the officers we had to deal with, or whether it was the fact of our neutrality, I cannot say, but from all, with very few exceptions—one at Balan, one at Versailles, and one at Orléans—we received the greatest courtesy and kindness. Still, we were more quiet before Dr. C— arrived. His little worrying ways annoyed us, and we felt, besides, how heavy a burden was the support of his staff on the already impoverished resources of the Sisters. At St. Marc lived one doctor and three or four clerks, with us three *infirmiers* and three servants, and they could not, or would not, rough it as we did.

Besides, men were sent in only fatigued and foot-sore, not wounded or really sick, and, being continually changed, imposed much additional labour and expense. The Sisters would never allow the sheets to be used a second time. This may seem an unnecessary piece of dandyism; but it was only a part of a system of exquisite cleanliness to which must be attributed the fact that we never had an epidemic in the Ambulance of St. Marc, and our death-rate was far the lowest in Orléans—not four *per cent*.

Every Saturday the wards and corridors were well scrubbed down. Sister St.-Antoine led the charge at the head of a band of French *in-*

firmiers, and the Germans, whose habits are of the dirtiest kind, looked on in wonder at the buckets of water thrown about, at the displacement of every bed and table, and at the carbolic acid mixed with the water. We had taken out carbolic acid in crystals; these were dissolved and mixed with water. Each bottle made twenty-five quart bottles strong enough for the dressings, and we used it much diluted to wash down the floors.

Every fever case was placed, as soon as discovered, in a separate building. Every case of wounds bad enough to be unpleasant was placed apart, and there was no ambulance smell in the house. The patients were never left, day or night. They had regular meals, and nothing between, except by special order, and then only a little good wine or a slice of bread and preserve. The Germans had newspapers. No French ones were allowed in Orléans, and we supplied the French with books, most kindly lent, without fee or reward, from the library of M. and Madame Blanchard, Rue Bannière. In all ways the citizens rendered us every possible assistance, furnishing us with many things concealed from German eyes, and we only regretted that our poverty prevented us availing ourselves more largely of their kindness, for rations often ran very short. We had about 500 men to feed, and that is no trifle with such a scarcity of provisions as existed.

But the French were so grateful and good tempered. 'What can we ask more?' they said. 'We have all you have. We have a good roof over our heads, good beds, clean shirts, kind words. What matter weak soup and small pieces of meat? we are happy here.' The Germans grumbled, and I had a process of reasoning to go through to convince them that out of nothing comes nothing; no bullocks, no beef; no flour, no bread; that we all fared alike, and we ought to be thankful we were not out in the snow, like the other poor creatures.

After which exertion of eloquence they usually agreed in my view of the case. Indeed, in no single instance had we to complain of the conduct of any one of them. Once one of the German servants got very tipsy and fell down in the garden, but the head *infirmier* came and kicked him so dreadfully, telling him he disgraced his great nation before the English ladies, that I should say he never did it again.

No difficulties ever arose as regarded difference of religious opinion, though we literally had in the ambulance Jews, Turks, heretics, and infidels—the *Turcos* being Mahometans, and, sad to say, many of the Germans utter unbelievers, while two of the officials were Jews. The Mother Superior herself offered every facility if a Protestant chaplain were appointed for the Prussians; and no objection whatever would have been made to his holding a service in the Salle Jeanne d'Arc, which was entirely for the Germans. One did come, saw and conversed with the Protestants, and indeed went over the ambulance. He paid a second visit, but that was all; and on my asking Herr Bon-bon why he did not come again, the *herr* replied that the men did not care to have him there; when they were well enough they went to service by order on Sunday morning, but it was holiday when they were in hospital.

Prussian *commandant* on one occasion asked one of the Sisters who had gone with an *infirmier* to get some requisition order signed, 'Do you try to convert the Protestants? Do you treat them just as you do the Catholics?

'Certainly,' she answered. 'Catholic or Protestant, they must eat, poor creatures; their religion is no business of mine. I do the cooking, not the conversions!'

But it was an extraordinary fact, that if ever there was any extra business, such as evacuating men, changing them from one ward to another, or making any fresh arrangements, it was always on a Sunday morning; so that it became a common saying amongst us, 'The pious king may look after his own soul; he does not give anybody else time to look after *theirs*.' And I must say that the needless work thus imposed upon all on the Sunday, the utter want of regard shewed for the day, set a very bad example to Catholics and Protestants alike, and certainly gave the French an odd idea of the Protestant religion.

Nor was it caused by the fact of a Jew being chief with us, for the orders came from the general in command as regarded the evacuation of prisoners; and he could certainly have issued a general order, or caused the Physician-in-chief to do so, that in large ambulances, where there were forty or fifty Protestants, service should be performed for them on Sunday, and some respect for the sacred day enforced. But in this, as in many other things, we found Prussian piety a very 'whited sepulchre.'

That second week of January was indeed a dreary one. Every day distant sounds of cannonade were heard and prisoners arrived, taken in the battles which resulted in the occupation of Le Mans by the Germans. On one of these days an order was received for one thousand coffins for the use of the Prussian Army, and I myself several times saw upwards of twenty large waggons in a line full of wounded, coming through the streets. The snow lay thick on the ground, a dense frost fog filled the air. Wood and provisions were scarcer than ever. The Prussians prevented all ingress to or egress from the towns. They had an idea that Bourbaki's army was coming on, and several times we were told of the French lancers being seen only three or four miles from the bridge over the Loire. Had the French come, there was not force enough to resist them, for even before the departure of Prince Frederick Charles the Germans were by no means easy as to their position.

So far back as New Year's Eve an alarm was given, which showed their consciousness of the likelihood of a surprise. At midnight the soldiers began to fire off their rifles, to salute the New Year. The prince and his staff were carousing at the *préfecture*, and hearing the sound, which indeed was exactly like the firing of the outposts when an attack commences, they decided that it must be the French, and hasty orders were given to saddle the horses. An enquiry, however, proved that it was only their own men; but we ascertained afterwards, in various places where the soldiers were quartered, that so deep were the potations they drank that night in honour of the New Year and '*Vaterland*,' that Bourbaki would have had a walk over the course 'if he had dashed in with some thirty thousand determined men.'

It was a very sad sight to see prisoners brought in. On the Thursday of that week there came through the Rue Bannière a strange procession—old men and women, little children, carried in their mothers' arms, or toddling, wondering, by their sides, a priest in his *soutane*, a lady well-dressed leading a child, several gentlemen, many artisans, labourers and domestic servants, male and female. Weary, foot-sore, half frozen, they had walked over twenty miles in the snow, their guards on either side urging them forward, and even in the street, as they lingered, looking wildly around for help or pity, blows and harsh words roused them to stumble on a little faster.

The poor lady, her rich black silk dress all draggled with mud, stopped to soothe her little daughter, who was crying with cold and pain, and a German guard roughly ordered her '*Vorwarts!*' A murmur of disgust rose from the bystanders, and a Hessian officer who was looking at the scene from a balcony rushed down into the street, put the soldier aside, and offering the lady his arm led her into his own rooms.

'They are prisoners!' shouted the captain of the guard.

'I will be responsible for them,' was the brave young fellow's reply; 'you will find them here, in my care.'

Several old German officers standing by applauded his conduct. '*Mein Gott!*' said one, 'what have these poor people done?' a question echoed around. It appeared that they were all the remaining inhabitants of a village where opposition had been offered to the advance of the troops, probably successful opposition; for this was sure to draw down summary punishment on such audacity. These poor people were therefore brought prisoners into Orléans, to be sent to Germany; but we heard that the feeling of the higher officials was so much against the proceedings of the colonel by whose orders the atrocity was committed, that they were shortly afterwards released. It is surely enough to have their homes entirely destroyed, to lose everything they had in the world, to be houseless in such cruel weather.

Whatever lesson was needed by upstart little villages that tried to bar the invaders' way, utter ruin might seem sufficient to teach non-combatants the doctrine of non-resistance. It is a splendid thing to fight for '*Vaterland,*' it is a noble deed to keep '*Die Wacht am Rhein,*' to guard that sacred stream against all foreign foes; but it is an act punishable with death in those who take up arms to watch beside the Loire—death to themselves, destruction to their homes.

Blot out that daring town or village from the map of France, burn down every humble homestead, bring out the petroleum casks to do the work more surely, drive old and young, weak women, little children, the priests of God and the helpless ones of their flock, through twenty miles of deep snow, at the bayonet's point, and then sit round the blazing fires piled high up with the remains of costly chairs and choice furniture, and sing '*Die Wacht am Rhein!*' When next English men and women hear that song, let them remember scenes like this, and ask, What is German consistency, and what her laws of war?

CHAPTER 13

Peace

As the hope of relief from the arrival of the French grew fainter and fainter, the distress all around deepened; the inhabitants of the Faubourg Olivet, just across the river, were driven out of their houses, which were required to be pulled down for the fortifications being constructed there, to prevent any sudden surprise by the French. There were large fruit gardens and orchards in this suburb the trees of which were cut down for firewood and military purposes, and the loss amounted to a couple of million of *francs*. Both bridges were mined afresh, and rumours were abroad every day that they were positively to be blown up that very afternoon.

The reports brought in by stray villagers, who occasionally got through the lines, ostensibly for the purpose of bringing fowls and vegetables for the hotels where were Prussian generals, spoke of the defeat of Chanzy's army and the march of Bourbaki into Germany. If so, he certainly was not coming our way, and Orléans was to be left in the hands of her conquerors.

On Thursday, the 12th, I was crossing the Place Martroi, laden with oranges and biscuits for the ambulance, when I was stopped by the passing of a crowd of French prisoners, some 1,500 in number. A scuffle took place just at the entrance of the Rue Bannière. A girl, looking out at a shop-door, recognised her brother in that miserable crowd, and darting out threw herself into his arms. The surprise was too much for the poor lad, worn out with his march from near Le Mans, and he fainted on the pavement. The guard kicked him to, make him get up, the crowd of lookers-on interfered, and an officer passing on horseback struck the brutal sentinel with his sword. The prisoner was carried into the shop, and probably transferred to an ambulance, as he was evidently much too ill to go farther.

As I was turning away to return home, I caught the words, '*Ambulance Anglaise! allez tout de suite.*' I stopped and saw several women, one of whom had a slip of paper in her hand, crowding round a stall on which were butter, *allumettes*, and biscuits.

'Did you want the *Ambulance Anglaise*?' I asked. 'Do you know where it is?'

'Yes,' said one woman; 'do you want to know? It is in the Faubourg St.-Marc'

'Thank you,'I answered; 'but I live there. Is there anything I can do?'

One woman seemed inclined to speak, the others checked her, thanked me, but said it was 'nothing.'

An hour or two after I reached home, one of the Sisters came up to our room with the Mother Superior, and showed a little note which had been brought by a stranger woman. During the passing of the prisoners up the Rue Bannière, this woman said, there had been a stop, owing to a confusion on the other side, and one of the prisoners had taken advantage of this to scribble half a dozen words on the leaf of his pocket-book. Calling to the woman, who kept the stall at the corner, he begged them to take it to his aunt, at the *Ambulance Anglaise*, directly. This was the mystery I had come upon, and it was most unfortunate that the woman was prevented telling me, for thus valuable time was lost. The note was to the Mother Superior, from her nephew; he was amongst the prisoners, very ill, and about to be sent to Germany. He begged her to find him out, and to get leave for him to remain in Orléans as a prisoner.

First, where to find this poor boy? Had I known of it when I was in the Rue Bannière, I should have followed the troop of captives, and watched into which churches they were put. Three churches were full of them, I knew—St.—Paterne, St.-Laurent, and St.-Paul—and probably others; but now it was dark, and the difficulty would be great. We must get an order from some chief to enable us to reclaim this poor boy. We remembered then the kind message of Prince Louis of Hesse, to apply to him in any case of difficulty. Cinq Francs was harnessed to the cart, and Louise being ill in bed with rheumatism, I started with La Mère Thérèse to the prince's headquarters on the Quai Cypierre.

We arrived. All was so lonely and quiet, I feared the prince was absent; but the porter, a civil old Frenchman, said he was at dinner. I told him I had a note I much wished the prince to get, and also to have a word of answer; but of course, I would wait to send it in till he had dined.

'My orders are,' said the porter, 'to take to the prince himself every letter as soon as it arrives. Ah heavens! how good and kind he is. No stealing here, no breaking up furniture; all quiet and respectable, like himself. But then he has an English princess for his wife. *Madame* is of that country. Ah, he will be delighted!!'

And off he trotted. We had not waited a moment, as it seemed, before an *aide-de-camp* came out, his dinner napkin in his hand, and most courteously led us into the salon behind the dining-room, which, apparently, was the prince's bedroom. His sword was hanging up, and some few coats and cloaks were lying about, a bright fire blazing, writing materials scattered about the table, and a large map open and thrown over a chair; but we remarked how neat and clean everything was, and, though the dining-room was only just beyond the folding-doors, how quiet; not the loud noise and shouting usually to be heard where Germans are congregated together. All bore the stamp of an orderly and gentlemanly establishment.

As we were looking round us and admiring the simplicity of the quarters, the door opened, and a fair, tall, pleasant-looking man came in, dressed in a plain dark blue uniform coat, with only the Iron Cross hanging from the button-hole. It was indeed Prince Louis. I apologised for thus disturbing his dinner, to which he replied he had quite finished, and we then discussed the business which had brought us there, and which I had explained in my note. The prince took the kindest interest in the case; he said he only regretted these prisoners belonged to Prince Frederick Charles, so that he had no power. Had they been his, he would have given the order directly consigning the lad to our guardianship, especially as he was not a regular soldier, had not even volunteered, but had been drawn three months before in the levy.

We thanked him, and regretted it, too, and were about to leave, when he said, 'Stay; let me see. I will tell you what I think will do. Go to the chief inspector of your ambulance, and ask him to claim this young man as *infirmier*. Tell him Prince Louis of Hesse advised you to do this, and I think, but I am not sure, that this will answer.' He then added, 'Do you know I passed you in the street the other day and bowed to you, but you did not see me?'

I replied that really, I had not recognised His Highness.

To which he answered, 'No, of course not; but I recognised you. I saw you before at Ste.-Marie-aux-Chênes. You had another lady with you; she had a grey hat like yours' (touching the brim of the one I wore). 'It is an English hat; I have seen my wife wear one.' After receiving a few more kindly assurances of his desire to assist us we took our leave, and la Mère Thérèse was full of delight at the prince's cordial, cheerful way of speaking and the graceful simplicity of his manner.

'He is good,' she said emphatically, 'and he looks so.' The queen ought to be very proud and pleased of the golden opinions won by her two German sons-in-law, in the midst of a savage war, and in the heart of an invaded country. Most fully were they at least acquitted from any share in, or even any knowledge of, the hardships and cruelties inflicted on the miserable people by some of their subordinates. Both the Prince Impériale of Germany and Prince Louis of Hesse bore the highest character, and were welcomed in the towns they entered as protectors rather than oppressors. If the enemy must occupy a city, it was well, the poor inhabitants thought, that their chiefs should be brave and good men, who would deal justly with them, and who had the will and the power to prevent unauthorised acts of plunder and wrong, and the laurels of the two princes are the proudest of all, for they are untarnished by the acts that too often disgraced the victors at this sad time.

When we left the prince, it was far too late to find our inspector. We called, but he was out, where no one knew, and it was only in early morning that the *Mère* sallied out again to find him. Then it was too late. The prisoners had started at daybreak on their way, but the poor lad did not long remain a prisoner, for, as we know, seven weeks after came the peace.

There was a large evacuation of French in the following week. We were very grieved to part with our men, but the weather was better, and no man was sent away who was really unfit to travel. Even rheumatism was accepted as an excuse, and several men went to bed and groaned piteously. One of them, when Dr. Kröner asked him if he was able to travel, said, 'Oh no; he was very ill with rheumatism.'

'Where?' asked the doctor.

'In my stomach, *monsieur*,' answered the patient.

'My friend,' said Dr. Kröner, 'if you had said anywhere else, I would have believed you; but it is impossible to accept this. Really you must go.'

The poor fellow had to get up and go, amidst the laughter of his companions, who called him 'pig' and 'wooden-head,' for not having 'put his rheumatism into his knees.' It was a sad sight to see the men who had been nursed and petted in warm, comfortable wards drawn up in line in the long corridor, with their knapsacks on their backs, ready to march away. Every man sent from the convent was duly provided with a flannel shirt and belt and a warm undervest, a good wrapper round his throat, and a thick pair of socks, a large loaf of bread, and a flask of wine and water. No men, it was said, were turned out so well as ours. Their coats and trousers had all been washed and repaired, their boots mended, their belts and buckles cleaned, and they presented a neat, smart appearance, very different from the poor fellows who had been in the military hospitals.

The French *intendance* had quite broken down; no attention was ever paid to the soldiers in ambulance. On the contrary, the very morning after a German came in, the chief clerk, 'Schwarzer Johann,' as he was called, from his black beard and gruff voice, came round and looked at every article of the man's dress, examining the soles of his boots and the buckles of his straps. Anything lost or worn out was replaced, ready by the time he left, so that he went out, as it were, repaired in health and equipment. The French had nothing but what we gave them, and the Sisters worked hard to patch their well-worn clothes. We had many little things to buy, buttons, buckles, tapes, and various odds and ends, and all trenched on our diminishing stock of gold, whilst we received daily appeals for assistance to the poor, who were actually starving. We wrote a letter which was published in the *Times*, and the kind response to the appeal for help enabled us, as soon as the peace was declared, to gladden many a heart.

Day after day passed on, and at last we heard that Paris had capitulated, and an armistice was arranged. After the first burst of anger and despair at the surrender of the capital, it was a relief to all to breathe tranquilly, as it were, for a time; but the relief came too late to heal one broken heart, that of M. Pereira, the *préfet* of the Loiret. Despairing of being able to alleviate the sufferings of the population from the ravages of war, he fell into a bad state of health, and indeed it was this which saved him from being sent prisoner into Germany. He was a marked man, from his proclamations and speeches, in which he had always encouraged the sternest resistance to the invader. He was detained a prisoner in his own house in Orléans, but, contrary to the report in the city, he was not treated with harshness, and was attended by one of the first German physicians with all possible care and skill.

His funeral was a most imposing sight. The Mass for the dead was celebrated in the cathedral, the bishop officiating. So universally respected and beloved was M. Pereira, that when the coffin was taken out and placed in the open hearse prepared to receive it, it was followed to the cemetery by more than 3,000 of his fellow-citizens, nobles, gentlemen, *bourgeois*, and artisans, all in mourning. As the coffin was carried out of the cathedral a German band was playing on the Place Ste.-Croix for the parade of some troops, but when it appeared. Prince Louis of Hesse ordered the music to cease, whilst himself and his staff stood bareheaded as the cortege passed down the Rue Jeanne d' Arc, amidst the mourning of all around; but there were many who felt as we did, that it was in mercy the dead man had been taken, that God Himself in His infinite love had broken the chain and set the prisoner free.

We had seen the good bishop several times during this sad month. Though no longer a prisoner, his palace was occupied as quarters by a Prussian general, and he himself had but two or three small rooms in which to live. Even his kitchen was taken possession of by the general's cooks, and his meals were prepared in a smaller one. On one occasion a German valet saw the bishop's dinner-tray ready prepared to be taken to him. There was a basin of soup, a little roast bird, and a decanter of Bordeaux. 'Stop!' he cried to the bishop's servant; 'I'll take that. My master has just come in, and is hungry; it will be a nice refreshment before his dinner;' and he actually walked off with it, the servant not daring to interfere.

But the noble old bishop bore all his sorrows and annoyances so gently, so patiently, so uncomplainingly, that even his oppressors learned to be ashamed of themselves, and owned that to be unkind to such a man was a hard service. Of one thing he could not complain, and that was any inequality in the disrespect with which religious edifices were treated; for if the cathedral and churches had been made into prisons, the Protestant 'Temple,' as it was called, had been turned into a Bavarian barrack. When we told the bishop of this, he looked sadder than ever, but simply said, 'What do these men respect? not even their own faith!'

The armistice was truly a relief to all, not that it made any difference with the Germans, except that there was no fighting. We had an old-fashioned idea, and so had several military friends, that during an armistice all things remained in *statu quo;* but now troops were moved in all directions, prisoners were sent off to Germany, and heavy requisitions made as before it began. We exchanged some prisoners; about fifteen French out of our houses were sent to Vierzon, the first French post, to form part of the number exchanged for Bavarian and Prussian prisoners at Pau. But on the French side the management was infamous. The poor fellows arrived at Vierzon, to wait for military passes to rejoin their depots; and there they were, no one to receive them, houseless and dinnerless, sleeping in barns and stables, and begging their daily bread, for several days, till at last they were sent on to their depots. Several of our men refused to go under such conditions and preferred taking their chance of peace setting them free.

After the surrender of Paris the *corps d'armée* of the Prince Impériale came to Orléans, ready to be sent on to the front if the war continued. The entrance was a sad sight for the Orleanais: for an hour and a half regiment after regiment poured down the street, amidst the triumphant music of their bands. There always was an idea that the Germans magnified their force, by marching their men out of one faubourg and in by another, and really we half believed that they had done so on this occasion, for there was a strange similarity between some of those who passed first and some who came last. The people stood by in stern silence, but oaths of vengeance were sworn that day which may yet have a dark fulfilment. 'Dogs! *canaille!*' were the muttered words around. 'See if we spare old or young, woman or child, when we ride through Berlin.' Many wept bitter tears, and surely in this hour of, at all events, temporary peace, this public entry was an unnecessary addition to their humiliation.

Some of the new generals, too, gave themselves great airs. One day we heard that two of our *infirmiers*, *Zouaves*, had been arrested for not saluting a certain gallant general, who shall be nameless, as he rode down the Rue Jeanne d'Arc. We started off directly to the city, found our two friends prisoners for twenty-four hours in the *mairie*, and looking piteously out of an attic window. From the third *infirmier*, who was with them (not a *Zouave*), we heard that really they had not seen the great gentleman, and also they did not know they were compelled to salute him, as they themselves were all *sous-officiers*, and the German privates did not salute them.

On enquiry of the *commandant de place* it appeared that the general had been hissed on the Quai du Chatelet by some *Zouaves*, and he had resolved not only to arrest them, but also every *Zouave* whom he could catch. The affair made a great deal of excitement and ill feeling, and as the *commandant's* secretary told me that an order from the general would obtain their release, I resolved to ask him for one. He was out. I waited an hour. On his arrival he went to his own room, and an *aide de-camp* asked me my business. I explained; said that my *infirmiers* begged to apologise, would not do so any more, had not seen the illustrious general, and were absolutely required for the service of the wards that night. He quite agreed, went in and spoke to the general, and coming back requested me to go in myself to see him.

Of that interview the less said the better. There was champagne on the table, and the general was very red in the face. He told me I might have two of his servants, and if they did not do the work properly, I might flog them! In short, he refused to release the men, and I left utterly disgusted with his conduct. They were released next day; but I should advise any office to decline taking an insurance on that general's life when next he meets the Third Zouaves, and I really must say he would be no loss to the German Army.

The armistice drew to its end, and there was no certain news of peace. On the morning of Sunday, 26th February, the 'Wandering Jew' arrived, and ordered every Frenchman in the ambulance to be ready to leave at three p.m. We found the *infirmiers* were included, and Dr. Kröner declared they should not and could not go. We should still have fifty sick and wounded left, and not a man to do the service of the wards; besides, several of them held Prussian commissions as *infirmiers*, and clearly had no right to be sent away as prisoners. All we could obtain, however, was that a list of ten should be taken, that the men named on it might be returned. Dr. Kröner was very vexed; but Dr. C— was imperative.

Dinner was ordered for noon precisely, but it had hardly been served up before orders came for every man except the *infirmiers* to go in marching order to Ste. Marie. We hurried them off, and went with them ourselves. Arrived there. Dr. C— asked, 'Where are the *infirmiers*? They must come, too.'

Dr. Kröner said to me, 'Send them over; it is only to take down their names.' I ran back and sent them. Then came fresh orders. They were to go with the rest to the *bureau* of the *commandant de place*; they must have their cloaks and knapsacks. We all ran about to collect them, and a most amusing scene it was to see the Sisters struggling across the garden, one with a knapsack, another with a great coat, another with a bundle.

About three all were assembled; the names of the *infirmiers* were taken down, and Dr. Kröner sent back every man he could on any excuse. I asked him what all this was for, and he told me the armistice ended at midnight. There were no tidings of peace, and a long train of prisoners was to start next day unless fresh news came; but what grieved him was that, the men were to be put in the Church of St. Euverte. This was the church which the Anglo-Americans had occupied. As predicted, both ventilation and means of warming it were deficient. The cold was intense, and the mortality very large. They had been obliged to evacuate it, by order, and it had been pronounced terribly infected.

Some prisoners had been put in, and several had been seized with fever. It was infested with vermin, which had made their appearance after the ambulance left, and the whole place was in a filthy state—most unfit for quarters for men fresh out of hospital. But there was no help for it, and our hearts were very heavy as we saw patients and *infirmiers* ranged in line, ready to start. Everyone had something to say. We had shared their joys and sorrows, had watched by their bedsides, and heard their tales of home. We had looked over their games of dominoes and *écarté*, and sympathised in their want of news and short commons, and they had given us all the help they could; some by content and patience in most trying circumstances, some by active service. They were friends now, each with his own individuality.

It was very sad to bid them thus goodbye, for ever, most probably; and, to add to the sadness, down came all the Germans who could walk, from St. Marc's, to shake hands with their French comrades, and give them addresses in far-away German towns of friends who would be kind to the prisoners. The guard had not arrived, and there they stood waiting, when one of them remembered a book he had left. I ran back to fetch it, and at the door of St. Marc's was nearly knocked over by a breathless Hessian, calling to me to stop. 'Peace! peace! the peace is signed!' he gasped out. 'They need not go; if they do, they'll all come back tomorrow.'

'Can it be true?' I asked; 'how do you know it?'

'*Madame*, I was lunching with my cousin, a Protestant pastor; I went with him to the general's; he was to say the service there; the general had just had the despatch from Versailles. It is true, but the official news is not here; that is, it will not be published till late tonight.' He gave me the names so truthfully, I could not doubt, and I ran back into the yard of Ste. Marie. The guard were there, the men from Pomme-du-Pin and the *bon pasteur* outside.

'The peace is signed!' I cried. My Hessian friend had followed, and we explained how the news had come to us.

A wild scene of joy occurred. The Germans shouted and embraced the French, the French screamed and hugged the Germans, and everybody cried for joy. But the 'Wandering Jew' was inexorable. He had been ordered to send in his prisoners that night, and go they should. Dr. Kröner subtracted several quietly, and at last the rest were marched off; but they went very gaily, for there was hope now. The *salles* looked very dreary that night. The Germans who could walk helped us to serve the dinners, but what with anxiety and fatigue, and uncertainty if the good news was really true, we had little or no sleep that night. Our poor boys, too, were in that miserable, infected church.

It was barely daylight before Sister Ste. Marthe brought our coffee and a message. 'The boys at St. Euverte were all waiting for "*Les dames anglaises.*" They had seen a little girl passing, and had sent her to say so.' We dressed directly, and, accompanied by the Sister, we started. The church was just over the railway-bridge, and in the yard around it we caught sight of 'our boys' looking out for us. They saw us, and a rush to the front gate ensued. Of course, we were let in, and were surrounded by a mob of soldiery, all friends of ours, and all exclaiming they were so tired and so hungry they had not slept, and they had said in the middle of the night they were sure we had not.

An officer had most kindly come at midnight and told them of the peace. Why were they kept prisoners there? We promised then to go and see about it, and first of all went and bought bread, wine, and tobacco. We called at the French *intendance*; they were utterly helpless. If we could get the men let out before next day, when the orders from Versailles would be there, well and good; *they* could not.

It was so evident there was no hope there that we resolved to go to the *commandant de place*; but first we took our stores to the church, and catching hold of the head *infirmiers* from St. Marc, Ste. Marie, and Pomme du-Pin, gave the wine and bread into their charge. The *infirmiers* called out for the men of their own ambulances to assemble by three pillars, and began to distribute provisions. A cry was raised, '*Vive Ste. Marie! Vive! Ambulance Anglaise!*' and the poor creatures from other houses crowded round. We were glad to see that our men gave liberally to all who asked, and presently after, the Little Sisters of the Poor brought some coffee and bread for their patients; and bread and coffee also came down from our convent, in charge of Sister Ste.-Helene, who, hearing of the distress of the men, had hastily made what coffee she could, and brought it to the church.

I went off and met our chief German *infirmier*, a very gentlemanly *sous-officier*, with warm French sympathies, looking for me. He said, 'Come with me. This will not do; the men will get furious. Come to the *commandant de place*.' We arrived, and the *commandant* quite agreed that, if we would be responsible for the men, till he gave them over to the French *commandant*, it would be better that they should go home to their various ambulances, but referred us to the Chief Director of Ambulances. To him we went, and I begged for the men of the ambulance Anglaise to be allowed to come back and remain with us till final orders were received transferring them once more to French rule.

He smiled and said, 'I would most willingly, for that ambulance has been very kind to our men; but if I give you all your men (you have about 200) I must let all the others go.'

'Then let them go,' I said; 'it is only the difference of half a dozen hours—very much to them, nothing to you. Please sign a little bit of paper, and let them all go back to their ambulances.'

The good old doctor laughed, signed a bit of paper, and gave it to my German attendant; he touched his cap and ran off. I began to thank the doctor; but he said, 'Run off, make haste, or you will miss a scene.' I did run, and arrived opposite the churchyard gate just as the German *sous-officier* rushed in telling the sentinels to stand aside. He ran into the church waving the paper, and before I could enter, I was all but carried away by the crowd as the French poured out of the gates in ecstasies of joy. I clung to the gateway, calling out, 'Men of St. Marc and Ste Marie, home to breakfast!' and every man obeyed. But it was a race; the German and myself headed it over the bridge, but were overtaken by a feather-weight *Chasseur d'Afrique* and a couple of *Gardes Mobiles,* who, arriving first at the convent door, thundered upon it.

Good Sister Ste-Marthe opened the wicket by the cord, as usual, and looked out, and when she saw the scene up the road she called out, 'They are all coming back!' and ran into the halls to summon everybody to welcome 'the boys.'. The *chasseur* helped to throw open the large doors, and in trooped the returning soldiers, met by a rush of the French and Germans still left, while good Sister St.-Antoine, standing in the middle of the road, extended her arms wide to receive her 'children,' crying out, '*Ah, mes enfants, mes enfants,* you are here! it is true!' Such a scene of honest, heartfelt joy I never saw; everybody had tears in their eyes. It was indeed the blessing of peace.

The days that followed were quiet and tranquil, and it now became our duty to try and relieve the sufferings of the peasantry around. We resolved, before the ambulance broke up, to revisit the places we had seen on those sad December days, and decided that our first excursion should be to Cercottes and Chevilly. The men in ambulance were allowed perfect liberty to walk about the city. We applied to the French *intendant* for boots, and with success; and now that the weary war was over, we gave every man as he left such clothes as he needed, the Germans too, but they were so well supplied that they rarely required anything. We had still many severely wounded, and to leave for a month or six weeks was impossible; but everything seemed changed and cheerful. Pretty things were to be seen once more in the shop windows, provisions and fuel were brought freely into the town, everybody was gay and good humoured. All around we saw and felt that it was PEACE.

CHAPTER 31

A German Funeral Pyre

The welcome help we had so earnestly prayed for had come. Kind hearts in England had responded to our appeals, and we resolved to commence our tour round the desolated villages of the Loiret by going to Cercottes and Chevilly on the direct road to Paris. The three days' battle had commenced at Artenay on the 1st of December, on the 2nd advanced to Chevilly, and on the 3rd to Cercottes, and all these villages had suffered fearfully. But things were very much changed on that sunny 4th of March from the sad winter day when we had gone out to seek the wounded there. It was peace now. Though German soldiers occupied the villages, and though the houses showed the ravages of war, the fields were cultivated, the little gardens being repaired, and women and children visible once more.

We took with us the young *Zouave* we had found in the farm at Cercottes, who was delighted to be our attendant, and with his crimson *fez* and embroidered jacket was quite a picturesque object. We drove slowly through the long faubourg and on the straight road leading from Les Aydes to Cercottes.

We did not stop there, but went straight on to Chevilly, and halted at the little house of the Sisters of St. Charles. There an English lady of a good Norfolk family, the friend I had met on the 6th of December, was still Superior of the Sisters. She was out, seeing some sick people in the village, but was sent for; and meantime one of the Sisters received us with most graceful cordiality, and showed us the ruin effected in their house by the Prussian soldiery. It was but a small building, with outhouses: added to it; a school for poor children; where the absolutely destitute are lodged, boarded, and clothed for nothing, and others for what they can pay, the average being about two pounds a year.

The good Superior had laid in her little winter stock. Butter being cheap in autumn, she had bought some and salted it down. She had made her store of preserves, and begged blankets and clothes for her little ones. Then came first the occupation of October. That was not so terrible. They had some sick in the house, and it was respected; besides, the Bavarians, who at that time took Orléans, were far gentler and kinder to the Sisterhoods than the Prussians. This may be accounted for by their being mostly Catholics, and naturally having a sympathy with the good works of their co-religionists.

On the 3rd of December the battle was close around them. Shot and shell passed over them, and one shell burst in a class-room, scattering some hundred bullets through the room. Fortunately, no one was there; the little children had fled with their parents into Orléans, and not a soul was hurt. But when the battle was over, and the French had retreated into the last trenches close by the city, the Germans occupied the village and took possession of the house. They cut down the doorways with their swords, to make them large enough for their horses to enter, and occupied the lower floor as stables. In vain the Sisters pleaded that something might be spared them; every single thing was taken, even the spectacles of the Superior, the scissors, boxes of cottons, and tatting materials of the Sisters.

All the blankets and counterpanes were stolen, and the black serge gowns of the nuns cut up for wrappers for the soldiers' throats. In one night, they consumed forty pounds of butter and nearly all the preserves. They tore off the leaves of the school desks and the doors for fuel, and burnt up the school benches. They even took the children's clothes, and when the Sisters begged them to spare these useless things, they would not hear a word, and actually took away the tiny socks and shoes.

'Spare these,' said the Sisters; 'these belong to the poor.'

'We are poor, too,' was the reply.

The Superior went to the *mairie*, where the commanding officer was installed, and prayed him to restrain his men. She was only met by a rough denial, and returned to her ruined home hopeless of redress or help. The windows were broken, the closets and drawers forced open with bayonets, and wanton and cruel damage committed, whilst the Sisters pleaded in vain that they would spare what was really the property of the poor of the village. For three days they had nothing to eat, except the broken bits of bread they picked up, and scraps of meat thrown away by the soldiers, which they washed and made soup of.

And now, though the worst was passed, poverty and destitution were their lot for many a long weary month. The children had come back to their home—for such it was—and it was a hard struggle to keep them, and surely the moderate assistance we could give was never more needed than here. To replace some of their bedding and children's clothes was indeed a great boon to them, and many a heart was gladdened by the assistance sent from England in time of need. The Sister produced some bread, wine, and preserve, and we did not like to refuse the hospitality so freely offered. We promised to return when we had visited the *mairie*, and there we accordingly went. It looked far brighter and more cheerful than on that terrible day in December when it was crowded with wounded. The rooms were still disarranged, the furniture strewed about here and there, and some few invalid soldiers had their beds in a salon. They had not forgotten us, nor how the *Ambulance Anglaise* brought them the first bread and wine after three days' living on rice.

From thence we walked with Madame H— through a pretty little wood, or rather shrubbery, where, as she told us, at this time last year, snowdrops, violets, and primroses carpeted the ground; but all were gone, and tramp of men and horse had trodden the earth into a hard, rough mass, like a dry ploughed field. We called at the house of Madame D'A—. It was still full of Prussians, and the family, fifteen in number, had only one sitting room. Though peace was signed and requisitions done away with, two German surgeons quartered there were most disagreeable, and claimed all kinds of provisions, whilst a major, also in quarter there, was very kind and considerate. All through the sad times at Orléans it seemed to depend entirely on the private character of the officers, rather than any settled rule, what the poor, wretched inhabitants had to supply to their conquerors.

The house had had a narrow escape, and a beautiful creeper in front had its stem severed by a ball. They spoke of the awful trial the last six months had been, and of the 2nd and 3rd of December, of the dead strewed about their garden and in the little wood, where the violets should be blooming now, and the dying who crawled into the village for shelter, from the bitter night and the falling snow. They told us how many a poor soldier, they feared, still lay unburied amongst the brushwood in the forest of Orléans, which extended behind and around the village. Hidden amongst the grass and shrubs many, doubtless, perished from cold; and they told us, too, how the wolves scented their prey, and, leaving the forest, prowled even almost into the village, adding to the terrors of the scene by their howls. God grant that hunger and frost had ended the agonies of the poor wounded in the forest before that savage pack tracked them in the recesses of the wood-paths.

When we returned to the house of the Sisters of St. Charles we found the Superior there, and having given the small sum intended for the repair of the schoolroom and the purchase of a few blankets and clothes, we were about to take leave, when she begged us not to go without having seen the farm of Andeglou. We walked with her up the village street. There were Prussians in every house, and all trade and employment was at a stand-still; but very few, if any, wounded were left there. We turned off to the right and came on the open country. The forest was close by in the background, and a level, open space before us, of what had once been cultivated fields.

To our left, the ground rose gently, and on it stood a roofless, lonely building, the gables clearly drawn out against the blue sky. It formed one side of a square enclosure. The central court, in the midst of which was a well, was entered by a large doorway, where once had been gates; to the left, the farmhouse, with stone steps up to it, and beyond it, forming the other side of the square, the stables. Facing us was a large barn, and the square was completed by another large barn, the buildings on our immediate right being also storehouses or barns. All was in ruins, and we picked up a bit of shell just by the entrance.

Unfortunately, the farm stood on the highest level of the plateau, directly, in the line of fire between the French and Prussian batteries, and the loss of men around it had been great on both sides. It had suffered much in October, but its utter ruin was only completed in December. The ravage and destruction in the house were frightful. Besides the shot which had entered, leaving gaps in the wall, pillage had done its worst. Not a single article of furniture was left; torn papers strewn about everywhere, the stair cases were nearly destroyed, not a window, and the marks of violence plainly to be seen all around.

The Germans had an idea that French soldiers were hidden in the farm, and they dashed open the doors to seek for them. Several shells had fallen on the house, and set fire to it here and there, but the flames had been extinguished by the farmer, who, with one or two of his men, had remained on the spot. The Germans, however, took entire possession of the buildings, and then came the saddest scene of all. Throughout the war we had always found how anxious the Germans were to conceal their enormous losses. Their published telegrams will prove this, as they always far understated the real loss both of killed and wounded. They always buried their dead instantly, and sent back their wounded to the ground in their own occupation, if not beyond the Rhine.

On this occasion there was no time to dig graves for the dead, and no means of sending large numbers of very badly or mortally wounded to the rear. The battle was not ended. It had gone forward, so to speak, sweeping over the country towards Orléans like an advancing wave, and every man was, pressed on to the front. The dead were therefore collected and placed in heaps in two of the barns, in which were still one thousand sacks of wheat, besides quantities of corn, hay, and mangoldwurzel. Many wounded had been placed there, and they were hurriedly removed, and the soldiers set fire to the barns. They did not burn quickly enough, and some casks of petroleum which they had with them, were broken open and poured upon those sad remains of humanity.

The flames roared fiercely, like a furnace; no one could approach the burning buildings that shot up columns of fire to the dark night sky; and that was a German funeral pyre!—that the dishonoured, unknown grave of upwards of three hundred of Germany's best and bravest soldiers. No word of prayer spoken above them, no stone to mark the spot. The roof that crashed in upon the dead was the substitute for the earth that should have been lightly and reverently piled over the remains of gallant men, who had fought and fallen for the glory of '*Vaterland*.' Nothing left but a huge mass of calcined ashes, showing too plainly the traces of human bones, mixed with fused metal, cloth, and grease. But a darker horror still is spoken of in hushed tones.

As the soldiers left the burning farm and went on their way, the farmer and his men crept out from their hiding-place. Something might yet be saved, but the flames beat them back, and they turned and fled in terror, for groans and shrieks were heard, and they knew that dead and dying were mingled together in that fiery furnace. Not all the wounded had been carried off. Many were doubtless insensible from loss of blood, and there was no time to look closely into all such cases. Would that we could hope that this was but an idle tale. It is a dark reality. We brought home with us some of the charred remains.

There were many things in the war, hearing of which and seeing which one could but feel that temporary success might follow; but no blessing could ever rest on emperor or king or nation, German or French, by whose soldiers such things were done. And surely the farm of Andeglou may be placed in the dark catalogue of such deeds. After this, all minor horrors seemed as nothing. The corpse of the sheepdog, wantonly shot in the stable, the stealing of thirty cows and six horses, these were merely accidents of war; but as we turned back and looked at the ruined farm, it seemed haunted by a hideous remembrance of wordless agony and crime, and to stand gaunt and blackened in the bright spring afternoon—a place stamped with a dark shadow that no sunshine can ever brighten.

We left Chevilly saddened and depressed, and drove back to Cercottes. The *curé* gave us a sad history of the sufferings of his little village since we had been there. The quartering of soldiery, and the constant requisitions, had crushed the poor to the earth. The love of the Germans for huge fires had brought about the burning of all palings, doors, even agricultural implements, of which 384 were destroyed in this village alone; and after three months of the misery entailed by an already impoverished commune having to feed and support many hundred soldiers, there arrived one day a commanding officer, with a demand for 12,000 *francs* (480*l.*), when certainly there were not 12,000 pence in the village.

The mayor was in Orléans, and had left his affairs in the hands of the *curé*, who was very busy preparing for the services of next day, which was Ash Wednesday. The *curé* was horrified, and told the officer it was utterly impossible to pay that sum. The officer said that something must be given to satisfy the *préfet*. What was the highest sum that Cercottes could pay? The *curé* said there were about a hundred houses. If, on an average, each family would pay ten *francs*, it was quite as much or more than they could do. That would be 1,000 *francs*.

The officer said it was not enough; more must be given. If not, there were three ways of compelling payment—firstly, pillage of the commune; secondly, the quartering of an additional number of soldiers; and thirdly, the taking the principal people of the village prisoners into Orléans as hostages for the whole sum. The *curé* remonstrated against any of these agreeable alternatives, and said that ever since October the village had been reduced to the greatest poverty. First, the French soldiers had been quartered there, then the Bavarians, then the French again, then the Prussians, but no one had ever been so hard before; and when the French were there they ate and drank much less than the others.

On this the officer was furiously angry, and proclaimed the *curé* his prisoner. The *curé* replied he was ready; but might he eat a morsel first? It was already prepared; and would the captain share it with him? It was indignantly refused, and the poor *curé*, hungry and tired, had to tramp three miles to Orléans by the side of the troopers' horses, and was shut up in the *mairie*. There he passed twenty-six hours. The *commandant de place*, before whom he was brought, said that probably there had been too much vivacity on both sides; however, he was not liberated till next day, when the captain himself came to let him out, saying that it was only a misunderstanding arising from too much vivacity.

The payment of the money was never enforced on Cercottes, and it is probable the vivacious captain had received a reprimand for a proceeding that looks exceedingly like buccaneering or highway robbery, and was perhaps a lively idea of his own, unauthorised by the *préfet* or any high military authority.

Cercottes was, perhaps, one of the most oppressed of all villages; always crowded with troops, on the high road to Paris, and in the midst of three or four battles. The list of destroyed blankets, clothes, sheets, and household goods is something almost incredible. A little assistance towards purchasing bread for the poor actually starving was most gratefully received, and we were assured that the *curé* and his flock would not forget to pray for the welfare of England.

We then drove on towards Orléans; we passed the lonely grave around which I had seen the bodies lying on the 6th December. No one had ever claimed that of the captain of the Foreign Legion, which the *curé* had placed so carefully on the top. Perhaps he is being waited for now in some far away country, and his near and dear ones do not know of his grave on the battle-ground of Orléans. We stopped at the farmhouse where Père Guerin and myself had found the young *Zouave*. How glad the good old couple were to see him, and how warmly they received us all! the farmer's wife saying in her graceful French way, 'Remember me well to thy mother, my boy, though I do not know her.' They were astonished to see how stout and rosy he had grown, and how actively the lad who had left them hardly able to crawl to the carriage, could help us in, shut the door, and jump upon the box, gaily waving his cap as we drove down the lane.

It was dark when we re-entered Orléans, but there was no being stopped by sentinels and asked all sorts of questions, no fear of gates being shut and our being left to pass the night in some miserable cabaret in the Faubourg. No fear, on our return, of finding that some of our poor fellows had been hurried away as prisoners. In every little detail it was Peace, not War; and what a difference that makes no one who has not lived amongst such scenes can tell. All was cheerful and quiet. Lights blazing from every window of the long corridors, the soldiers passing up and down, carrying the supper into the halls, and our own cheerful little room ready to receive us.

CHAPTER 32

A Gallant Little Town

If Bazeilles was the saddest scene of the war, in its entire destruction, the fate of Châteaudun will excite even warmer sympathy. Place that brave little town in the midst of our English land, picture to yourselves Englishmen defending wife and child, hearth and home, against a foreign invader, and the name of Châteaudun would never be heard in any public assembly ungreeted by those ringing cheers that meet the recital of acts of heroism and self-devotion whenever they are told to our countrymen and women. It was early in the autumn when this sad scene occurred. Bazeilles was burned on the 1st of September, Châteaudun on the 18th of October; yet in a letter, signed R. Loyd Lindsay, dated January 2, and published in the '*Standard*' January 3, 1871, we read as follows:—

> A number of English gentlemen of high character, some of them soldiers, are acting as reporters to the English press at the seat of war, and, like their brethren at home, are not only keen to mark anything that may be done amiss, but also prompt and ready to place on record the good deeds which may come under their notice. Thus, like the bards of the Middle Ages, who, while they incited the Knights to do their utmost, gave them a place and a name to be remembered in history. *While the keenest eyes that can be found have been watching the war, there has not been detected any act of wanton barbarity or premeditated cruelty during the whole of this invasion of France by the Germans.* But though England has not had cause to cry shame upon anything which the writers at the seat of war have made public, she has been called upon to point out that much which ought to be done in civilised warfare remains on both sides undone.

But let us see how, in reality, the bards of the nineteenth century write of the colonel's German friends. They time their minstrel harps, and chant the following lay to the glory of the Teuton Knights. Mr. W. H. Bullock, writing to the *Daily News* on the 9th of November, 1870, says:

> The burning of Bazeilles was an act of vengeance wreaked on victims of whose innocence I have been at the utmost pains to convince myself.

He goes on to speak of Beaurepaire, a little hamlet burnt by the German troops that:

> Women and little children were unhoused at the beginning of winter, besides losing the bulk of their linen, clothes, and bed furniture, which is, as a rule, plundered first by the German soldiers, and then sold by them to the Jews and others who are reported to follow the camp.

An admirable article in the *Quarterly* of January, 1871, gives also extracts from the letter of a French pastor, for whose credibility the writer can vouch, first published in the *Times*, whose sickening details of cruelty and barbarity in the neighbourhood of Dreux can be well corroborated by our own researches in and around Orléans. In one sentence he says, 'So great is the terror they inspire, that we hear on all sides of suicides.'

But to return to Châteaudun—and we here by beg Colonel Loyd-Lindsay and all who may read this work to take notice that we relate no single occurrence that cannot be vouched for on official authority, and we give our authors' names for all details of the October massacre. 'Châteaudun,' saith Murray, 'is a town of 6,781 inhabitants, on the banks of the Loire.'

It is a station on the line from Paris to Tours, *via* Vendôme, and, with its old castle crowning it, stands picturesquely, where the gradual rise of the flat land around it slopes perpendicularly down on the north side to the river, beyond which is the Faubourg of St. Jean. The Prussian attack was from the south and east sides, where they took advantage of rising ground to plant their batteries.

The history of the defence, written by L. D. Coudray, of Châteaudun, from his own personal experience and official documents, gives many interesting details, and commences by showing the unblushing falsehood of the account given in the *Times* by its Berlin correspondent. From the first incursions of the invader over the fertile plains of the Beauce Châteaudun prepared to give them a warm reception. The National Guard was organised and armed, and a body of *francs-tireurs* arrived from Tours. One word as to these *francs-tireurs*, so detested by the Prussians. They were men recruited from all ranks and classes, nobles and their servants, farmers and their labourers, gamekeepers, soldiers, '*en retraite*,': country gentlemen, clerks, mechanics, and artisans. Most of them were splendid shots, and the guerilla system of warfare they adopted is the very one so often pointed out as the way in which our Rifle Volunteers, sheltered behind the numerous hedges of Old England, could hold a foreign foe in check, and carried out exactly the orders given by the '*Landsturm-Ordnung*' of 1813, as published in Prussia.

This orders them to shoot at their enemies from behind houses and hedges, and inflict every possible injury on them; but the French did not go as far as these orders authorise the Prussians to do, for they always retained their uniform, and did not, as the *Landsturm* are ordered to do, lay aside their distinctive caps and belts; when the enemy appears in force, and 'assume to be simple inhabitants.' These orders are still in force in Prussia, (1871) yet the Germans on all occasions treated the *francs-tireurs* as brigands, and a general order was published forbidding the German Army to take them prisoners, but to shoot there down whenever they showed themselves.

However, a small body of this dreaded force, about 900 men, under a Polish colonel named Lipowski, arrived in Châteaudun on the 29th of September. On the 10th of October the first *Uhlans* were seen, and on this day a small detachment of Prussian cavalry was attacked at Varize, a small village near Châteaudun, and put to flight. On the 14th 200 Prussian troops returned and were again defeated, and whilst retreating through Civry, a neighbouring village, were attacked, and left many men dead. Next day 800 Prussian cavalry arrived at Varize by the only road which traverses the marshes around it.

They prevented all escape, and the frightened women and children hid amongst the tall grass of the marshes whilst the few National Guards still held bravely out, and fifty Prussians were put *hors de combat*. The Prussians forced their way in, pillaged every house in the town, and then set fire to them, aided by petroleum, which they seem always to have carried about with them, and, having thus punished Varize, proceeded to Civry, and did the same there. Of the sixty-two houses which composed the little town of Varize only two houses and the church remain, and these are damaged by fire.

Unwarned by the fate of these villages, Châteaudun resolved to defend itself, in spite of the decision of the commanders of the hussars. *Gardes Mobiles,* and *francs-tireurs* quartered there, that defence was impossible; but the inhabitants and the National Guard considered this declaration as unnecessary, and Colonel Lipowski submitted a proposition to the *sous-préfet* to defend the town to the last extremity. The municipality would have declined the proposal, to save the town from pillage; but it was otherwise settled, and the preparations for defence were commenced. Barricades were erected at the entrance of the streets and walls pierced for musketry, and 1,300 National Guards and *francs-tireurs*, with no cannon, prepared to hold Châteaudun to the death against General Von Wittich with 12,000 men and numerous artillery.

This general's name should be well remembered. He bore the reputation, and not unjustly, of one of the fiercest and most merciless of the Prussian commanders, and went in France by the name of the 'Butcher of Châteaudun.' It is this very general whose enthusiastic thanks to Surgeon Manley, of the War Office Ambulance, are quoted by Colonel Loyd-Lindsay in his letter of the 3rd January. He says:

'The work during all this period was most severe, and Surgeon Manley gives great credit to all there, both officers and men, who worked under him. The message which he received on one occasion from General Von Wittich shows that the services rendered by his ambulance were thankfully accepted and appreciated by the *Prussian commanders.* "Receive," said the general, "our heartfelt thanks for your most valuable aid, given to *us in the moment of our great need, when our own ambulances were not forthcoming!*"'

Thank God that when the bloody scene was over there was another ambulance who came with help and protection to the poor citizens to work amidst the smouldering ruins 'to feed the hungry, and clothe the naked, to visit the sick and the prisoner'; and though no Prussian thanks record its noble service, the little children of Châteaudun have learned to lisp a prayer for the Irish Ambulance and the good Dr. Baxter and Arthur Picard. We shall speak of them by and by.

To resume the sad story—At noon on the 18th of October the cry was raised, 'The Prussians, the Prussians!' and whilst the little garrison flew to arms the German Army appeared on the south side of the town. The attack commenced at one o'clock by the firing of a shell, which struck the town-hall, and immediately afterwards a hail of shot and shell fell around it, and in the very heart of the place. The noise of falling chimneys and crashing roofs, the roar of cannon, the rattle of musketry, and the shrieks of women filled the air, whilst clouds of smoke and dust arose. The bombardment from that time never ceased till darkness closed in, and the Prussians meantime tried to force their way past the barricades.

About two in the afternoon the Prussian batteries were firing on the Convent of the Dames Blanches, the *sous préfecture*, the Church of the Madeleine, and even the hospital, though the Geneva flag, displayed from its highest roof, was visible to every battery. About three p.m. a shell fell on the roof and penetrated to a hall full of wounded. One of these, who had suffered amputation only a quarter of an hour before, was so terrified that he fled, dragging himself down the staircase to the cellars, his wound bleeding afresh. Several of the shells were filled with petroleum and other explosive matters, and set fire to the houses as they fell.

About four o'clock nearly twenty houses were blazing, yet it was seven o'clock in the evening before the Prussians entered the town. A strong column forced their way up the Rue de Chartres, on their way to the Grande Place, and at eight o'clock the whole division marched in. Then began the deplorable scene that must for ever tarnish the laurels of the Emperor of Germany. All resistance had ceased, they were masters of Châteaudun, but the gallant little town had dared to resist, and its punishment must be such as to be a warning to other impertinent little places, that would not throw open their gates and welcome their cruel foe. Over some scenes it is well to pass lightly. The shooting of *Gardes Nationaux* and *francs-tireurs* taken red-handed in the fight was, perhaps, a natural consequence of war.

They claimed no immunity as 'simple inhabitants,' and met the fate of soldiers, but petroleum and pine-torches did the work of destruction too surely in the private houses of unoffending women and old men. One Andre Martin, aged and bedridden, could not rise when the Prussian soldiers entered the room, ordering him to get up and leave the house, as they intended to burn it. His wife pleaded in vain that, being paralysed from head to foot, he could have taken no part in the battle. She was torn away from his bedside, fire was brought and piled under the bed, and the miserable victim expired in the midst of frightful torture; his charred remains were found, and bear witness to a deed the very savages would blush to own.

Close by lived an old officer who in youth had fought in the

Grande Armée of the First Napoleon. Still suffering from a wound which had crippled him, he too had taken no share in the defence. The Prussians entered his house, ordered him to leave it, as it must be burnt, and he remonstrated with them that this was not war; in all his campaigns he had never seen such things done. The answer was a blow from the butt end of a musket. He was shot down on the threshold of his home, *unarmed* and unoffending, and his bleeding corpse thrown into the flames of his house. The '*Echo Dunois*,' in the first number published after the peace dated the 9th of May, thus gives their deaths amongst a list of those who perished on the 18th and 19th of October, 1870:

> *Andre Martin, rentier, veuf, brûlé vif dans son lit par la main des Prussians, 69 ans.*
> *Casimir-Etienne Michau, capitaine de cavalerie en retraite, chevalier de la Légion d'honneur, veuf, 73 ans: tué sur le seuil de sa maison.*

Can these things be read, attested as they are by those who saw them done, and yet men talk of 'no act of wanton barbarity or premeditated cruelty during the war!' The Hotel of the Grand Monarque was fired, the Prussians setting fire first to the long dining-room; in short, that night two hundred houses were blazing, whilst the wretched inhabitants fled across the river, and took refuge in the suburb of St. Jean. The victory cost the Prussians dear; they lost from 2,000 to 2,500 killed and wounded, as acknowledged by their own officers, whilst the defenders amounted only to 1,300, and the town was held for eight hours against such enormous odds.

At break of day a few of the most courageous citizens crept back. Their return was unopposed, but what a sight met them! From every house that had been spared all its contents had been taken: wine, liqueur, linen, furniture, all were gone. Soldiers were quartered in the empty rooms, and demanded dinner and wine when there were none to give. Meantime General von Wittich was resolved that prisoners should grace his triumph, and about one hundred citizens were made captive and taken away to Germany. A list of their names is given in the '*Echo Dunois*,' and not one is a soldier or *franc-tireur*.

They were brought to Orléans, where the citizens, seeing them faint and weary, prepared some refreshment for them. It was immediately consumed by the German soldiery, who threw the broken pieces to their prisoners, and when the indignant Orleanais brought a fresh supply, they were met with threats and menaces. The inhabitants who remained were treated with insult and oppression. The halls of the college were turned into stables, the officer remarking to one of the professors, 'Don't you feel very humiliated at seeing horses in your class-rooms?'

The Jews who accompanied the division stabled their heavy waggons in the factory Rainville, where they were loaded with the booty bought from the soldiery, and were then sent away to Germany. After the pillage came the demand for a money contribution. General von Wittich fixed it at 200,000 *francs* (8,000*l*.), an enormous sum for a half-burned and wholly ruined town, 1,500 blankets, 200 pounds of salt, 200 pounds of coffee, 400 litres of brandy, and 20,000 litres of hay. The poor people got together 30,000 *francs*, 110 blankets, the coffee and salt, and, finding it impossible to *screw* out more, the general was obliged to be contented with this.

The day after the battle, amidst smoking ruins and unburied bodies, the German bands played one of Strauss's *valses*, an air by Weber, and an overture by Wagner! How bitterly must the mourners have felt this mockery of their sorrow and desolation! the greater part of the German troops left on the 20th, but the town remained occupied by a small garrison. Several houses were fired just before they left, and one instance more may be given of wanton mischief. A German surgeon quartered in the house of a French resident medical man not only carried off the best of the surgical instruments of his unfortunate host, but broke those he did not care to take away. On the 20th also thanks were voted to the town of Châteaudun by the government at Tours, and 100,000 *francs* were granted to aid in repairing the damages, whilst nine of the heroic defenders, including Colonel Lipowski, received the Legion of Honour, and a street in Paris had its name changed from Rue Cardinal Fesch to Rue Châteaudun. 285 houses were completely destroyed; twelve only by shell, 193 were fired by hand, and the rest caught fire from the proximity of burning buildings. The entire loss of house property and furniture amounted to 5,000,000 *francs*.

The list of innocent victims amounts to twenty-eight civilians, five of whom were men in the prime of life, who perished in the burning buildings. One was a blacksmith, shot the day after the battle in the street because he did not answer a sentinel's challenge given in German, and one paragraph from the death list will tell its own tale how father, mother, and children died together:—

Saillard, carrossier, marie, 42 ans: asphyxie.

Estelle-Uranie Menant, femme Saillard, 38 ans environ: asphyxie.
Marie-Lucie Saillard, 13 ans 4 mois asphyxie.
Louise-Uranie Saillard, 2 ans 4 mois asphyxie.

Three servant-girls of one family were smothered in a cellar.

We had always had a great desire to visit this place, and one fine bright morning in March, the 8th, Louise and myself started for Châteaudun. It is about twelve leagues from Orléans; the country, a flat level, gave the exact impression of a brown sea with islets rising out of it, in the shape of small villages and isolated farms. Nothing could be drearier. We left Orléans by the long suburb leading to Les Ormes. The Germans had attacked on this side, and many houses were much damaged, especially at Les Ormes, which had suffered heavily from pillage and requisition. Traces of earthworks were still visible, and it seemed to us, as we journeyed around Orléans and looked at the lines of defence, that a far more desperate resistance might have been made.

Beyond Les Ormes we came on the open country, leaving about a mile on our left the village of Ingres, which, being unable to pay a heavy money requisition, had been given up to pillage, and where many acts of cruelty had been perpetrated.

We halted at Tournoisie, a little village half-way, to rest the horses, and entering the principal *auberge*, we asked for some *déjeuner*. The poor woman assured us that German troops had passed the night in the village, and eaten and taken everything away. Not a truss of hay was left, all had been carried off, and not one farthing paid for it; and this was after the peace was signed, when it had been specially arranged that no requisitions were to be made without payment. But resistance was useless against armed and unscrupulous men, and the system was carried on to the last. Even the knives and forks had been stolen, and all we could have was some eggs and bread. We had some wine with us, and there was a little coffee.

We gave something to replace the knives, and the poor woman said she hoped their troubles were nearly over now. The corps expected every moment to arrive in the village would be the last to pass through, and as they were Hessians, she hoped they would behave more mercifully than the Prussians. Everywhere we found it the same. The Prussians proper were considered by the French as the most cruel and the most detested of all the 'people and tribes' who made up the German Army. Each of these 'tribes' disliked the others, and only agreed in one thing, jealousy of their head, Prussia; but this jealousy and dislike were far stronger on the part of the Bavarians than on that of any of the others.

We left Tournoisie after a rest of an hour and at four o'clock entered Châteaudun. It had changed masters twice since the day of its first capture, but on the 28th of November had been finally reoccupied by the Germans, and, to our surprise, was still in their hands, the evacuation not having been yet carried out. As this meant the occupation of every available quarter by soldiers, it was far from an agreeable discovery. It is a luckless little town. It was burned by the Orleanais in the sixth century, by the Normans in the ninth, was the centre of a war against robber hordes in the twelfth, was nearly destroyed by fire in 1783, and again, as we know, in 1870. Its old castle escaped through all these troubles; it was built in the tenth century, and was the residence of the Comtes de Dunois. It is now (1871) the property of the Duc de Luynes, and was being restored when the war broke out. It presents no appearance of decay, and as it stands, with its huge pile overlooking the town, is the very picture of a feudal castle.

As we drove slowly up the slope, we passed the railway station; it had been much injured, and a very large white building close by had been destroyed by fire, and was a mere empty shell. We proceeded up the Rue d'Orléans, and here burnt houses were visible on every side, and piles of ruins still encumbered the streets. We made our way to the Place Royale, or central square, and to the hotel whose sign-board announced it as Hôtel de la Place. It had been Hôtel Impériale, but that word was erased, and the host was waiting a permanent change of government, or dynasty, to replace it. Will it be '*Republique*,' or '*Royale*,' or '*Impériale*' again? The hostess came out to greet us, and one word—that we were friends of M. Arthur Picard—secured us a warm reception. She had no room for us; but the head groom had a nice little house, not burned down, and we could have a room there. Meantime she would prepare our dinner. We should have it quietly before those noisy Germans came in.

One word as to M. Picard, and the great service he rendered to Châteaudun, as our kind landlady told us the tale, whilst waiting on us at dinner. He was the '*comptable*' or manager of the Irish Ambulance, which he had joined in company with Dr. Ryan shortly after our being at Tours where we met them. This Irish Ambulance was formed in Dublin and sent out to aid the French. It had no connection whatever with the so-called Irish Ambulance formed in London and dissolved at Havre, but it originally consisted of far too many dressers and *in-*

firmiers, and its chief. Dr. Baxter, sent back two-thirds of them when he joined at Havre, where they had arrived from Cork. They entered Châteaudun when the Germans evacuated it, at the time the French retook Orléans, and were there on the re-entrance of the Germans, having some of their surgeons at Patay and other villages.

During this time a very strange event occurred. The Church of the Madeleine was once more used for Divine worship. The Host was in the shrine, one solitary French National Guard kneeling in the aisle, and a few humble inhabitants. A German soldier—let us charitably hope, the worse for wine or brandy—mounted the altar steps, and was in the act of climbing upon the altar itself, to desecrate most shamefully the sacred place, when the revolver in his belt caught some projection, turned upwards, one of the barrels was discharged, and the ball lodged so close to his heart, that his death followed instantaneously.

General Von Wittich immediately demanded 20,000 *francs* fine. He could not prove the murderer was that National Guard, nor could he identify him; but he was convinced a French hand had done the deed, and he threatened to bombard the town afresh if the fine was not paid. It could not be raised, and things were looking desperate, when Arthur Picard, accompanied by one of the Sisters of Mercy nursing in the Irish Ambulance, sought out the general at his quarters, about a mile out of town, to plead for mercy. M. Picard offered to pay down at once 5,000 *francs* on condition that the body of the dead German was given up to him for examination, that two German surgeons should be present, and that on the result of this examination future proceedings should depend.

The general consented; the examination took place. The ball was found; it was the ball of the soldier's own revolver. The general was convinced and the fine remitted; but the 5,000 *francs* were retained. Such is the tale that has made Arthur Picard's name known in Châteaudun; but of one and all we heard high praise. Their skill, their courage, their unselfish devotion, their kindly sympathy, not only with the sick but the sorrowing, were the theme of every tongue, and that we were friends of theirs was our sufficient passport. They did splendid service, though no official thanks have ever been given to them. However, two days before we arrived, they had left, and only a waggon with '*Ambulance Irlandaise*' painted on it, and standing in the yard of a factory, remained to testify of their presence there.

Before dinner we strolled about the town. It was a sad sight of wreck and ruin. The back of our hotel was entirely destroyed, and next door a range of buildings, once a splendid shop, was in ruins. The other side of the Place Royale had escaped better, but the windows were starred with bullet holes. When the Prussians stormed the barricades and entered the town a great deal of random firing took place in the streets, to the destruction of the windows. We heard sad tales from one and all of the terror and distress in the town on that October night; how when the Prussians entered—*'comme des sauvages'*—women and children fled down the steep path that led to the river banks, and so escaped by the *faubourg*.

The shops were broken open and their contents strewed about the street; sugar, rice, coffee, pieces of silk, muslin, and linen, books, furniture, bacon, butter, cheese, very conceivable article, were heaped together in the streets and trodden under foot. Many inhabitants were utterly ruined, and it will be years, if ever, before Châteaudun recovers the effect of that day's work. The hundred citizens sent away as prisoners passed several months in Germany, and the entire suspension of trade and business had been the consequence.

The next morning, after a walk about the town, we ordered breakfast, and prepared to leave on our return to Orléans. When we went down to the *salle-à-manger*, we found a very fat, red-faced officer there, who was giving directions for his breakfast in bad French. After him entered two or three others, and they began to eat their cutlets and salad with good appetites. Just as they had finished the landlady came in, and, addressing the first officer, asked him if he were the general who had sent to command a *déjeuner*. '*Ja*,' answered the individual in question.

'Then, *Monsieur*,' said the good woman, 'your *déjeuner* is prepared in the small *salle*. I apologise that I did not recognise Your Excellency.'

'Bring the breakfast here,' replied His Excellency; 'I can eat a second, but I shall not stir from here.'

All persuasions were vain, so the second breakfast was brought, and devoured with equal appetite; and the general began to converse. He spoke in German, and was telling the others how, where he had been quartered, he had been called a tyrant; but he only wished he could do twice as much to crush the *'canaille of France.'* As for sparing men, women, and children, it was all nonsense. The Germans should have rule over all, to do as they pleased with them. The rest of the chivalrous warrior's ideas, as regarded his captives, had best be omitted.

I suppose our faces showed the disgust we felt, for one of the officers tried to silence him, and he said, still in German, looking at us,

'They are brave women to travel about in this country just now.' We resolved to show him that we were not unguarded, and, calling the landlady, I whispered to her to send in Louis, our chief *infirmier*, who had accompanied us, telling her why. Louis came in, the very picture of a bright, intelligent French soldier, in the neat dress of the marine infantry. He was nearly six feet high, with a bright, blue eye, fair hair, and neatly-trimmed moustache. He stood behind our chairs as Louise and I turned and spoke to him, giving him some directions about the carriage, whilst a sudden silence fell on the noisy group of Germans, and the general let fall his knife and fork, and sat as if thunderstruck.

To have a French private, free and happy, travelling about in their lines, and actually introduced into his august presence, was a fact he could not realise. Louis left, touching his *kepi* as he went; and the general, drawing a long breath, said emphatically, '*Ach Himmel!* but they *are* brave indeed to dare to do *this!*'

The rest of his party thoroughly enjoyed the scene, and as for the landlady and the various inhabitants who were lounging about, their delight was excessive, and if it had been possible to give us a French guard of honour out of the town's precincts, I really believe it would have been done, they were so pleased at what they considered the compliment paid to their nation, and in speaking in a friendly manner, before the general, to a French soldier, and showing that we had confidence in his fidelity and good-will to act as our guard. Trifles like these go very far in war time. There are two generals we met whose lives are not worth an hour's purchase when the next war comes between Prussia and France, and this blustering bully is one of them.

We reached Orléans in safety, and the story, as related by Louis, was the amusement of the ambulance. One of the Germans told me the general was a well-known man, very harsh to his own men, and probably very cruel to his enemies. Characters vary in all men, but the difference in German officers was extraordinary. I never could account for it, on any settled principle, except that they differed much in themselves at various times, and that often champagne had a great deal more to do with it than natural character.

It was an invariable rule with us never to have any conversation with them after 7 p.m.; and though I do not go so far as some people do who say that three parts of the officers in the German Army were drunk all day, except during a few hours in the morning, I am quite sure that very many drank very hard, and many things were done in consequence which could not be recalled, and which were bitterly regretted in the cooler judgment of the early morning.

This fact is another proof of the terrible demoralisation of war. These gentlemen were not habitual drunkards, were not wild boys, were, at least many of them, steady-going citizens, fathers of families, and respectable members of society. It may be feared that the habits acquired in this miserable war will cling to them through life, and be handed down to their children; and this fear should be a strong motive to promote peace by every honourable means, so that our own land may, in God's mercy, be spared from the awful scourge of war.

Chapter 33

The Loiret

Our last expedition before we left Orléans was to the villages of Artenay, Beaune-le-Rolande, and Lorcy, all the sites of fierce contest. Artenay especially had suffered. It was on the high road to Paris, and round it and in it several conflicts had taken place. Like all other towns in the neighbourhood, it had been full of wounded, and had been heavily oppressed by requisitions. The *curé* showed us where a shell had exploded in his garden, and the church had been struck by several. We heard one strange and true thing there.

A tricolour flag was displayed side by side with a Red Cross one, from the window of a respectable house which was pointed out to us in the main street, and this had been stolen by some German soldiers, a gilt eagle was fitted upon it, and it was taken away to figure in the triumphal entry to Berlin as a regimental standard. A second instance of this occurred in the same town. So, if a vast number of captured flags are borne through the streets of Berlin, we may fairly entertain some doubt as to their authenticity.

Artenay must always be a very dull little place, and was of course now a very depressed one. We visited the branch house of the St. Aignan Sisterhood. The poor things had but little left. Their bedding was spoiled by the use of the wounded, and their chairs had been burnt for firewood; but they had reassembled their poor children, and the school was going on as usual. Relief was sadly needed, and some was given by the kindness of two gentlemen we met in the inn, agents for the distribution of the American fund, to whom we mentioned their case, and we cannot speak too highly of the thorough manner in which these gentlemen discharged their duty, examining personally into the cases, and using their own good judgment, not trusting to the reports of others, or leaving their work to be done second-hand.

The road to Beaune-le-Rolande ran through the forest. We passed over several huge trenches with stakes at the bottom, very nasty if man or horse fell into them. They were bridged now with planks, and it was rather nervous work passing over in a carriage. Various earth-banks had been thrown up amidst the brushwood for riflemen to hide behind; and certainly it would have been impossible for an enemy to pass in face of an opposing force; but unluckily the enemy, in this instance, did not come that way. We stayed at a way side inn to lunch, and early in the afternoon reached Beaune-le-Rolande. The battle here had been a very severe one; several houses were destroyed by shell, and several more had been burnt.

We went to the *curé* to enquire into the state of the poor, and were surprised, on announcing ourselves as English, to be received with the greatest coldness and suspicion. 'English, are you?' said the *curé*; 'then why did you not accompany your ambulance? they went to Beaugency with the Prussians, they came here with them in the first instance, stayed here a little while, and then went to rejoin them.'

'Very likely,' we said. 'But we do not belong to that ambulance. They are with the Prussians; but they never worked in Orléans. They sent a messenger to us to know if we had any work for them; but we did not want them, and said 'No. We are of the *Ambulance Anglaise* in the Convent of St. Marc, Orléans, under Monseigneur Dupanloup.'

This simple explanation changed all. We were requested to sit down and share what dinner there was. We complained of having been followed and unkindly spoken to as we came, and the *curé* said he would explain to the people that we did not belong to the great English Ambulance that had gone with the Prussians. Justly or unjustly, I know not, as we never came across them; but from first to last the War Office Ambulance was considered by the French as merely supplementing the regimental ambulances of the German Army, and they had the same idea that I had been told of in England as being the boast of a Prussian officer—that the assistance given to the Germans enabled them to send 20,000 more men to the front than could otherwise have been spared.

We left Beaune-le-Rolande next day, and by that time the news had been spread that we were not English like the English who had been there, who had lived hand-in-glove with the German officers. They had nursed the wounded certainly, but the fact of intimate acquaintanceship with the invaders, could not be forgiven by the people. In any future war this rock must be avoided; neutrals should be really neutral. The great ambulances occupied a prominent place, but their help would have been gladly dispensed with by the French because they were distrusted. It was the case with the Anglo-American at Orléans, popular as it had been at Sedan, and more particularly so during the whole career of the War Office Ambulance; but the experience we gained of practical ambulance work will be better given hereafter in a separate form.

We drove to Lorcy to see the branch house of our convent there. The Sisters told us of the day when the fighting was near them, and the balls were whistling up the street. The children they taught were all in class, but, as the Sister Superior remarked, 'they could not attend to their lessons,' so the shutters were closed to prevent the balls coming in, and they tried to amuse the poor little things. Imagine the difficulty of playing a children's game, with shot and shell falling around they told us a sad tale, too, which we heard confirmed in the villages named. The combat commenced around Ledon on the 24th October, but neither party seems to have gained a decided advantage, and the Prussians encamped at a little distance from Lorcy, which is four miles from Ledon and four miles farther from Orléans.

On the 25th a peasant went to the French *commandant* at Ledon and told him that there were only a couple of hundred Prussians at Lorcy. Seventeen mounted *Chasseurs d'Afrique* and three hundred infantry instantly started for that place. The Prussians were there; not two hundred, as the peasant said, but between two and three thousand. The poor French fought with all the courage of despair, fifteen German officers were killed and nearly five hundred men, but at last the French were obliged to surrender. They were summoned to do so, and to throw down their arms; resistance was hopeless, and they did lay down their arms, and gave themselves up prisoners.

Then came a scene which surely is a disgrace to the German name: helpless and disarmed, they were made to kneel down, the poor wounded remnants of that gallant band, a file of Prussian soldiers was marched in front of them, a volley was fired, and all was over. They had dared to fight as brave men should, in an unequal contest, and they paid the penalty with their lives. But the story will never be forgotten by those who saw the execution, and before long the place of their burial will be marked by some memorial of their sad fate.

We drove back through several villages, all showing traces of war, to Châteauneuf. Here we found a very good hotel but lately evacuated by the Germans; and the landlady showed us into a room, apologising for its being not yet in order, for a mechanic was repairing the locks of the drawers, which had been forced open with their swords by the Prussian officers who had lodged in that room, and everything had been plundered. There had been no resistance in Châteauneuf, and this had been done *since the armistice*.

Whilst our dinner was preparing, we tried to get the workman into a chat, but he was exceptionally silent and, as it seemed, sulky. At last he unbent. Our sympathy with the poor people of the district was too evident not to win his confidence, and he told us his tale. It came out in short sentences, with long intervals of silence between. He had been a soldier in early life, and when his time of service expired, became a whitesmith in a village hard by; being married, with one young child, he had not been drawn in the first levies. Many Prussians were quartered on him at one time. They ate and drank all he had. He had not even bread to give his wife and child; but a sergeant, who saw the state to which they were reduced, insisted on his men sharing their rations with the family.

'We lived like brothers,' said the poor fellow; 'he was a good man, Prussian though he was. I pray God to bless him. It was through him we did not die of starvation.'

He went on to say that he was drawn in the last levy; but before he joined, the second taking of Orléans occurred, and he went back to his ruined home. He found his wife there, and his only child dying. There was nothing to give them; no food, no medicine, no help, for the enemy were all around, and 'at even the child died.' They laid the body decently on the only mattress left them, and covered it with the poor fellow's coat. But that night more Prussians came by, and demanded food, and fire, and lodging.

Of the first two there was none, the last was there, but no beds, only that one mattress with its sacred burden. But even this was not respected; the body of the child was flung out into the roadway, and a Prussian soldier threw himself down upon the mattress. The father took up the corpse of his child, and as he carried it in his arms to the woods hard by, where at least its bed of dry leaves would not attract a Prussian soldier, he swore a deep oath of vengeance, and when the French cross the Rhine (and the day may come, for none can tell what is in the future), that oath will be fearfully kept.

As he took up his basket of tools with a stern, sad, absent air, we looked at his white, fixed face and the pitiless expression round his set lips, and said to each other, 'God forbid we should be Germans in a

German village when that man comes by, on his way to Berlin!' He touched his cap gravely, 'Good evening, *Mesdames*; you are kind, you can feel for us. It was my only child,' and so left the room. Many such a tale can be told. The Germans have sown the wind, they will reap the whirlwind; and none know this better than their leaders. France must be utterly crushed, that the day of vengeance for 1870-71 may never dawn; but she has a power of elasticity left that may defy them yet.

We returned next day to Orléans. A visit to Coulmiers concluded our work in the Loiret. We saw the battlefield where the only real French victory of the war was won which had any important results, for it was after this battle that Orléans was evacuated by the Germans, and the *château* which had been the headquarters of Von der Tann. Like all others it had been completely pillaged. We heard here from the peasants who had buried the dead, that the German killed and wounded were that day six to one of the French. Wherever we went this was the case, and during our excursion to Artenay and Beaune we were shown a farm near Artenay, called 'Arblay,' where the Germans had burned their dead, as at Andeglou.

We saw where a huge pile of wheat-straw and human remains had been; the charred relics were still left there. It was in the midst of a courtyard surrounded by farm buildings. It burned for two days, and when the farmer, who had gone into Orléans, returned to his farm to see what he could save, he found smoke and flames ascending from the courtyard, but was prevented from entering it by German sentinels. We heard of several similar cases in various villages.

That it was not done from sanitary motives is evident by the fact that very few French were missing; most of those absent from their regiments were accounted for. They were buried on the field, taken into ambulance, or sent away prisoners; besides, the buttons and scraps of singed clothing found were all German. There is no doubt it was done to conceal their losses, especially as the fact is not recorded, I believe, in any of their medical or military reports, and was indignantly denied by those in our ambulance, till we produced convincing evidence in portions of the charred remains, buckles, buttons, and other little proofs of our statement. We have these things still.

Our work was now done, and we prepared to leave; but before concluding this simple relation of our experiences in the war, I will add a few words as to the domestic state of Orléans in that sad time. The inhabitants were well aware that to have soldiers quartered upon them was the fate of war; but they did feel it hard that there were no rules as to what quantity of meat and wine they must be furnished with, and that no complaints of excess ever met with any redress. How hopeless complaint was, may be seen from the fact that a lady presented herself before the *commandant de place*, to request that some orders might be given to the soldiers in her house to conduct themselves with common decency. His answer was, 'Madame, you appear to forget that you are lodging with the Prussians, not the Prussians with you. If you do not like your hosts, you can leave.'

The requisitions for forage made on the villagers were ruinous; not only was sufficient taken to supply the daily wants of the cavalry and train horses, but the demand was only limited by the supply, and all was carried off for future use. The same with stores of wine, flour, potatoes, rice, and groceries. Nothing was left, and too often clothes useless to the soldiery, were cut into ribands, whilst every little ornament was taken to send as a present to some German fair one, and furniture was recklessly burned for firewood.

It was not only the soldiers but the officers who acted with positive dishonesty. There seemed to be an utter demoralisation amongst them. Two instances may here be given. A colonel was quartered in the house of a retired officer of good family in Orléans. He lived with the gentleman and his daughter on the most friendly terms; they gave him up the *salon* for his sleeping apartment, and treated him as an honoured guest. In the *salon* was a *secretaire*, locked, and the key in the possession of the old officer. This *secretaire* contained family papers and some jewels of value. After the departure of the German colonel the officer inspected the *secretaire*; it was apparently untouched. He opened it; it was empty!

The mystery was soon explained; for, by a strange mischance, the colonel had omitted to search his room for anything he had forgotten to pack up, and there, under his mattress, was an instrument for picking locks. A German Catholic chaplain was quartered in the humble presbytery of the *curé* of Les Aydes, a suburb of Orléans. Will it be credited, yet it is strictly true, that the reverend gentleman actually robbed his poor host, his brother priest, of all his linen and clothes, and carried away sundry small articles which he found about!

It is a well-known fact that many officers, as well as privates, had with them complete sets of housebreaking instruments, whilst a number of Jews followed the army, under pretext of selling tobacco, and bought the plunder from the thieves. I doubt if Frenchmen would have condescended to this meanness. The loss of the papers and jewels will form the subject of a suit at Berlin for their restitution, as well as the little bill of 8,000 *francs* for extras which Prince Frederick Charles ran up at Montargis, and forgot to pay. Story after story of this kind could be related. The dishonest propensities of the Germans, their enormous appetites, their love of comfort, and their entire disregard of decency in their habits, will remain impressed on the minds of the French as the leading characteristics of their invaders.

With the coming of peace our ambulance was broken up—the still uncured men being sent to the hospitals of their depots, whilst the rest and the *infirmiers* rejoined their regiments. The German doctors and *infirmiers* left early in March, and Matthias returned to his convent. The 'Wandering Jew' said he should close the ambulance. To this we demurred. It had been opened before his coming; it should be continued after his departure. They had all been there on sufferance, and because we were glad of their services; but they could neither open nor close an English Ambulance. M. de Capes sent us in some fresh French wounded from private houses, now cleared of their patients, and the ambulance remained open till late in April, though we left on the 28th of March. The good bishop, who in February had been elected a deputy, was at Versailles, but sent us a warm letter of thanks.

What the state of Orléans was during that wretched winter may be judged from a few statistics. It is a town of 50,000 inhabitants. Over 50,000 troops were quartered there at intervals, for two or three days at a time, whilst the permanent garrison was 10,000 men; but the passing and repassing of large bodies of soldiers often swelled this number, and during the months of December and January there were more than 30,000 wounded in the city, the majority Germans. There were 360 ambulances in private houses, none with less than six men in them, many with 20 or 30, and besides these, every barrack and public building, every convent and manufactory, were converted into hospitals.

Four hundred Sisters of various orders were employed nursing the wounded, besides a staff of ladies of Orléans, and some Protestant deaconesses with the Hessian *corps d'armée*. In the large buildings from 200 to 400 wounded were received at one time. The *évêché*, three churches, the college, the seminary, were all ambulances. The Hôtel-Dieu and the Caserne St.-Charles were reserved for small-pox cases, of which there were 4,000 at one time during the winter, including civilians. Typhus and scarlet fever were also terribly prevalent.

Several German papers unblushingly propagated the falsehood that the German wounded were ill-treated, even mutilated, in the ambulances of Orléans. This was positively and indignantly denied in a letter from the German general in command. The chief medical Inspector bore witness that 'in no place were the German wounded so well treated.' One German officer told the bishop that he felt such false assertions dishonoured his country. Another wrote to Monseigneur Dupanloup, 'We cannot go on making war as we are doing now.'

A most emphatic denial was given in a letter published by the bishop. Hardly treated as were the people of Orléans, no single act of unkindness, far less cruelty, has been proved against any one of them. And yet they *were* hardly treated. It was said by the *commandant de place* that a quarrel had taken place in a very low house, between a German soldier and a citizen of Orléans, and that the soldier had been stabbed. Prince Frederick Charles imposed a fine of 600,000 *francs* on the city for this murder. The authorities offered to prove that no such event had taken place, and requested an inquest on the body. The body was never produced, and all enquiry into the matter refused.

There was not one word of truth in the statement, but the fine had to be paid, and the transaction left a feeling of uncertainty as to the probability of the proceeding being repeated whenever Prince Frederick Charles fell short of ready money. He was the most unpopular of all the German commanders, and women used the name of the Red Prince to frighten their rebellious children. He was decidedly the Ogre of the War, but as we never received from himself and his staff anything but kindness and good-will, it would be a very ungracious act on our parts to repeat the many tales we heard to his disadvantage.

Besides money, perpetual requisitions were made in kind. Once, leather enough for 100,000 pair of half-boots! or money to the same value. Nothing could be more crushed and miserable than the population of this town under the Prussian rule, and the harshness had its usual recoil—the victims had resort to a system of deceit, for self-preservation, in itself destructive of all fair dealing. To cheat a German was a justifiable, nay, further, a praiseworthy act, and the old example of 'spoiling the Egyptians' was quoted in proof of its having the sanction of Scripture; but here and there a singular trait of honesty cropped up. I met a peasant woman in a bookseller's shop, buying a German grammar of the most puzzling description.

'Why do you buy that?' I asked; 'why not have one of these simple phrase-books? They give you all necessary to know when soldiers are quartered in your house.'

'*Madame*' she replied gravely, 'that is not what I want. I have a little boy of eight years old. I must teach him German.'

'But why?' I asked.

"Because, *Madame*, the Prussians have stolen everything I had in the world, and when our soldiers go to Berlin, my boy may be old enough to go with them, and then (as I am honest) I should wish him to take from some poor place like ours, only just what they took from us; so he must know German well.'

This cool, determined spirit of revenge will be more dangerous to the peace of Europe, in future years, cultivated as it is in the rising generation, than all the passionate threats of the present one. The French of twenty years hence may be a sadder and a wiser people. Taught by the follies, the madness, and the misfortunes, of the France of the Second Empire, they may avoid the errors which brought about the ruin of their country; but one thing they will never learn—to forgive the Germans.

One of the grand vicars said to us, 'Yes, it is true we hated the English nation as a nation, though we loved and esteemed individuals; but we, have changed our hatred now, and Waterloo is forgotten in Sedan.'

It has become a sacred duty to detest the Prussians, and to train up the young in this spirit. Even the priests share in this feeling, and look forward, and lead their flocks to do so too, to the time when victory on the other shore of the Rhine shall efface the disgrace and humiliation of this war.

It must be confessed, too, that the insolent manner of the Germans, their boasts and threats, stimulated this evil feeling. The noblest and the gentlest natures were stung by it into deep resentment. One of the *abbés* in Orléans is a man renowned for the sanctity of his life and the eloquence of his preaching. He is the head of a college for junior boys, intended for the *Grand Seminaire*. He himself told me that on one occasion, accompanied by a servant, he went to the forest, to cut wood for the fires in his house, which he had made into an ambulance. At the entrance of the wood he met a young German officer, who stopped and insulted him in the grossest way.

The *abbé* turned to him, saying in German, 'You ought to be more courteous, sir, to a fallen foe. You are the victors now; but the day may come when we, in our turn, shall stand in the position you hold now, lords of an invaded country. You have taught us lessons we shall not forget. From the seed you have sown, a bitter harvest shall be reaped. Yes, sir, in ten years' time, I shall accompany our army across the Rhine. I myself—and why? To plead with the avengers, for your wives and your children, to save your homes from fire and pillage, to tell our soldiers that the noblest revenge will then be to show how victories can be won, and yet the laws of God and man be respected.'

The German turned sulkily away, saying, 'Don't trouble yourself, old gentleman; I shall never live to see that.'

'No, you will not,' answered the *abbé*; 'you will leave your bones here in France, to fertilise the soil you have invaded. I shall go to tell your countrymen how the graves of those who sleep in France are respected, even by their enemies!' and raising his hat, he walked off. The officer died, and was buried in Orléans about a month afterwards.

Many a time it has been difficult for us to suppress our feelings of indignation, at being told by Prussian officers, that they all looked forward to the day when they should invade and conquer England; that it was a thing arranged already, when Holland and Belgium were added to the German Empire, and that the quarrel would begin about Heligoland. They did not speak of our nation with the insolent contempt with which they treated the French, but with an amount of jealousy and hatred that they could not conceal. They told us, too, that the wonderful system of espionage which had been carried on for years in France was being practised in England.

It is a fact that they had plans of every house and garden in Orléans, even of the convent where we were, and knew the way up the path and through the paddock to Ste.-Marie, before they had seen it in reality. A party of *Uhlans* entered a brewer's office in Orléans. He gave them beer; but one, raising his helmet, said, 'Don't you know me. *Monsieur?* Give us some of the good beer in cellar five.' It was his head clerk, who had left about two years ago!

For five years a shepherd lived in a small farmhouse close by one of the great forts near Paris. There he kept the sheep, and led the hard life of a peasant. It was an engineer officer who in this disguise took maps of the fort and the country around. Instance after instance could be adduced of men who had passed years as clerks, servants, and tutors in various families, coming back to the places where they had resided at the head of the *Uhlans*, sent on before the main body of the army.

No wonder the French desire to expel every German from their land. If would be well if England would make sure, that in her peaceful homes, in her busy warehouses, in farmhouse or lordly hall, she is not nursing vipers that may turn round and sting her. We heard and knew so much of this system and its terrible results that we never hear of

German servants, or even governesses, without a fear that their master's secrets are being recorded at Berlin—the amount of his property and the value of his plate.

But it is time to conclude this simple sketch of our life in an invaded country. A few passing remarks I would make as regards ourselves personally. We had to lament the death in our ambulance at Ste.-Marie of the young German student I named as Dr. Kröner's assistant. He caught the smallpox, and died of it, after an illness of four days. He received from Mère St -Joseph and her Sisters the kindest and tenderest of nursing, and was buried with military honours only a few days before the peace was signed. With the coming in of peace we received our letters and papers, and found Dr. Pratt had not sent his promised apology to the '*Times*.' He called at our request, and promised to do it.

He left next day for Paris, and it has remained undone; but the full and truthful statement we have made will quite explain the state of the case as it stands between ourselves and the National Committee, and we leave the verdict to the justice of our countrymen and women. If only the National Society had aided us out of their ample resources, we might, indeed, have done in Orléans a work that would have made their names honoured not only in the city, but throughout France itself. As it is, the deep gratitude and the public thanks which have been bestowed upon us are given to ourselves alone; but as Englishwomen we feel that we share those thanks with all who bear the English name. Many gave us substantial aid, many more, true sympathy and hearty prayers for our welfare; and much of our safety and success was, under Providence, owing to the Union Jack that floated bravely over our convent home.

Our tale has been a sad yet a true one We saw the *domestic* horrors of war, and turned in sadness from its so-called glories. We looked on happy homes, ruined and desolated, on the fair land of France laid waste, and we heard the mourning and lamentation for the dear ones fallen in fight, or led away captives to a strange land. But we sorrowed most of all, over the demoralisation of character in two great nations—a demoralisation which has stamped its ineffaceable brand on the men who fought in the campaigns of 1870-71, and which will be handed down to the next generation: the brand of licentiousness, brutality, dishonesty, untruthfulness, hatred, and revenge.

May God in His mercy save England from things like these, for He alone can guard us in the hour of danger, national or personal. We trust and believe that when the storm-clouds are gathering as now around us, 'The Lord shall give strength to His people: the Lord shall give His people the blessing of peace.'

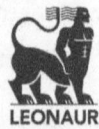

ALSO FROM LEONAUR
AVAILABLE IN SOFTCOVER OR HARDCOVER WITH DUST JACKET

THE WOMAN IN BATTLE by *Loreta Janeta Velazquez*—Soldier, Spy and Secret Service Agent for the Confederacy During the American Civil War.

BOOTS AND SADDLES by *Elizabeth B. Custer*—The experiences of General Custer's Wife on the Western Plains.

FANNIE BEERS' CIVIL WAR by *Fannie A. Beers*—A Confederate Lady's Experiences of Nursing During the Campaigns & Battles of the American Civil War.

LADY SALE'S AFGHANISTAN by *Florentia Sale*—An Indomitable Victorian Lady's Account of the Retreat from Kabul During the First Afghan War.

THE TWO WARS OF MRS DUBERLY by *Frances Isabella Duberly*—An Intrepid Victorian Lady's Experience of the Crimea and Indian Mutiny.

THE REBELLIOUS DUCHESS by *Paul F. S. Dermoncourt*—The Adventures of the Duchess of Berri and Her Attempt to Overthrow French Monarchy.

LADIES OF WATERLOO by *Charlotte A. Eaton, Magdalene de Lancey & Juana Smith*—The Experiences of Three Women During the Campaign of 1815: Waterloo Days by Charlotte A. Eaton, A Week at Waterloo by Magdalene de Lancey & Juana's Story by Juana Smith.

NURSE AND SPY IN THE UNION ARMY by *Sarah Emma Evelyn Edmonds*—During the American Civil War

WIFE NO. 19 by *Ann Eliza Young*—The Life & Ordeals of a Mormon Woman During the 19th Century

DIARY OF A NURSE IN SOUTH AFRICA by *Alice Bron*—With the Dutch-Belgian Red Cross During the Boer War

MARIE ANTOINETTE AND THE DOWNFALL OF ROYALTY by *Imbert de Saint-Amand*—The Queen of France and the French Revolution

THE MEMSAHIB & THE MUTINY by *R. M. Coopland*—An English lady's ordeals in Gwalior and Agra during the Indian Mutiny 1857

MY CAPTIVITY AMONG THE SIOUX INDIANS by *Fanny Kelly*—The ordeal of a pioneer woman crossing the Western Plains in 1864

WITH MAXIMILIAN IN MEXICO by *Sara Yorke Stevenson*—A Lady's experience of the French Adventure

AVAILABLE ONLINE AT **www.leonaur.com**
AND FROM ALL GOOD BOOK STORES

www.ingramcontent.com/pod-product-compliance
Lightning Source LLC
Chambersburg PA
CBHW031618160426
43196CB00006B/178